The Impact of Altered Timing of Eating, Sleep and Work Patterns on Human Health

Special Issue Editors

Siobhan Banks
Alison M. Coates
Jillian Dorian

MDPI • Basel • Beijing • Wuhan • Barcelona • Belgrade

MDPI

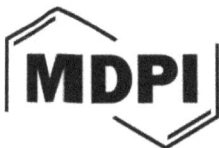

Special Issue Editors
Siobhan Banks
University of South Australia
Australia

Alison M. Coates
University of South Australia
Australia

Jillian Dorian
University of South Australia
Australia

Editorial Office
MDPI AG
St. Alban-Anlage 66
Basel, Switzerland

This edition is a reprint of the Special Issue published online in the open access journal *Nutrients* (ISSN 2072-6643) from 2016–2017 (available at: http://www.mdpi.com/journal/nutrients/special_issues/eating_sleep_work_pattern).

For citation purposes, cite each article independently as indicated on the article page online and as indicated below:

Lastname, F.M.; Lastname, F.M. Article title. *Journal Name*. **Year**. Article *number*, page range.

First Edition 2018

ISBN 978-3-03842-759-9 (Pbk)
ISBN 978-3-03842-760-5 (PDF)

Table of Contents

About the Special Issue Editors

Siobhan Banks, is Co-Director of the Behaviour-Brain-Body Research Centre at the University of South Australia. Siobhan's research examines the impact of sleep deprivation and shift work on psychological and physiological functioning and how countermeasures may be used to prevent the deleterious effects of disturbed sleep, in particular dietary interventions, napping and caffeine. She has expertise in the objective measurement of fatigue and with designing tools and protocols to investigate the biological and behavioural responses to sleep deprivation, irregular work hours and stress. Her research has been funded by the NHMRC, NIH, The US Air Force Office of Scientific Research, NASA, Beyond Blue, SA Department of Health and Aging and DST-Group. She has received over $6M in research funding during her career, ranging from basic to applied research. This work has been cited over 3700 times (GoogleScholar). She is on the editorial board of the specialty journal SLEEP, has been awarded a South Australian Young Tall Poppy Science Award (2010) and the Sleep Research Society Young Investigator Award (2011) and she also serves on the Sleep Health Foundation Board of Directors.

Alison M. Coates, is a lecturer and researcher in the School of Health Sciences at the University of South Australia. As a nutritional scientist, Alison is interested in how bioactive compounds from food can impact risk factors for obesity, cardiometabolic diseases and impact sleep and cognitive function. Alison has been involved in numerous clinical trials using nutritional supplements and whole foods over the past 20 years sponsored by industry partnerships and through government grants. Alison is a Registered Nutritionist and has written over 95 peer-reviewed journal articles and book chapters. Her contribution to the area of cardiometabolic health and nutrition has been recognized by a South Australian Tall Poppy Award and the Nutrition Society of Australia Mid-Career Research Award. She is President-Elect of the Nutrition Society of Australia.

Jillian Dorian is Co-Director of the Behaviour-Brain-Body Research Centre (BBB) at the University of South Australia. She has a PhD in Psychology and a Master of Biostatistics. Her primary research experience is in human sleep, biological rhythms and performance. She also studies alcohol consumption, dependence and abuse. She works primarily with the Australian Healthcare and Rail and Industries investigating fatigue, workload, operational performance, safety and health. She also works with mining, construction, and manufacturing, providing research and education to promote fatigue management, worker health, and safety. Jillian has written over 100 peer-reviewed journal articles and book chapters, and is heavily involved with research student supervision and training in publishing and other forms of research communication. She has been recognised by the Australian Graduate Research Council for her excellence in graduate research supervision.

Preface to "The Impact of Altered Timing of Eating, Sleep and Work Patterns on Human Health"

Some 20% of the population is required to work outside the regular 9:00 a.m.–5:00 p.m. working day, and this number is likely to increase as economic demands push work hours into the night for many companies. Long and irregular work hours mean workers are often sleep deprived, with working and sleeping hours that deviate from our diurnal biology. This causes a misalignment between normal daylight entrained internal physiological processes, such as metabolism and digestion, and the external environment. As a direct consequence of sleep loss and disturbed circadian rhythms, workers on long and/or irregular schedules are at increased risk of chronic illness, even after controlling for lifestyle and socioeconomic status. Issues associated with sleep loss and circadian misalignment are not limited to populations working these schedules, they are also experienced by the broad population across development as a consequence of biological and social changes, and sleep disorders.

The purpose of this book, compiled from a Special Issue of the journal Nutrients, is to consider the relationship between eating, sleep and circadian disruption. The book contains 14 chapters, with contributions from Australia, Brazil, China, Finland, Germany, Japan, Korea, Norway, and the U.S.A. There are 12 original research contributions and two reviews in research involving humans and rodent models, conducted in the laboratory and the field. Implications of these relationships are considered across the lifespan, with different models of sleep and circadian disturbance.

The book is organised in three sections. The first section focuses on sleep deprivation and restriction, with three studies conducted with very different methods—one with humans in a laboratory (Dennis et al. 2016), one with humans in the field (Doo et al. 2017), and one that included a combination of animal and human laboratory studies (de Oliveira et al. 2017). These studies demonstrate that insufficient sleep adversely affects metabolic health and is an independent predisposing factor for obesity and insulin resistance.

The second section focuses on changes in timing of daily rhythms. Two studies in human shiftworkers (Heath et al. 2016 and Bonnell et al. 2017) and one in rodent model of shiftwork (Marti et al. 2016) demonstrate that long and irregular hours are associated with diet-related chronic conditions such as obesity and cardiovascular disease and that dietary profile/choices have differing effects. One study shows that food timing is related to body composition in adolescents (Diederichs et al. 2016). There are also two reviews in this section—one showing the link between food timing and weight (Hutchison et al. 2017), and the other looking at the impact of typical shiftwork consequences on drivers of skeletal muscle health (Aisbett et al. 2017).

The third section focuses on interactions between sleep and diet. Komada et al. (2017) demonstrate the that sleep duration was associated with specific nutrients and foods in Japanese men, but not in women. Han et al. (2017), highlight the association between vitamin D and sleep disturbance, and Watson et al. (2016), show greater caffeine intake in those with shorter and poorer quality sleep. Two intervention studies (Scholey et al. 2017 and Tan et al. 2016) explore whether dietary and supplement interventions can improve sleep quality.

It is our hope that this book will strengthen our understanding of the importance of considering the interactions between diet, sleep and circadian patterns on health outcomes. We acknowledge the excellent work of the authors and thank the reviewers who contributed their time to review each paper, without whom this book would not be possible.

Siobhan Banks, Alison M. Coates and Jill Dorrian

Special Issue Editors

nutrients

MDPI

Article

Phenotypic Stability of Energy Balance Responses to Experimental Total Sleep Deprivation and Sleep Restriction in Healthy Adults

Laura E. Dennis [1], Andrea M. Spaeth [2] and Namni Goel [1,*]

[1]   Division of Sleep and Chronobiology, Department of Psychiatry, Perelman School of Medicine at the University of Pennsylvania, Philadelphia, PA 19104, USA; ledennis@mail.med.upenn.edu
[2]   Center for Obesity Research and Education, College of Public Health, Temple University, Philadelphia, PA 19122, USA; andrea.spaeth@temple.edu
*   Correspondence: goel@mail.med.upenn.edu; Tel.: +1-215-898-1742; Fax: +1-215-573-6410

Received: 15 November 2016; Accepted: 16 December 2016; Published: 19 December 2016

Abstract: Experimental studies have shown that sleep restriction (SR) and total sleep deprivation (TSD) produce increased caloric intake, greater fat consumption, and increased late-night eating. However, whether individuals show similar energy intake responses to both SR and TSD remains unknown. A total of $N = 66$ healthy adults (aged 21–50 years, 48.5% women, 72.7% African American) participated in a within-subjects laboratory protocol to compare daily and late-night intake between one night of SR (4 h time in bed, 04:00–08:00) and one night of TSD (0 h time in bed) conditions. We also examined intake responses during subsequent recovery from SR or TSD and investigated gender differences. Caloric and macronutrient intake during the day following SR and TSD were moderately to substantially consistent within individuals (Intraclass Correlation Coefficients: 0.34–0.75). During the late-night period of SR (22:00–04:00) and TSD (22:00–06:00), such consistency was slight to moderate, and participants consumed a greater percentage of calories from protein ($p = 0.01$) and saturated fat ($p = 0.02$) during SR, despite comparable caloric intake ($p = 0.12$). Similarly, participants consumed a greater percentage of calories from saturated fat during the day following SR than TSD ($p = 0.03$). Participants also consumed a greater percentage of calories from protein during recovery after TSD ($p < 0.001$). Caloric intake was greater in men during late-night hours and the day following sleep loss. This is the first evidence of phenotypic trait-like stability and differential vulnerability of energy balance responses to two commonly experienced types of sleep loss: our findings open the door for biomarker discovery and countermeasure development to predict and mitigate this critical health-related vulnerability.

Keywords: individual differences; sleep restriction; total sleep deprivation; recovery; caloric intake; late-night intake; macronutrients; gender differences

1. Introduction

Experimental studies have demonstrated causal mechanisms between short sleep duration and obesity risk. In healthy adults, sleep restriction (curtailed sleep across multiple consecutive days) leads to increases in caloric intake [1–10], snacking [7,11], fat and carbohydrate consumption [2,5,7,8,10,11], late-night eating/delayed meal timing [1,2,10] and weight gain [1–3]. Similarly, during total sleep deprivation (one night of continuous wakefulness), adults consume a large number of calories during the overnight period [12], consume more fat the following day [12], make more food purchases [13], consume larger portion sizes [14] and eat more calories from snacks [14].

This increased consumption of energy (via food/drink) [9] exceeds the additional energy required to sustain the extended wakefulness associated with either type of sleep loss [1,15–17]. Notably, the additional energy cost differs by sleep loss type: approximately 100 additional calories are required during sleep restriction [1,15], while 135 additional calories are required during total sleep deprivation [16], suggesting that intake amounts may differ during and following these sleep loss types to compensate for differential increases in energy expenditure.

Studies have found neurobehavioral vulnerability to sleep loss shows individual differences and is trait-like and stable within individuals across sleep restriction and total sleep deprivation [18,19]. Previously, we observed individual differences in the increased caloric intake, late-night eating and weight gain responses to sleep restriction but stability in the responses within individuals during two sleep restriction exposures separated by long time intervals [20]. However, it remains unknown whether energy balance responses are also trait-like and stable within individuals across different types of sleep loss, namely sleep restriction and total sleep deprivation.

Separate studies of sleep restriction [1–3,21,22] and total sleep deprivation [16] have demonstrated energy balance responses to sleep loss return to baseline levels after one or more nights of recovery sleep. Whether this recovery and its time course is similar following sleep restriction and total sleep deprivation remains unknown. Although the time course for recovery for some objective and subjective measures of sleepiness and cognitive performance from sleep restriction and total sleep deprivation is similar [23–30], this is not true for all tests [30,31]. Thus, it is possible that recovery of energy balance measures may differ depending on the type of sleep loss experienced.

Gender differences also have been observed in the energy balance response to sleep loss. During sleep restriction, men exhibit lower subjective ratings of fullness [5] and greater increases in caloric intake [1,10,21], consume more calories during late-night hours [10], and gain more weight than women [1,2]. Furthermore, these energy balance responses are more stable across repeated exposures to sleep restriction in men than women [20]. Notably, evidence for gender differences in objective energy balance responses during total sleep deprivation is limited since the majority of such studies either have used only men or used sample sizes precluding reliable gender comparisons [32]. Thus, additional research is needed to identify gender differences in energy balance responses during total sleep deprivation, and moreover, to compare such responses to those observed during sleep restriction.

In the current study, we examined daily and late-night caloric and macronutrient intake responses to one night of sleep restriction and one night of total sleep deprivation, as well as intake responses during subsequent recovery from both types of sleep loss. Given the stability of neurobehavioral responses across sleep restriction and total sleep deprivation and the stability of energy balance responses across two separate sleep restriction exposures, we hypothesized intake responses would be consistent across one night of sleep restriction and one night of total sleep deprivation. We also hypothesized recovery intake responses would be similar after sleep restriction or total sleep deprivation, given prior neurobehavioral response findings. Finally, we predicted men would exhibit greater late-night and caloric intake responses to both sleep restriction and total sleep deprivation, given prior reports of gender differences in energy intake.

2. Materials and Methods

2.1. Participants

Healthy individuals between the ages of 21 and 50 years old were recruited in response to study advertisements. Participants reported habitual nightly sleep durations between 6.5 h and 8.5 h, with habitual bedtimes between 22:00 and 00:00 and habitual awakenings between 06:00 and 09:30; these were confirmed via wrist actigraphy. Chronotype was determined via the Morningness–Eveningness Composite Scale [33]. Participants did not engage in habitual napping and did not present with sleep disturbances (i.e., no complaints of daytime sleepiness, insomnia, or other sleep–wake disturbances). They did not have any acute or chronic psychological and medical conditions, as determined by questionnaires, interviews, physical exams, clinical history, and urine and blood tests (including a fasting blood glucose test). They were not taking any regular medications (except oral contraceptives) and were nonsmokers with body mass indices (BMIs) between 17.3 and 30.3 kg/m^2. They did not participate in transmeridian travel or shift work, or have irregular sleep–wake routines in the 60 days before the study. Participants were monitored at home with actigraphy, sleep–wake diaries, and time-stamped call-ins to determine bedtimes and waketimes during the 7–14 days before the laboratory phase and the 7 days following the laboratory phase. Sleep disorders were excluded on the first laboratory night by oximetry and polysomnography measurements. Participants were not allowed to use tobacco during the 7 days before the study, as verified by blood and urine screenings. The protocol was approved by the University of Pennsylvania's Institutional Review Board (IRB number: 812523). All participants provided written informed consent in accordance with the Declaration of Helsinki. They received compensation for participation.

2.2. Procedure

Participants engaged in a 13-day laboratory study in which they were studied continuously, and received daily checks of vital signs and symptoms by nurses (with a physician on call). All participants experienced two types of sleep loss during the protocol—sleep restriction (SR) and total sleep deprivation (TSD)—with the order of sleep loss exposures counterbalanced across conditions. Participants were randomized as a group (N = 4 per group) to one of the two conditions after two initial nights of baseline sleep (BL1-2) of 10 h (22:00–08:00) and 12 h (22:00–10:00) time in bed (TIB) respectively, and were blinded to condition assignment until after the second night of baseline sleep. Participants randomized to Condition A (N = 34) underwent five consecutive nights of sleep restricted to 4 h TIB per night (SR1-5, 04:00–08:00) followed by four consecutive nights of 12 h recovery sleep (R1–R4, 22:00–10:00), one night of total sleep deprivation (TSD, 0 h TIB) during which they were kept awake for 36 h (10:00–22:00 the following day), and then a final night of recovery sleep (R5, 22:00–10:00). Participants randomized to Condition B (N = 32) underwent one night of total sleep deprivation (TSD, 0 h TIB) during which they were kept awake for 36 h (10:00–22:00 the following day), followed by four consecutive nights of 12 h recovery sleep (R1–R4, 22:00–10:00), five consecutive nights of sleep restricted to 4 h TIB per night (SR1-5, 04:00–08:00) and then a final night of recovery sleep (R5, 22:00–10:00). Participants were discharged from the study on the day following R5.

Participants were ambulatory and were permitted to perform sedentary activities such as watching television, reading, and playing video or board games between cognitive test bouts (completed while seated at a computer); however, they were not allowed to exercise. Ambient temperature was maintained between 22 °C and 24 °C. Laboratory light levels remained constant at <50 lux during scheduled wakefulness and <1 lux during scheduled sleep periods. Participants were monitored continuously by trained staff throughout the study to ensure adherence.

2.3. Measures

Participants chose their meals/snacks from various menu options, and selected additional food/drink (including chips, cookies, fruit, low-fat yogurt, caffeine-free soda and juices) available in the laboratory kitchen, which included an industrial-size refrigerator, microwave, and toaster oven. They could also make requests to the study coordinator and study monitors. To ensure participants had sufficient time to eat each day, three 30 to 45-min meal opportunities were specified in the study during days with a 22:00 bedtime and one additional 30-min meal opportunity was specified at 00:45 during SR and TSD. Beyond these allotted meal times, participants could also consume food/drink at any time during the study during wakefulness except when they were performing cognitive tests. Participants were not told they must eat/drink and they were instructed to eat/drink whenever they desired as long as doing so did not interfere with cognitive testing. Furthermore, participants could eat the items they had ordered or could select from other foods available in the laboratory kitchen, and could eat as much or as little as they desired. Participants retrieved their own food/drink from the laboratory kitchen when they wanted to eat/drink and had the choice of eating at a table in the common area or privately in their bedrooms. Participants were not permitted to consume caffeinated beverages or chocolate during the protocol.

All food was weighed and recorded before being given to the participants. Food items were served in individual containers to increase the measurement accuracy of each item's weight. Each day, trained monitors recorded a detailed description, the amount consumed and the intake time of the items. In addition, any left-over food/drink after each meal was weighed and recorded. The intake data were entered into The Food Processor SQL program (version 10.11; ESHA Research, Salem, OR, USA), a validated [34] professional nutrition analysis software and database program that generates food/drink intake components including calories and macronutrients.

2.4. Statistical Analyses

Mixed-model ANOVAs evaluated condition and sleep loss exposure type effects for late-night intake during the first night of SR and during TSD (SR: 22:00–04:00; TSD: 22:00–06:00) as well as for daily intake following the first night of SR (SR1: 08:00–22:00) and following TSD (06:00–22:00) for calories, macronutrients, saturated fat, sugar, and fiber. Mixed-model ANOVAs assessed gender and sleep loss exposure type effects for both late-night intake during and daily intake following sleep loss.

Between-subjects ANOVAs, covarying baseline intake, compared intake on the day following recovery sleep from either SR or TSD (R1, recovery sleep between sleep loss exposures) for each intake variable. Mixed-model ANOVAs, covarying baseline intake, compared the time course of intake across the four recovery days (R1–R4) following consecutive recovery sleep nights from either SR or TSD for each intake variable. Intraclass correlation coefficients (ICCs) examined consistency in intake responses between SR and TSD. The following ranges characterize ICCs and reflect the stability of interindividual differences: 0.0–0.2 (slight); 0.2–0.4 (fair); 0.4–0.6 (moderate); 0.6–0.8 (substantial); and 0.8–1.0 (almost perfect) [35]. Statistical analyses were conducted using IBM SPSS Statistics for Windows (version 21).

3. Results

3.1. Participant Characteristics

Sixty-six participants (aged 21–50 years, 72.7% African American; 48.5% female) participated in the study, with $N = 34$ randomly assigned to Condition A (experienced five consecutive nights of SR first) and $N = 32$ randomly assigned to Condition B (experienced one night of TSD first). There were no significant differences between conditions in age ($p = 0.28$), BMI ($p = 0.60$), the percentage of participants who were African American ($p = 0.69$) or women ($p = 0.81$), or in chronotype ($p = 0.07$), pre-study sleep duration ($p = 0.74$) or midpoint ($p = 0.26$) (Table 1). Participants also did not differ significantly in caloric, macronutrient (protein, carbohydrate, fat), fiber, sugar or saturated fat intake (p's > 0.08) during the first baseline day (08:00–22:00), which occurred prior to randomization.

Table 1. Participant characteristics (Mean ± SD).

	N	Age (Years)	BMI (kg/m²)	Women	African American	Chronotype [a]	Sleep Duration (h) [b]	Sleep Midpoint (Time ± h) [b]
All Participants	66	34.4 ± 9.0	24.4 ± 3.2	32 (48.5%)	48 (72.7%)	42.1 ± 5.9	8.0 ± 0.5	03:34 ± 0.8
Condition A (SR first)	34	33.2 ± 8.9	24.6 ± 3.0	16 (47.1%)	24 (70.6%)	40.9 ± 6.1	8.1 ± 0.4	03:41 ± 0.8
Condition B (TSD first)	32	35.6 ± 9.1	24.2 ± 3.3	16 (50.0%)	24 (75.0%)	43.6 ± 5.3	8.0 ± 0.6	03:27 ± 0.8

[a] Morningness–Eveningness Composite Scale [33]; [b] Determined by wrist actigraphy (one week prior to study entry).

3.2. Late-Night Intake during Sleep Restriction and Total Sleep Deprivation

For late-night caloric intake, there was a significant sleep loss exposure (SR and TSD) × condition (A and B) interaction ($F(1, 64) = 18.05$, $p < 0.001$) but no main effect of sleep exposure type ($p = 0.12$) or condition ($p = 0.85$). In both conditions, participants consumed more late-night calories during their first sleep loss exposure than during their second (Figure 1); however, this was only statistically significant for participants in Condition B ($F(1, 31) = 18.49$, $p < 0.001$) and not for those in Condition A ($F(1, 33) = 3.37$, $p = 0.08$). When examining late-night macronutrient, sugar, saturated fat and fiber intake, there were no significant sleep loss exposure × condition interactions (p's > 0.11) or condition main effects (p's > 0.20). There were significant sleep loss exposure main effects for protein and saturated fat: participants consumed a significantly larger percentage of calories from protein ($F(1, 64) = 6.79$, $p = 0.01$) and saturated fat ($F(1, 64) = 5.79$, $p = 0.02$) during SR late-night hours than during TSD late-night hours. By contrast, there were no significant sleep loss exposure main effects for caloric, carbohydrate, sugar, fat, or fiber intake (p's > 0.17) (Figure 2).

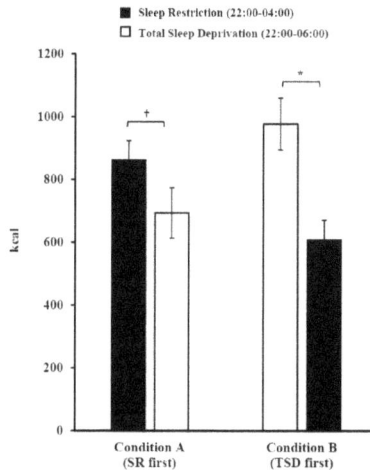

Figure 1. Mean ± SEM late-night caloric intake during sleep restriction (SR) and total sleep deprivation (TSD). There was a significant sleep loss exposure type (SR and TSD) × condition (A and B) interaction ($p < 0.001$), but no main effect of condition ($p = 0.85$). In both conditions, participants consumed more late-night calories during their first sleep loss exposure; however, this was statistically significant for Condition B (* $p < 0.001$), but not for Condition A († $p = 0.08$).

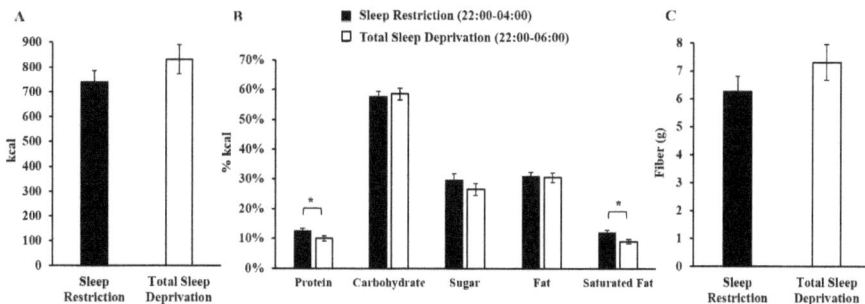

Figure 2. Mean ± SEM late-night intake during sleep restriction (SR) and total sleep deprivation (TSD). (**A**) Late-night caloric intake during SR and TSD did not significantly differ ($p = 0.12$); (**B**) During late-night hours, participants consumed a significantly larger percentage of calories from protein (* $p = 0.01$) and saturated fat (* $p = 0.02$) during SR, but there were no differences in carbohydrate, sugar, fat, or fiber (**C**) intake (p's > 0.17).

For late-night caloric intake, while there was no significant sleep loss exposure (SR and TSD) × gender interaction effect ($p = 0.24$), there was a significant main effect of gender ($F(1, 64) = 6.40$, $p = 0.01$), whereby men consumed more late-night calories than women during both types of sleep loss (men: 878.4 ± 369.5 kcal, women: 687.5 ± 220.3 kcal). There were no significant sleep loss exposure (SR and TSD) × gender interactions (p's > 0.07) or gender main effects (p's > 0.19) for late-night macronutrient, sugar, saturated fat or fiber intake.

ICC analyses, which examined the consistency in the late-night intake response between SR and TSD, ranged from slight to moderate: caloric intake: 0.18 (women: −0.42; men: 0.28); carbohydrate (%kcal): 0.18 (women: 0.31; men: 0.08); fat (%kcal): 0.03 (women: 0.14; men: −0.15); protein (%kcal): 0.55 (women: 0.59; men: 0.51); sugar (%kcal): 0.16 (women: 0.34; men: −0.06); saturated fat (%kcal): −0.25 (women: −0.90; men: −0.01); and fiber (g): 0.21 (women: 0.25; men: 0.19).

3.3. Daily Intake Following Sleep Restriction and Total Sleep Deprivation

For protein intake, there was a significant main effect of condition ($F(1, 64) = 4.83$, $p = 0.03$): participants in Condition A consumed a greater percentage of calories from protein during the day following SR and TSD compared to participants in Condition B (A: 13.3%, B: 11.9%). However, there was no significant sleep loss exposure × condition interaction effect ($p = 0.33$) or main effect of sleep loss exposure type ($p = 0.58$). In addition, for saturated fat, there was a significant main effect of sleep loss exposure ($F(1, 64) = 5.09$, $p = 0.03$): participants consumed a greater percentage of calories from saturated fat during the day following SR than TSD ($p = 0.03$; Table 2). However, there was no significant sleep loss exposure × condition interaction effect ($p = 0.09$) or main effect of condition ($p = 0.11$). There were no significant sleep loss exposure (SR and TSD) × condition (A and B) interaction effects (p's > 0.16) or main effects of sleep loss exposure type (p's > 0.11, Table 2) or condition (p's > 0.11) for caloric (Figure 3), carbohydrate, fat, sugar or fiber intake.

Table 2. Mean ± SD daily intake during the day following sleep restriction (SR) and the day following total sleep deprivation (TSD).

	Day Following SR (08:00–22:00; N = 66)	Day Following TSD (06:00–22:00; N = 66)	*p* Values
Kcal	2326.6 ± 811.1	2178.9 ± 793.7	0.11
Protein (%kcal)	12.4 ± 3.3	12.8 ± 3.4	0.50
Carbohydrate (%kcal)	58.4 ± 7.3	59.0 ± 8.6	0.56
Fat (%kcal)	31.2 ± 7.1	30.4 ± 8.1	0.31
Sugar (%kcal)	28.7 ± 7.5	28.4 ± 8.8	0.94
Saturated Fat (%kcal)	11.0 ± 3.5	10.0 ± 3.5	0.03
Fiber (g)	19.6 ± 9.6	18.5 ± 10.0	0.38

While there were no significant sleep loss exposure (SR and TSD) × gender interactions for any intake variables (p's > 0.12), there were main effects of gender for caloric intake ($F(1, 64) = 14.09$, $p < 0.001$) and protein intake ($F(1, 64) = 5.02$, $p = 0.03$). Compared to women, men consumed more calories and a greater percentage of calories from protein during the day following SR and TSD (Mean ± SD; men: 2546.4 ± 802.2 kcal, 13.3% ± 2.7% protein; women: 1940.8 ± 448.0 kcal, 11.9% ± 2.4% protein). There were no significant main effects of gender for carbohydrate, fat, sugar, saturated fat, or fiber intake (p's > 0.22).

ICC analyses, which examined the consistency in daily intake following SR and TSD, ranged from fair to substantial (Figure 4): caloric intake: 0.75 (women: 0.54; men: 0.74); carbohydrate (%kcal): 0.54 (women: 0.45; men: 0.64); fat (%kcal): 0.54 (women: 0.54; men: 0.57); protein (%kcal): 0.34 (women: 0.24; men: 0.34); sugar (%kcal): 0.70 (women: 0.61; men: 0.77); saturated fat (%kcal): 0.59 (women: 0.52; men: 0.66); and fiber (g): 0.65 (women: 0.62; men: 0.67).

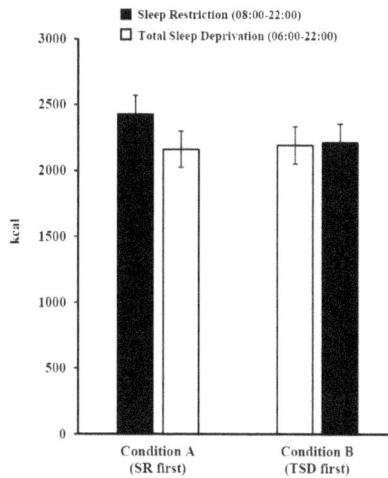

Figure 3. Mean ± SEM daily caloric intake following one night of sleep restriction (SR) and one night of total sleep deprivation (TSD). There was no significant sleep loss exposure type (SR and TSD) × condition (A and B) interaction effect ($p = 0.16$), and no significant main effects of sleep loss exposure type ($p = 0.11$) or condition ($p = 0.61$).

3.4. Recovery Sleep Following Sleep Restriction or Total Sleep Deprivation

Because some participants received an Ensure nutrition shake during a metabolic testing procedure on the first recovery day, recovery data analyses were conducted only in the subset of participants who did not receive this nutrition shake ($N = 24$; Condition A: $N = 12$, Condition B: $N = 12$). In this subset, there were no significant differences between conditions in age ($p = 0.15$), BMI ($p = 0.49$), or in the percentage of participants who were African American (Condition A: 58.3%, Condition B: 41.7%; $p = 0.51$) or women (Condition A: 50.0%, Condition B: 50.0%, $p = 1.0$). Participants in each condition also did not differ in chronotype ($p = 0.08$) or pre-study sleep duration ($p = 0.86$) or midpoint ($p = 0.14$).

Between-subjects ANOVAs, covarying baseline intake for each variable, compared intake during the day following the first recovery sleep night from either SR or TSD. Participants on the first day of recovery from TSD consumed a greater percentage of calories from protein than those on the first day of recovery from SR ($F(1, 21) = 32.64$, $p < 0.001$, Table 3). Participants on the first day of recovery from SR tended to consume more calories than those on the first day of recovery from TSD; however, this did not reach statistical significance ($F(1, 21) = 3.80$, $p = 0.07$, Table 3). There were no differences between conditions in carbohydrate, fat, saturated fat, sugar or fiber intake (p's > 0.08).

Mixed-model ANOVAs, covarying baseline intake for each measure, compared the time course of intake across four recovery days following consecutive recovery nights (R1–R4, 10:00–22:00) from either SR or TSD. There were no recovery day main effects (p's > 0.10) or recovery day × condition interaction effects for any intake measure (p's > 0.06). There were no main effects of condition for daily caloric, carbohydrate, fat, saturated fat, sugar, or fiber intake (p's > 0.11); however, participants across the four days of recovery from TSD consumed a greater percentage of calories from protein than those across the four days of recovery from SR ($F(1, 21) = 19.00$, $p < 0.001$).

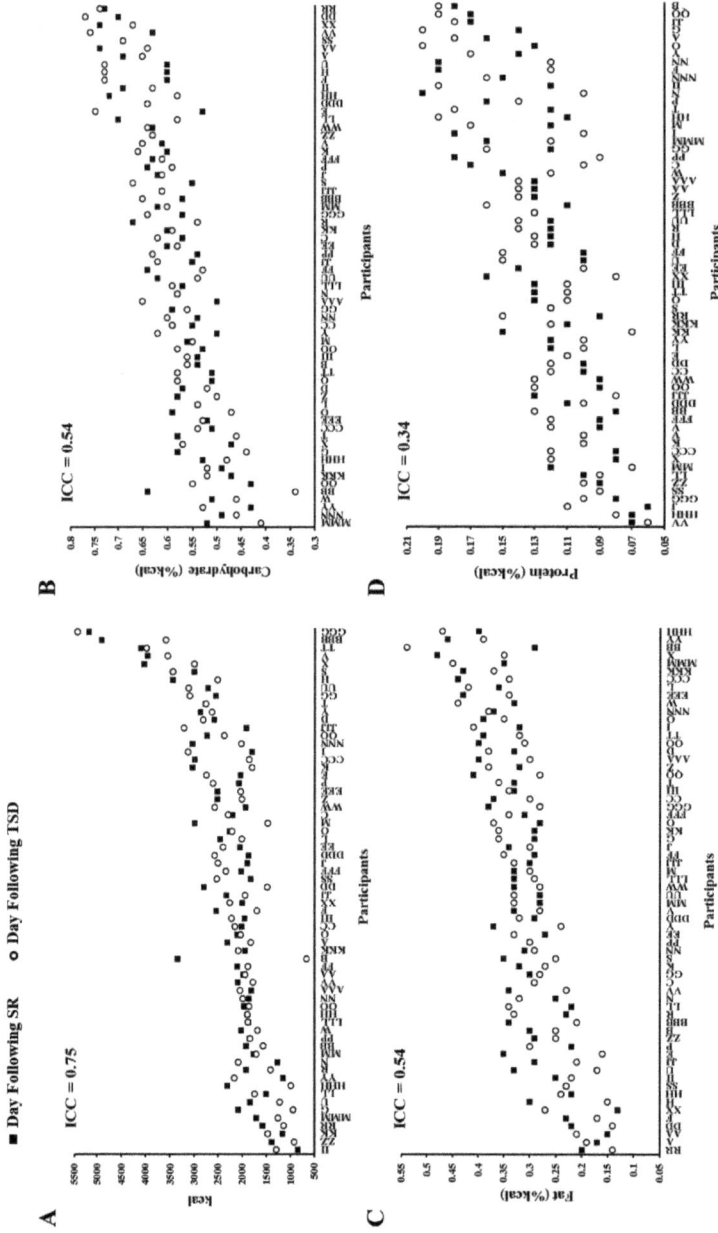

Figure 4. Individual differences and substantial phenotypic stability of caloric and macronutrient intake measures to sleep restriction (SR) and total sleep deprivation (TSD). Stability of caloric and macronutrient intake during the day following SR (08:00–22:00) and TSD (06:00–22:00) for (**A**) total caloric intake; (**B**) percentage of caloric intake from carbohydrates; (**C**) percentage of caloric intake from fat; and (**D**) percentage of caloric intake from protein. Participants (denoted individually with letters) are plotted in ascending order based on the mean intake of both sleep loss exposures (SR and TSD). See text for ICC ranges.

Table 3. Mean ± SD intake for each of the four days following recovery sleep (12 h TIB from 22:00–10:00, R1–R4, $N = 24$) from sleep restriction (SR; $N = 12$) or total sleep deprivation (TSD: $N = 12$).

	R1		R2		R3		R4	
	SR	TSD	SR	TSD	SR	TSD	SR	TSD
Kcal	2307.9 ± 615.0 [†]	2007.4 ± 659.0	2055.3 ± 607.7	2060.1 ± 654.0	2096.2 ± 761.6	2018.7 ± 751.9	2026.6 ± 863.8	1861.2 ± 630.0
Protein (%kcal)	10.8 ± 3.3	16.2 ± 5.0 *	12.7 ± 4.8	17.6 ± 3.3	11.8 ± 3.8	16.2 ± 5.0	15.0 ± 7.8	15.1 ± 3.8
Carbohydrate (%kcal)	63.1 ± 6.0	55.2 ± 10.0	61.4 ± 10.2	52.7 ± 11.1	62.6 ± 8.6	57.8 ± 8.0	56.7 ± 13.0	53.0 ± 9.5
Sugar (%kcal)	31.2 ± 6.9	24.1 ± 9.6	29.0 ± 9.9	23.2 ± 4.6	34.9 ± 12.6	27.7 ± 7.2	26.8 ± 7.6	26.9 ± 6.6
Fat (%kcal)	28.1 ± 5.6	30.0 ± 7.6	27.8 ± 7.3	31.8 ± 8.8	27.4 ± 7.6	28.3 ± 7.7	31.7 ± 6.8	33.5 ± 7.6
Saturated Fat (%kcal)	10.4 ± 3.1	11.9 ± 3.4	10.1 ± 4.1	12.7 ± 4.5	8.5 ± 2.9	11.5 ± 4.4	10.7 ± 3.4	12.6 ± 4.2
Fiber (g)	20.7 ± 7.1	21.4 ± 9.3	17.7 ± 11.1	19.0 ± 10.4	12.0 ± 5.7	21.1 ± 15.5	15.1 ± 6.3	16.8 ± 9.2

[†] $p = 0.07$: Participants tended to consume more calories on the first day of recovery (R1) from SR than from TSD; however, this did not reach statistical significance. * $p < 0.001$: Protein intake was significantly higher on the first day of recovery (R1) from TSD than from SR.

4. Discussion

In this study, we found caloric and macronutrient intake during the day following one night of SR and one night of TSD were moderately to substantially consistent within individuals and showed differential vulnerability between individuals. During the late-night period of one night of SR and one night of TSD, consistency was slight to moderate; furthermore, although caloric intake did not differ, participants consumed a greater percentage of calories from protein and saturated fat during SR. Similarly, participants also consumed a greater percentage of calories from saturated fat during the day following SR than following TSD, despite comparable caloric intake. Notably, participants consumed a greater percentage of calories from protein during recovery after TSD. Caloric intake was greater in men during late-night hours and the day following sleep loss. These findings highlight the critical relationship between energy balance and sleep, and underscore the need to identify biomarkers and countermeasures to predict and mitigate energy balance vulnerability to sleep loss. Our findings are of timely importance, given recent, marked escalations in nighttime and overall caloric consumption, and the increased prevalence of both obesity and sleep loss in the population.

Caloric and macronutrient intake during the day following one night of SR and one night of TSD showed moderate to substantial consistency within individuals and differential vulnerability between individuals. Thus, if an individual was vulnerable to increased caloric and macronutrient intake in one type of sleep loss, he/she was also remarkably vulnerable to this eating behavior in the other type of sleep loss. These findings are in line with our prior study of the stability of energy balance responses across two separate sleep restriction exposures [20], and with studies showing stability of neurobehavioral responses across SR and TSD [18,19]. Future studies should examine the stability and individual differences of responses for another key component of energy balance—energy expenditure—as this measure differs between SR and TSD [1,15,16].

During the late-night period of one night of SR and one night of TSD, consistency was slight to moderate. These findings are in agreement with our prior study examining the stability of late-night responses across two separate sleep restriction exposures [20], which used comparable late-night eating intervals. Interestingly, although caloric intake did not differ, participants consumed a greater percentage of calories from protein and saturated fat during the late-night hours of SR than TSD, despite similar time intervals for eating. Participants also consumed a greater percentage of calories from saturated fat during the day following SR than following TSD, even though caloric intake was comparable. Our findings are consistent with other research showing increased protein and saturated fat intake during the SR period [36]. These macronutrient differences may be due to minor variations in late-night or daytime food selection and consumption, which could lead to differences in salt intake or other factors, by participants during SR and TSD.

Of interest, participants consumed more late-night calories during their first sleep loss exposure. There are several possible explanations for this finding. Participants may have overindulged in the first session due to the initial novelty of available food selections from the hospital menu and from the laboratory kitchen. In addition, the recovery sleep between sleep loss periods (12 h TIB for four nights) may have served as a partial buffer against the increase in late-night eating during the second sleep loss period. There is evidence that "banking" sleep can mitigate some of the neurobehavioral deficits resulting from sleep loss [37], and such banking may serve a similar purpose in regulating intake behaviors. Further research is needed to explore these possibilities.

Although most intake variables did not differ during recovery from TSD or SR—as we had hypothesized—participants consumed a greater percentage of calories from protein on the first day of recovery from TSD, and tended to consume more calories on the first day of recovery from SR. These findings are in line with studies showing most [23–30], but not all [30,31] neurobehavioral responses recover similarly after TSD or SR. Intake differences following recovery sleep may be due to variations in sleep duration, timing, quality and architecture. Notably, these sleep parameters, which may differ when recovering after TSD versus SR, have been shown to modulate the percentage of caloric intake derived from protein as well as other energy balance measures [35,38–43]. Future studies are needed to explore this and other possible mechanisms underlying recovery intake differences between SR and TSD.

As predicted, in men, late-night caloric intake was nearly 200 kcals higher and caloric intake the day following sleep loss was more than 600 kcals higher (with a 1.4% protein intake increase), across SR and TSD. Our results are in concordance with prior studies showing marked gender differences in energy intake with sleep loss [1,10,21]. In this study, daily caloric intake was also more stable in men, consistent with our prior findings [20]. A number of reasons may explain these gender differences, including differences between men and women in sex and metabolic hormones, peripheral controls of eating, or in eating behaviors and attitudes about food [10].

Our study had a few limitations. The participants were all healthy, and between the ages of 21 and 50 years old with BMIs in the normal to overweight range. As such, our results may not be generalizable to other groups, such as adolescents, obese individuals, or the elderly. In addition, we examined only healthy adult sleepers with habitual sleep durations of approximately 8 h per night. A recent study found habitually long sleepers had a higher sweet taste preference and decreased activity following sleep restriction, whereas habitually short sleepers did not experience such changes, suggesting the former group may be more vulnerable to energy balance changes following sleep loss [44]. Thus, future research should determine the stability of caloric and macronutrient intake, and late-night eating responses to sleep restriction and total sleep deprivation in normal weight, overweight and obese individuals of varying ages and with varying habitual sleep durations.

5. Conclusions

Caloric and macronutrient intake during the late-night period of sleep loss and during the day following one night of SR and one night of TSD were consistent within individuals with differential vulnerability between individuals. Caloric intake did not differ during the late-night period of one night of SR and one night of TSD, although participants consumed a greater percentage of calories from protein and saturated fat during SR. Participants also consumed a greater percentage of calories from saturated fat during the day following SR than following TSD, and a greater percentage of calories from protein during recovery after TSD. Caloric intake was greater in men during the sleep loss period. We show, for the first time, robust differential vulnerability and phenotypic stability of energy balance responses to two commonly experienced types of sleep loss, heralding the use of biomarkers and countermeasures for prediction and mitigation of this critical vulnerability. These novel findings are timely, given worldwide increases in nighttime and overall caloric consumption, and in the prevalence of obesity and sleep loss.

Acknowledgments: The authors thank the participants and the faculty and staff of the Division of Sleep and Chronobiology who helped acquire the data. This research was performed at the Division of Sleep and Chronobiology, Department of Psychiatry, Perelman School of Medicine, University of Pennsylvania, Philadelphia, PA. This research was supported by the Department of the Navy, Office of Naval Research Award No. N00014-11-1-0361 (N.G.); National Aeronautics and Space Administration NNX14AN49G (N.G.); Clinical and Translational Research Center (CTRC) grant UL1TR000003; and NIH grant F31 AG044102 (A.M.S.). None of the sponsors had any role in the following: design and conduct of the study; collection, management, analysis, and interpretation of the data; and preparation, review, or approval of the manuscript. No funds were received to cover publication costs.

Author Contributions: All authors played a role in the conduct of the study; Namni Goel conceived and designed the study; Andrea M. Spaeth collected the data; Laura E. Dennis, Andrea M. Spaeth and Namni Goel performed management, analysis, and interpretation of the data; and Laura E. Dennis, Andrea M. Spaeth, and Namni Goel played a role in the preparation, review, and approval of the manuscript. Laura E. Dennis and Andrea M. Spaeth had full access to all the data in the study and take responsibility for the integrity of the data and the accuracy of the data analysis. All authors have read and approved the final manuscript.

Conflicts of Interest: The authors declare no conflict of interest.

References

1. Markwald, R.R.; Melanson, E.L.; Smith, M.R.; Higgins, J.; Perreault, L.; Eckel, R.H.; Wright, K.P., Jr. Impact of insufficient sleep on total daily energy expenditure, food intake, and weight gain. *Proc. Natl. Acad. Sci. USA* **2013**, *110*, 5695–5700. [CrossRef] [PubMed]
2. Spaeth, A.M.; Dinges, D.F.; Goel, N. Effects of experimental sleep restriction on weight gain, caloric intake, and meal timing in healthy adults. *Sleep* **2013**, *36*, 981–990. [CrossRef] [PubMed]
3. Bosy-Westphal, A.; Hinrichs, S.; Jauch-Chara, K.; Hitze, B.; Later, W.; Wilms, B.; Settler, U.; Peters, A.; Kiosz, D.; Muller, M.J. Influence of partial sleep deprivation on energy balance and insulin sensitivity in healthy women. *Obes. Facts* **2008**, *1*, 266–273. [CrossRef] [PubMed]
4. Brondel, L.; Romer, M.A.; Nougues, P.M.; Touyarou, P.; Davenne, D. Acute partial sleep deprivation increases food intake in healthy men. *Am. J. Clin. Nutr.* **2010**, *91*, 1550–1559. [CrossRef] [PubMed]
5. St-Onge, M.P.; Roberts, A.L.; Chen, J.; Kelleman, M.; O'Keeffe, M.; RoyChoudhury, A.; Jones, P.J. Short sleep duration increases energy intakes but does not change energy expenditure in normal-weight individuals. *Am. J. Clin. Nutr.* **2011**, *94*, 410–416. [CrossRef] [PubMed]
6. Calvin, A.D.; Carter, R.E.; Adachi, T.; Macedo, P.G.; Albuquerque, F.N.; van der Walt, C.; Bukartyk, J.; Davison, D.E.; Levine, J.A.; Somers, V.K. Effects of experimental sleep restriction on caloric intake and activity energy expenditure. *Chest* **2013**, *144*, 79–86. [CrossRef] [PubMed]
7. Broussard, J.L.; Kilkus, J.M.; Delebecque, F.; Abraham, V.; Day, A.; Whitmore, H.R.; Tasali, E. Elevated ghrelin predicts food intake during experimental sleep restriction. *Obesity* **2016**, *24*, 132–138. [CrossRef] [PubMed]
8. Spiegel, K.; Tasali, E.; Penev, P.; van Cauter, E. Brief communication: Sleep curtailment in healthy young men is associated with decreased leptin levels, elevated ghrelin levels, and increased hunger and appetite. *Ann. Intern. Med.* **2004**, *141*, 846–850. [CrossRef] [PubMed]
9. Capers, P.L.; Fobian, A.D.; Kaiser, K.A.; Borah, R.; Allison, D.B. A systematic review and meta-analysis of randomized controlled trials of the impact of sleep duration on adiposity and components of energy balance. *Obes. Rev.* **2015**, *16*, 771–782. [CrossRef] [PubMed]
10. Spaeth, A.M.; Dinges, D.F.; Goel, N. Sex and race differences in caloric intake during sleep restriction in healthy adults. *Am. J. Clin. Nutr.* **2014**, *100*, 559–566. [CrossRef] [PubMed]
11. Nedeltcheva, A.V.; Kilkus, J.M.; Imperial, J.; Kasza, K.; Schoeller, D.A.; Penev, P.D. Sleep curtailment is accompanied by increased intake of calories from snacks. *Am. J. Clin. Nutr.* **2009**, *89*, 126–133. [CrossRef] [PubMed]
12. Fang, Z.; Spaeth, A.M.; Ma, N.; Zhu, S.; Hu, S.; Goel, N.; Detre, J.A.; Dinges, D.F.; Rao, H. Altered salience network connectivity predicts macronutrient intake after sleep deprivation. *Sci. Rep.* **2015**, *5*, 8215. [CrossRef] [PubMed]
13. Chapman, C.D.; Nilsson, E.K.; Nilsson, V.C.; Cedernaes, J.; Rångtell, F.H.; Vogel, H.; Dickson, S.L.; Broman, J.E.; Hogenkamp, P.S.; Schiöth, H.B.; et al. Acute sleep deprivation increases food purchasing in men. *Obesity* **2013**, *21*, E555–E560. [CrossRef] [PubMed]
14. Hogenkamp, P.S.; Nilsson, E.; Nilsson, V.C.; Chapman, C.D.; Vogel, H.; Lundberg, L.S.; Zarei, S.; Cedernaes, J.; Rångtell, F.H.; Broman, J.E.; et al. Acute sleep deprivation increases portion size and affects food choice in young men. *Psychoneuroendocrinology* **2013**, *38*, 1668–1674. [CrossRef] [PubMed]
15. Shechter, A.; Rising, R.; Albu, J.B.; St-Onge, M.P. Experimental sleep curtailment causes wake-dependent increases in 24-h energy expenditure as measured by whole-room indirect calorimetry. *Am. J. Clin. Nutr.* **2013**, *98*, 1433–1439. [CrossRef] [PubMed]
16. Jung, C.M.; Melanson, E.L.; Frydendall, E.J.; Perreault, L.; Eckel, R.H.; Wright, K.P. Energy expenditure during sleep, sleep deprivation and sleep following sleep deprivation in adult humans. *J. Physiol.* **2011**, *589*, 235–244. [CrossRef] [PubMed]
17. Al Khatib, H.K.; Harding, S.V.; Darzi, J.; Pot, G.K. The effects of partial sleep deprivation on energy balance: a systematic review and meta-analysis. *Eur. J. Clin. Nutr.* **2016**. [CrossRef] [PubMed]
18. Rupp, T.L.; Wesensten, N.J.; Balkin, T.J. Trait-like vulnerability to total and partial sleep loss. *Sleep* **2012**, *35*, 1163–1172. [CrossRef] [PubMed]
19. Van Dongen, H.P.A.; Baynard, M.D.; Maislin, G.; Dinges, D.F. Systematic interindividual differences in neurobehavioral impairment from sleep loss: Evidence of trait-like differential vulnerability. *Sleep* **2004**, *27*, 423–433. [PubMed]

20. Spaeth, A.M.; Dinges, D.F.; Goel, N. Phenotypic vulnerability of energy balance responses to sleep loss in healthy adults. *Sci. Rep.* **2015**, *5*, 14920. [CrossRef] [PubMed]
21. Spaeth, A.M.; Dinges, D.F.; Goel, N. Resting metabolic rate varies by race and by sleep duration. *Obesity* **2015**, *23*, 2349–2356. [CrossRef] [PubMed]
22. Buxton, O.M.; Cain, S.W.; O'Connor, S.P.; Porter, J.H.; Duffy, J.F.; Wang, W.; Czeisler, C.A.; Shea, S.A. Adverse metabolic consequences in humans of prolonged sleep restriction combined with circadian disruption. *Sci. Transl. Med.* **2012**, *4*. [CrossRef] [PubMed]
23. Banks, S.; Van Dongen, H.P.A.; Maislin, G.; Dinges, D.F. Neurobehavioral dynamics following chronic sleep restriction: Dose-response effects of one night for recovery. *Sleep* **2010**, *33*, 1013–1026. [PubMed]
24. Axelsson, J.; Kecklund, G.; Åkerstedt, T.; Donofrio, P.; Lekander, M.; Ingre, M. Sleepiness and performance in response to repeated sleep restriction and subsequent recovery during semi-laboratory conditions. *Chronobiol. Int.* **2008**, *25*, 297–308. [CrossRef] [PubMed]
25. Haavisto, M.L.; Porkka-Heiskanen, T.; Hublin, C.; Härmä, M.; Mutanen, P.; Müller, K.; Virkkala, J.; Sallinen, M. Sleep restriction for the duration of a work week impairs multitasking performance. *J. Sleep Res.* **2010**, *19*, 444–454. [CrossRef] [PubMed]
26. Sallinen, M.; Onninen, J.; Tirkkonen, K.; Haavisto, M.L.; Härmä, M.; Kubo, T.; Mutanen, P.; Virkkala, J.; Tolvanen, A.; Porkka-Heiskanen, T. Effects of cumulative sleep restriction on self-perceptions while multitasking. *J. Sleep Res.* **2013**, *22*, 273–281. [CrossRef] [PubMed]
27. Philip, P.; Sagaspe, P.; Prague, M.; Tassi, P.; Capelli, A.; Bioulac, B.; Commenges, D.; Taillard, J. Acute versus chronic partial sleep deprivation in middle-aged people: Differential effect on performance and sleepiness. *Sleep* **2012**, *35*, 997–1002. [CrossRef] [PubMed]
28. Pejovic, S.; Basta, M.; Vgontzas, A.N.; Kritikou, I.; Shaffer, M.L.; Tsaoussoglou, M.; Stiffler, D.; Stefanakis, Z.; Bixler, E.O.; Chrousos, G.P. Effects of recovery sleep after one work week of mild sleep restriction on interleukin-6 and cortisol secretion and daytime sleepiness and performance. *Am. J. Physiol. Endocrinol. Metab.* **2013**, *305*, E890–E896. [CrossRef] [PubMed]
29. Carskadon, M.A.; Dement, W.C. Cumulative effects of sleep restriction on daytime sleepiness. *Psychophysiology* **1981**, *18*, 107–113. [CrossRef] [PubMed]
30. Lamond, N.; Jay, S.M.; Dorrian, J.; Ferguson, S.A.; Jones, C.; Dawson, D. The dynamics of neurobehavioural recovery following sleep loss. *J. Sleep Res.* **2007**, *16*, 33–41. [CrossRef] [PubMed]
31. Belenky, G.; Wesensten, N.J.; Thorne, D.R.; Thomas, M.L.; Sing, H.C.; Redmond, D.P.; Russo, M.B.; Balkin, T.J. Patterns of performance degradation and restoration during sleep restriction and subsequent recovery: A sleep dose-response study. *J. Sleep Res.* **2003**, *12*, 1–12. [CrossRef] [PubMed]
32. St-Onge, M.P. Impact of sleep duration on food intake regulation: Different mechanisms by sex? *Obesity* **2016**, *24*, 11. [CrossRef] [PubMed]
33. Smith, C.S.; Reilly, C.; Midkiff, K. Evaluation of three circadian rhythm questionnaires with suggestions for an improved measure of morningness. *J. Appl. Psychol.* **1989**, *74*, 728–738. [CrossRef] [PubMed]
34. Hise, M.E.; Sullivan, D.K.; Jacobsen, D.J.; Johnson, S.L.; Donnelly, J.E. Validation of energy intake measurements determined from observer-recorded food records and recall methods compared with the doubly labeled water method in overweight and obese individuals. *Am. J. Clin. Nutr.* **2002**, *75*, 263–267. [PubMed]
35. Landis, J.R.; Koch, G.G. The measurement of observer agreement for categorical data. *Biometrics* **1977**, *33*, 159–174. [CrossRef] [PubMed]
36. Dashti, H.S.; Scheer, F.A.; Jacques, P.F.; Lamon-Fava, S.; Ordovás, J.M. Short sleep duration and dietary intake: Epidemiologic evidence, mechanisms, and health implications. *Adv. Nutr.* **2015**, *6*, 648–659. [CrossRef] [PubMed]
37. Rupp, T.L.; Wesensten, N.J.; Bliese, P.D.; Balkin, T.J. Banking sleep: Realization of benefits during subsequent sleep restriction and recovery. *Sleep* **2009**, *32*, 311–321. [PubMed]
38. McNeil, J.; Doucet, É.; Brunet, J.F.; Hintze, L.J.; Chaumont, I.; Langlois, É.; Maitland, R.; Riopel, A.; Forest, G. The effects of sleep restriction and altered sleep timing on energy intake and energy expenditure. *Physiol. Behav.* **2016**, *164*, 157–163. [CrossRef] [PubMed]
39. Baron, K.G.; Reid, K.J.; Kern, A.S.; Zee, P.C. Role of sleep timing in caloric intake and BMI. *Obesity* **2011**, *19*, 1374–1381. [CrossRef] [PubMed]

40. St-Onge, M.P.; Bormes, A.; Salazar, I. The role of sleep duration on energy balance: An update. *Curr. Nutr. Rep.* **2016**, *5*, 278–285. [CrossRef]
41. St-Onge, M.P.; Roberts, A.; Shechter, A.; Choudhury, A.R. Fiber and saturated fat are associated with sleep arousals and slow wave sleep. *J. Clin. Sleep Med.* **2016**, *12*, 19–24. [CrossRef] [PubMed]
42. St-Onge, M.P.; Mikic, A.; Pietrolungo, C.E. Effects of diet on sleep quality. *Adv. Nutr.* **2016**, *7*, 938–949. [CrossRef] [PubMed]
43. Spaeth, A.M.; Dinges, D.F.; Goel, N. Objective measurements of energy balance are associated with sleep architecture in healthy adults. *Sleep* **2016**, in press.
44. Smith, S.L.; Ludy, M.J.; Tucker, R.M. Changes in taste preference and steps taken after sleep curtailment. *Physiol. Behav.* **2016**, *163*, 228–233. [CrossRef] [PubMed]

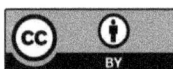

nutrients

MDPI

Article

The Risk of Being Obese According to Short Sleep Duration Is Modulated after Menopause in Korean Women

Miae Doo and Yangha Kim *

Department of Nutritional Science and Food Management, Ewha Womans University, Ewhayeodae-gil,
Seodaemun-gu, Seoul 03760, Korea; miae_doo@ewha.ac.kr
* Correspondence: yhmoon@ewha.ac.kr; Tel.: +82-2-3277-3101; Fax: +82-2-3277-2862

Received: 30 November 2016; Accepted: 21 February 2017; Published: 27 February 2017

Abstract: We previously reported that women with short sleep duration consumed more dietary carbohydrate and showed an increased risk for obesity compared to those who slept adequately, but not for men. Using a cross-sectional study of 17,841 Korean women, we investigated the influence of sleep duration on obesity-related variables and consumption of dietary carbohydrate-rich foods in relation to menopausal status. Premenopausal women with short sleep duration had significantly greater body weight ($p = 0.007$), body mass index ($p = 0.003$), systolic and diastolic blood pressures ($p = 0.028$ and $p = 0.024$, respectively), prevalence of obesity ($p < 0.016$), and consumption of more carbohydrate-rich foods such as staple foods ($p = 0.026$) and simple sugar-rich foods ($p = 0.044$) than those with adequate sleep duration after adjustment for covariates. Premenopausal women with short sleep duration were more obese by 1.171 times compared to subjects adequate sleep duration (95% confidence interval = 1.030–1.330). However, obesity-related variables, dietary consumption, and odds of being obese did not differ according to sleep duration for postmenopausal women. The findings suggest that the increased risk for obesity and consumption of dietary carbohydrate-rich foods with short sleep duration appeared to disappear after menopause in Korean women.

Keywords: menopausal status; sleep duration; carbohydrate-rich foods; obesity; Korean national health and nutrition examination survey

1. Introduction

Sleep duration is regarded as a risk factor for obesity. It is generally accepted that poor sleep duration is associated with higher obesity-related variables and an increased risk for developing obesity as well as being associated with dietary consumption patterns [1–3]. However, poor sleep duration is more prevalent in women, and these associations are not comparable between men and women. Interestingly, our previous study reported these associations only for women, and not for men [3]. Women with poor sleep duration were particularly associated with increased odds of being obese among women who consumed more dietary carbohydrate (CHO) than subjects with adequate sleep duration [3].

Unlike men, women are greatly affected by hormone fluctuations during the menstrual cycle, which regulate dietary consumption and metabolic and physiological conditions [4]. Menopause is the cessation of reproductive ability in a woman's life and is associated with a decrease in hormone production [4,5]. The decrease in estrogen levels is known to be associated with behavioral changes such as stress, nervousness, depression, and poor sleep as well as physiological changes [6]. Postmenopausal women tend to show an increased prevalence for poor sleep compared with premenopausal women [7]. However, some studies have reported that poor sleep is not primarily attributed to decreases in the production of estrogen [8,9].

Therefore, we hypothesized that the gender differences in the interaction between short sleep duration and dietary consumption in relation to obesity in our previous study was caused by differences in reproductive hormones. To determine this hypothesis, we conducted a study in which menopausal status was divided into two categories, premenopausal and postmenopausal women, by considering the data of women who participated in the Korean National Health and Nutrition Examination Survey (KNHANES). Further, we investigated the influence of sleep duration on obesity-related variables and consumption of dietary CHO-rich foods in relation to menopausal status.

2. Subjects and Methods

2.1. Study Population and Subject Selection

The study was based on data from the KNHANES VI (2007–2009) and V (2010–2012), which is a national representative and cross-sectional survey carried out by the Korea Centers for Disease Control and Prevention (KCDC). The KNHANES was conducted to investigate the health and nutritional status of selective participants from a non-institutionalized civilian Korean population. The survey used a complex and stratified multi-stage probability clustered sampling design and consisted of a health interview, a physical health examination, and a nutritional survey. Detailed information can be found elsewhere [10]. From a total of 50,405 participants (22,926 men and 27,479 women) in the KNHANES IV–V (2007–2012), 21,620 women over the age of 19 years were selected for this study. Women with missing and inadequate sleep duration ($n = 1690$) and menopausal status ($n = 850$) data were excluded. Additionally, women who reported an implausible daily total energy consumption of ≤ 500 kcal or ≥ 3500 kcal ($n = 1239$) were excluded. Finally, 17,841 women were selected for the final analysis (Figure 1). Analysis before and after excluding missing and inadequate data showed no significant differences in sleep duration and energy consumption compared with menopausal status. All participants signed the provided written informed consent, and the survey protocol was approved by the Institutional Review Board of the KCDC.

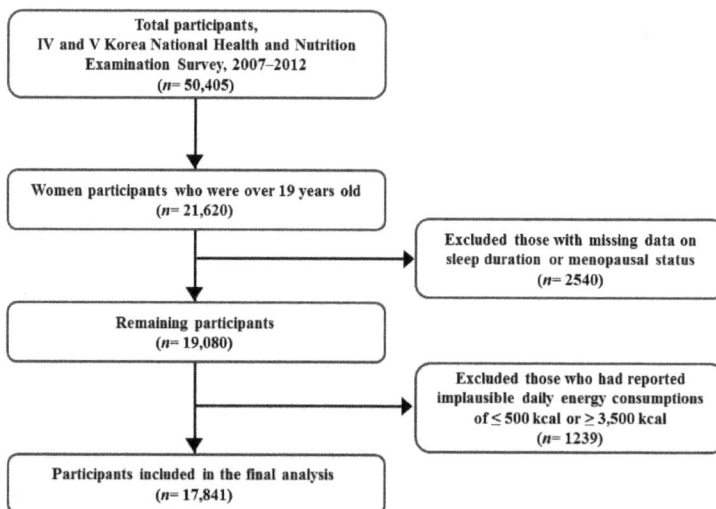

Figure 1. Framework of participants' selection.

2.2. Measurements

Menopausal status, anthropometric and blood biochemical factors, sleep duration, and dietary consumption were collected from the KNHANES data. Menopausal status and sleep duration data from the health interview and dietary consumption data from the nutritional survey were collected by trained specialists using questionnaires. Anthropometric and blood biochemical variables were obtained from the health examination using a direct measurement method.

2.3. Menopausal Status

Menopausal status was determined based on the following question: "Have you menstruated for the past 12 consecutive months?" If "yes", participants were defined as premenopausal, and if "no", participants were defined as postmenopausal.

2.4. Anthropometric Variables and Obesity Definition

Anthropometric variables were measured directly as part of the health examination [11]. Height and body weight were measured with participants wearing light clothing and no shoes to the nearest 0.1 cm using a stadiometer (SECA 225; seca GmbH, Co., KG., Hamburg, Germany) and 0.1 kg using an electronic scale (GL-6000-20; G-tech, Seoul, Korea), respectively. Body mass index (BMI) was calculated by dividing weight (kg) by height squared (m^2). The definition of obesity (based on criteria from the International Obesity Task Force of adults in the Asia-Pacific region) was BMI > 25 kg/m^2 [12]. Waist circumference (WC) was measured at the narrowest point between the lower borders of the rib cage and the uppermost borders of the iliac crest at the end stage of a normal expiration to the nearest 0.1 cm using a measuring tape (SECA 200; seca GmbH, Co., KG., Hamburg, Germany).

2.5. Biochemical Variables

Blood pressure (BP) was measured using a mercury sphygmomanometer (Baumanometer; WA Baum, Co., Copiague, NY, USA) and an average of three readings with 5-min rest intervals in the sitting position was used for the analysis [11]. Blood samples were collected after an overnight fast. Fasting glucose (FG), total cholesterol (TC), triglycerides (TG), and high-density lipoprotein (HDL-C) were analyzed using a Hitachi 7000 automatic analyzer (Hitachi, Tokyo, Japan) in a certified clinical laboratory [11].

2.6. Sleep Duration Assessment

Sleep was assessed using a self-reported questionnaire about average sleeping hours per day. Participants were divided into two categories according to their sleep duration: short sleep duration (≤6.9 h/day) and adequate sleep duration (≥7.0 h/day). A sleep duration of 7–8 h/day was taken as the recommended time for sleeping in accordance with previous studies [13,14].

2.7. Dietary Consumption Assessment

Assessment of dietary consumption was conducted by face-to-face interviews by trained dietitians. A single 24-h recall record method was used to obtain food items, which were categorized into 18 food groups based on common food groups classified in the Korean Nutrient Database [15]. Among 18 food groups, the drink group was divided into three subgroups: sweet; non-sugar (e.g., green tea, black tea, pure coffee); and alcohol. Consumption of CHO-rich foods as the staple foods or dessert foods is considered to be generally high in Korean women and to be influenced by sleep duration [3]. As a result, CHO-rich foods were defined as either staple foods such as a combination of grain and potato products or simple sugar-rich foods such as a combination of sugary products and sweet beverages.

2.8. Statistical Analyses

To reflect estimates of the entire Korean population, sample weights were applied in all analyses. To evaluate general characteristics and food group consumption by menopausal status, categorical variables, such as obesity prevalence, physical activity, current smoking, and drinking status were analyzed by Pearson's Chi-square test. Continuous variables, such as age, height, weight, BMI,

BP, FG, TG, TC, HDL-C, sleep duration, and dietary consumption were analyzed by independent *t*-tests. Because data were divided by menopausal status, generalized linear models were used to analyze the effects of sleep duration on anthropometric and biochemical variables and on food-group consumption as well as the interaction between menopausal status and sleep duration with respect to the anthropometric and biochemical variables and on food-group consumption after adjustment for covariates. Socioeconomic variables (age, education level, and monthly household income), disease prevalence-related variables (hypertension, cardiovascular disease, and diabetes), and health-related variables (age, smoking status, alcohol drinking status, and physical activity) were adjusted to prevent confounding effects. The interaction between menopausal status and sleep duration on the risk for being obese was determined using a multivariable logistic regression model. According to menopausal status, the odds ratio (OR) and 95% confidence intervals (CI) for the risk for being obese were estimated in reference to sleep duration of ≥ 7.0 h/day. A *p*-value < 0.05 was considered statistically significant. All statistical analyses were performed using SPSS (version 21.0; IBM Corp., Armonk, NY, USA) software for Windows.

3. Results

The general characteristics stratified by menopausal status are shown in Table 1. The average age was 35.71 and 62.85 years for premenopausal and postmenopausal women, respectively, and the percentage of women participating with each menopausal status was 51.9% and 48.1%, respectively. There were significant differences between menopausal statuses for all anthropometric and blood biochemical variables except for weight. BMI, WC, systolic blood pressure (SBP), diastolic blood pressure (DBP), FG, TG, and TC were significantly higher in postmenopausal women, but height and HDL-C were significantly higher in premenopausal women ($p < 0.001$ for all). Postmenopausal women showed higher prevalence of obesity than premenopausal women ($p < 0.001$ for both). Among health-related habits, premenopausal women showed a higher proportion who currently smoked and drank alcohol compared with menopausal women ($p < 0.001$ for both). Sleep duration was significantly higher in premenopausal compared with postmenopausal women (7.06 and 6.47 h, respectively, $p < 0.001$).

Table 1. General characteristics of Korean women study participants.

	Premenopausal (*n* = 9268)	Postmenopausal (*n* = 8573)	*p*-Value *
Age (years)	35.71 ± 0.14	62.85 ± 0.15	<0.001
Height (cm)	159.46 ± 0.08	153.34 ± 0.09	<0.001
Weight (kg)	57.38 ± 0.13	57.24 ± 0.14	0.460
BMI (kg/m^2)	22.58 ± 0.05	24.31 ± 0.05	<0.001
WC (cm)	75.37 ± 0.14	82.51 ± 0.17	<0.001
Obesity prevalence (%)	21.0	38.2	<0.001
SBP (mmHg)	108.39 ± 0.18	126.83 ± 0.30	<0.001
DBP (mmHg)	71.68 ± 0.14	77.13 ± 0.15	<0.001
FG (mg/dL)	91.06 ± 0.21	101.50 ± 0.39	<0.001
TG (mg/dL)	96.29 ± 0.99	138.29 ± 1.22	<0.001
TC (mg/dL)	179.34 ± 0.42	201.93 ± 0.55	<0.001
HDL-C (mg/dL)	56.06 ± 0.20	51.43 ± 0.20	<0.001
Sleep duration (h/day)	7.06 ± 0.02	6.47 ± 0.02	<0.001
Physical activity (%)	49.4	47.6	0.050
Current smoking (%)	6.8	4.7	<0.001
Alcohol drinking (%)	49.8	26.1	<0.001

BMI, body mass index; WC, waist circumference; SBP, systolic blood pressure; DBP, diastolic blood pressure; FG, fasting glucose; TG, triglycerides TC, total cholesterol; HDL-C, high density lipoprotein cholesterol. Values are means ± SE or %; * *p*-values calculated using *t*-test or chi-square test.

Among the different food groups, consumption of grains, potatoes, sugar, nuts, vegetables, fruit, eggs, fish, seaweed, milk, oil, seasoning, sweet drinks, tea, and alcohol were significantly different according to menopausal status (Table 2). The staple foods (177.49 ± 3.61 g vs. 166.43 ± 2.77 g, $p < 0.001$) were consumed more, but simple sugar foods (84.95 ± 4.67 g vs. 79.95 ± 2.92 g, $p < 0.001$) were consumed less in postmenopausal women compared with premenopausal women.

Table 2. Food group consumption in Korean women participants.

	Premenopausal (n = 9268)	Postmenopausal (n = 8573)	p-Value *
Grains and products (g)	134.79 ± 1.69	155.82 ± 2.30	<0.001
Potatoes and products (g)	42.23 ± 1.28	63.69 ± 1.98	<0.001
Sugar and products (g)	4.98 ± 0.12	4.63 ± 0.13	0.034
Tofu and products (g)	30.02 ± 0.74	29.82 ± 0.83	0.844
Nuts and products (g)	2.64 ± 0.13	3.08 ± 0.17	0.030
Vegetables and products (g)	144.29 ± 2.64	159.60 ± 3.23	<0.001
Mushrooms and products (g)	10.65 ± 0.37	10.45 ± 0.57	0.765
Fruits and products (g)	158.49 ± 2.67	169.06 ± 3.16	0.006
Meats and products (g)	54.49 ± 1.05	51.85 ± 1.48	0.122
Eggs and products (g)	22.57 ± 0.44	20.60 ± 0.53	0.003
Fish and shellfishes (g)	29.68 ± 0.59	24.91 ± 0.66	<0.001
Seaweed and products (g)	5.20 ± 0.22	6.81 ± 0.34	<0.001
Milk and products (g)	123.18 ± 2.18	132.71 ± 2.68	0.003
Oil (g)	4.03 ± 0.07	2.83 ± 0.07	<0.001
Seasoning (g)	36.30 ± 2.01	25.21 ± 1.46	<0.001
Sweet beverages (g)	79.48 ± 2.36	45.18 ± 2.05	<0.001
Tea (g)	89.14 ± 4.18	46.01 ± 6.26	<0.001
Alcohol drinks (g)	174.97 ± 6.85	122.77 ± 7.44	<0.001
Staple foods (g)	169.96 ± 2.49	207.29 ± 3.26	<0.001
Simple sugar-rich foods (g)	81.50 ± 2.51	53.20 ± 2.67	<0.001

Values are means ± SE represented as grams per 1000 kcal. * p-values calculated using t-test.

Significant differences in obesity-related variables and BP by sleep duration were observed in premenopausal women after adjustment for age, education level, monthly household income, hypertension, cardiovascular disease, diabetes, smoking status, alcohol drinking, and physical activity (Table 3). Premenopausal women with short sleep duration had significantly higher body weight (58.09 ± 0.22 kg vs. 57.04 ± 0.15 kg, $p = 0.007$) and BMI (22.96 ± 0.08 kg/m^2 vs. 22.39 ± 0.06 kg/m^2, $p = 0.003$) compared with those with adequate sleep duration after adjustment for the covariates. Moreover, SBP (109.68 ± 0.28 mmHg vs. 107.76 ± 0.21 mmHg, $p = 0.028$) and DBP (72.54 ± 0.21 mmHg vs. 71.26 ± 0.16 mmHg, $p = 0.024$) were higher among premenopausal women with short sleep duration compared with those with adequate sleep duration. All anthropometric and blood biochemical variables by sleep duration were not significantly different for postmenopausal women, except for HDL-C ($p = 0.005$). Significant interactions between menopausal status and sleep duration were observed for body weight, BMI, SBP, DBP, TC, and HDL-C (p-interaction < 0.001 for all), WC (p-interaction = 0.008), and TG (p-interaction = 0.015). The prevalence of obesity according to sleep duration was significantly different only for premenopausal women and not for postmenopausal women; premenopausal women with short sleep duration showed a higher proportion with obesity after adjustment for the covariates (24.1% vs. 19.5%, $p = 0.016$, Figure 2).

Table 3. Anthropometric and biochemical variables for different sleep duration in participating Korean women.

| | Premenopausal (n = 9268) | | | | Postmenopausal (n = 8573) | | | | |
	≤6.9 h (n = 2960)	≥7.0 h (n = 6308)	p-Value *	p-Value **	≤6.0 h (n = 4297)	≥7.0 h (n = 4276)	p-Value *	p-Value **	p-Interaction †
Age (years)	37.28 ± 0.22	34.94 ± 0.16	<0.001	-	63.63 ± 0.21	62.07 ± 0.21	<0.001	-	-
Height (cm)	159.08 ± 0.13	159.64 ± 0.09	<0.001	0.641	153.14 ± 0.12	153.54 ± 0.12	0.019	0.398	0.061
Weight (kg)	58.09 ± 0.22	57.04 ± 0.15	<0.001	0.007	57.20 ± 0.17	57.28 ± 0.20	0.718	0.186	<0.001
BMI (kg/m²)	22.96 ± 0.08	22.39 ± 0.06	<0.001	0.003	24.36 ± 0.06	24.27 ± 0.07	0.313	0.374	<0.001
WC (cm)	76.10 ± 0.22	75.02 ± 0.16	<0.001	0.186	82.57 ± 0.20	82.44 ± 0.23	0.633	0.981	0.008
SBP (mmHg)	109.68 ± 0.28	107.76 ± 0.21	<0.001	0.028	126.89 ± 0.37	126.79 ± 0.38	0.844	0.053	<0.001
DBP (mmHg)	72.54 ± 0.21	71.26 ± 0.16	<0.001	0.024	76.99 ± 0.20	77.28 ± 0.19	0.255	0.381	<0.001
FG (mg/dL)	91.67 ± 0.36	90.77 ± 0.24	0.032	0.735	100.90 ± 0.46	102.14 ± 0.58	0.080	0.138	0.059
TG (mg/dL)	96.70 ± 1.37	96.11 ± 1.27	0.746	0.104	136.97 ± 1.70	139.68 ± 1.73	0.260	0.102	0.015
TC (mg/dL)	179.64 ± 0.67	179.21 ± 0.53	0.611	0.071	201.45 ± 0.69	202.42 ± 0.81	345	0.344	<0.001
HDL-C (mg/dL)	56.13 ± 0.28	56.03 ± 0.23	0.737	0.131	51.73 ± 0.26	51.13 ± 0.26	0.071	0.005	<0.001

BMI, body mass index; WC, waist circumference; SBP, systolic blood pressure; DBP, diastolic blood pressure; FG, fasting glucose; TG, triglycerides TC, total cholesterol; HDL–C, high density lipoprotein cholesterol. Values are means ± SE. * p-values were calculated using general linear model. ** p-values were calculated using general linear model after adjustment for age, education level, monthly household income, hypertension, cardiovascular disease, diabetes, smoking status, alcohol drinking, and physical activity. † p values were obtained in interaction between menopausal statues and sleep duration using general linear model after adjustment for age, education level, monthly household income, hypertension, cardiovascular disease, diabetes, smoking status, alcohol drinking, and physical activity.

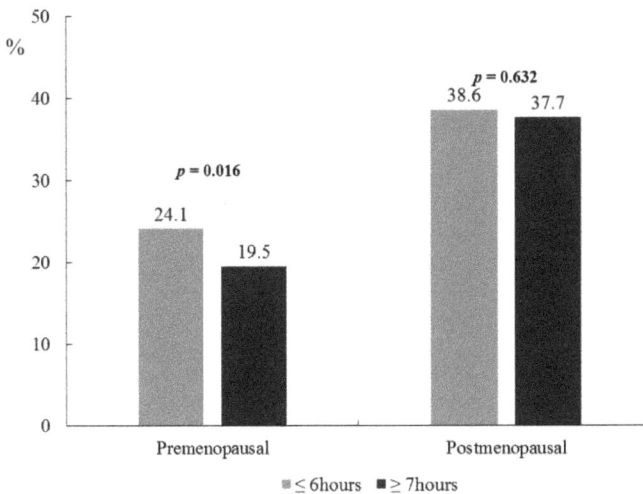

Figure 2. Prevalence of obesity and metabolic syndrome by sleep duration in participating Korean women. Premenopausal, n = 2906 for ≤6 h, n = 6308 for ≥7 h. Postmenopausal, n = 4297 for ≤6 h, n = 4276 for ≥7 h. p-values were calculated using a general linear model test after adjustment for age, education level, monthly household income, hypertension, cardiovascular disease, diabetes, smoking status, alcohol drinking, and physical activity

Significant differences in food-group consumption by sleep duration were observed only for premenopausal women, but not for postmenopausal women after adjustment for the covariates (Table 4). Among premenopausal women, those with short sleep duration showed significantly higher consumption of milk and milk products (p = 0.042), seasoning (p = 0.020), sweet beverages (p = 0.027), and tea (p = 0.013) compared with those with adequate sleep duration. Only among premenopausal women was short sleep duration associated with the consumption of CHO-rich foods in the adjusted model. In other words, premenopausal women with short sleep duration consumed more CHO-rich foods with respect to the staple foods (177.49 ± 3.61 g vs. 166.43 ± 2.77 g, p = 0.026) and simple sugar-rich foods (84.95 ± 4.67 g vs. 79.95 ± 2.92 g, p = 0.044) compared with those with adequate sleep duration. Interactions between menopausal status and sleep duration with respect to food-group consumption were found to be significant after adjustment for the covariates (p-values for the interaction for potatoes and products, vegetables and products, milk and products, seasoning, sweet drinks, and tea were 0.025, 0.031, 0.038, 0.025, <0.001, and 0.006, respectively). Furthermore, significant interactions between menopausal status and sleep duration by CHO-rich food consumption were observed (p-interaction for staple foods and simple sugar-rich foods were 0.028 and <0.001, respectively).

Adjusted OR for the risk for being obese and the interaction between menopausal status and sleep duration were examined using a multivariate logistic regression model after adjustment for age, education level, monthly household income, hypertension, cardiovascular disease, diabetes, smoking status, alcohol drinking, and physical activity (Figure 3). A significant interaction between menopausal status and sleep duration was found to be associated with the risk for being obese (p-interaction = 0.002). However, among postmenopausal women, no significant association was observed between obesity and sleep duration (p = 0.632). On the other hand, only among premenopausal women with short sleep duration, the adjusted OR for the risk for being obese significantly increased (p = 0.016). After adjusting for covariates, premenopausal women with short sleep duration showed a significantly increased risk for being obese (1.171 times) compared with women with adequate sleep duration (95% CI = 1.030–1.330).

Table 4. Food group consumption according to sleep duration in participating Korean women.

	Premenopausal (n = 9268)				Postmenopausal (n = 8573)				p-Interaction†
	≤6.9 h (n = 2960)	≥7.0 h (n = 6308)	p-Value*	p-Value**	≤6.0 h (n = 4297)	≥7.0 h (n = 4276)	p-Value*	p-Value**	
Grains and products (g)	137.50 ± 1.96	133.43 ± 1.88	0.032	0.188	156.39 ± 2.47	155.24 ± 2.68	0.622	0.863	0.198
Potatoes and products (g)	44.67 ± 2.52	41.10 ± 1.42	0.213	0.448	62.45 ± 2.69	65.09 ± 2.85	0.496	0.496	0.025
Sugar and products (g)	5.19 ± 0.22	4.88 ± 0.13	0.199	0.148	4.55 ± 0.16	4.72 ± 0.19	0.472	0.491	0.200
Tofu and products (g)	31.31 ± 1.37	29.38 ± 0.85	0.222	0.317	30.65 ± 1.27	28.97 ± 0.99	0.282	0.478	0.074
Nuts and products (g)	2.75 ± 0.22	2.58 ± 0.16	0.545	0.717	2.93 ± 0.20	3.23 ± 0.27	0.350	0.441	0.405
Vegetables and products (g)	152.09 ± 4.18	140.50 ± 2.77	0.006	0.102	161.16 ± 3.82	157.89 ± 3.82	0.422	0.351	0.031
Mushrooms and products (g)	10.94 ± 0.69	10.51 ± 0.46	0.618	0.670	11.45 ± 0.90	9.52 ± 0.69	0.089	0.143	0.286
Fruits (g)	159.91 ± 4.27	157.83 ± 3.17	0.679	0.794	168.58 ± 4.24	169.54 ± 4.04	0.858	0.848	0.611
Meats and products (g)	55.31 ± 1.67	54.10 ± 1.20	0.518	0.331	52.16 ± 2.11	51.60 ± 1.93	0.839	0.778	0.772
Eggs and products (g)	22.57 ± 0.66	22.57 ± 0.54	0.999	0.719	20.86 ± 0.73	20.35 ± 0.77	0.633	0.677	0.851
Fish and shellfishes (g)	30.30 ± 0.96	29.40 ± 0.69	0.419	0.711	25.18 ± 0.87	24.63 ± 0.87	0.625	0.551	0.152
Seaweed and products (g)	5.21 ± 0.39	5.20 ± 0.24	0.984	0.773	6.48 ± 0.46	7.15 ± 0.45	0.261	0.221	0.612
Milk and products (g)	129.36 ± 3.60	120.36 ± 2.58	0.035	0.042	131.87 ± 3.62	133.45 ± 3.91	0.765	0.725	0.038
Oil and products (g)	3.91 ± 0.10	4.09 ± 0.09	0.113	0.501	2.84 ± 0.08	2.82 ± 0.09	0.853	0.510	0.256
Seasoning (g)	40.44 ± 3.12	34.30 ± 2.08	0.045	0.020	23.92 ± 1.44	26.54 ± 2.26	0.276	0.505	0.025
Sweet beverages (g)	82.23 ± 4.27	78.24 ± 2.67	0.408	0.027	46.19 ± 3.03	44.04 ± 2.76	0.599	0.383	<0.001
Tea (g)	99.58 ± 7.60	83.29 ± 4.74	0.063	0.013	38.68 ± 4.34	53.16 ± 11.55	0.239	0.507	0.006
Alcohol drinks (g)	186.05 ± 11.44	169.12 ± 8.64	0.242	0.559	117.61 ± 8.55	126.66 ± 12.08	0.543	0.287	0.098
Staple foods (g)	177.49 ± 3.61	166.43 ± 2.77	0.004	0.026	205.54 ± 4.17	209.20 ± 4.14	0.477	0.255	0.028
Simple sugar-rich foods (g)	84.95 ± 4.67	79.95 ± 2.92	0.358	0.044	56.23 ± 4.26	50.08 ± 3.13	0.240	0.148	<0.001

Values are means ± SE. * p-values were calculated using a general linear model. ** p-values were calculated using a general linear model after adjustment for age, education level, monthly household income, hypertension, cardiovascular disease, diabetes, smoking status, alcohol drinking, and physical activity. † p values were obtained in interaction between menopausal statues and sleep duration using a general linear model after adjustment for age, education level, monthly household income, hypertension, cardiovascular disease, diabetes, smoking status, alcohol drinking, and physical activity.

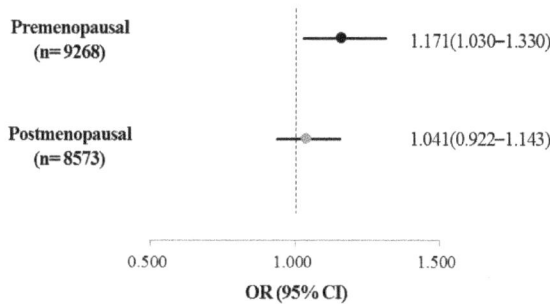

Figure 3. Adjusted odds ratio for obesity and for sleep duration in participating Korean women. OR, odds ratio; CI, confidence interval. The ORs (95% CI) were calculated in reference to sleep duration ≥7.0 h/day using multivariate logistic regression after adjustment for age, education level, monthly household income, hypertension, cardiovascular disease, diabetes, smoking status, alcohol drinking, and physical activity (*P*-interaction between menopausal status and sleep duration = 0.002).

4. Discussion

In this study, which was based on a national representative Korean women population, obesity-related variables and consumption of CHO-rich foods were found to be different according to menopausal status. Among premenopausal women, sleep duration appeared to influence obesity-related variables, consumption of CHO-rich food, and the risk for being obese in the model adjusted for age, education level, monthly household income, hypertension, cardiovascular disease, diabetes, smoking status, alcohol drinking, and physical activity.

Associations between sleep duration and obesity-related variables in women but not men are reported to be because of hormone differences [3]. In the current study, to investigate hormonal effects, a large population of women was divided by menopausal profile, which was considered to be a critical contributing factor in determining hormonal differences in women. Our finding was consistent with previous studies [16–18], which reported an increased trend in the prevalence of obesity after menopause. It is possible that the findings are associated with changes in reproductive hormones, such as estrogen, follicle stimulating hormone (FSH), and luteinizing hormone (LH) as well as melatonin secretion after entering menopause [15,16]. These changes lead to metabolic changes such as increases in appetite, dietary consumption, and adiposity as well as alternation in energy homeostasis [19–21]. A study of a population of Brazilian females reported that postmenopausal women with higher BMI levels had high levels of TG and FG but low levels of HDL-C [22].

Generally, for Koreans, the traditional main meal consists of rice and potatoes, and these products, which are consumed two to three times per day as staple food, provide about 37.9% of the total daily energy [23]. In the current study, postmenopausal women consumed more staple food and less simple sugar food compared with premenopausal women. Premenopausal women, who were mostly younger, had a higher consumption of simple sugar food and consumed more grams of food in the form of snacks than as the main meal when compared with postmenopausal women.

Interestingly, after adjustment for age, education level, monthly household income, hypertension, cardiovascular disease, diabetes, smoking status, alcohol drinking, and physical activity, premenopausal women with short sleep duration showed a significant association with both higher obesity-related variables and the risk for being obese, but this was not found for postmenopausal women. Previous clinical studies [24–26] have reported that a shorter sleep duration is associated with increases in the intake of dietary CHO or CHO-rich foods, which is consistent with our results in premenopausal women, and may be associated with decreased leptin and increased ghrelin levels [24–26].

In our previous study, we reported that increased dietary consumption of CHO-rich foods in relation to short sleep duration potentially induced obesity in women, but not in men [3]. The correlation was explained by the combination of appetite controlling hormones such as leptin and ghrelin as well as the reproductive steroid hormones. When circulating estrogen levels decrease, levels of FSH and LH increase [27]. Increases in FSH and LH are reported to be associated with a low blood melatonin level, and injection of melatonin has been shown to reinforce the effects of FSH and LH [28]. Low levels of blood melatonin in the fall–winter period [29], which is a main marker of the circadian system, are reported to increase appetite and influence poor sleep duration [29,30]. Normal levels of estrogen, FSH, and LH in premenopausal women may affect the levels of blood melatonin, which controls adequate sleep duration and status. Moreover, melatonin regulates appetite controlling hormones such as leptin and ghrelin, which are associated with the consumption of CHO-rich foods. It is suggested that the increased risk for obesity caused by short sleep duration in premenopausal women might decrease in postmenopausal women due to abnormal changes in the levels of reproductive hormones, such as estrogen, FSH, and LH.

These interesting data suggest that menopausal status may be related to the consumption of CHO-rich foods, and may therefore influence obesity. However, this study has several limitations. First, the data that is used in this study is from a cross-sectional study. Consequently, the results of this study, per se, could not explain the sequence of associations between variables. Second, the age of the postmenopausal women was substantially higher compared to the premenopausal women. Although age as a confounding factor was adjusted, physical and psychological changes related with age may influence obesity status and dietary intake in addition to menopausal status. Third, we classified two categories for sleep duration; "short" and "proper". Although some studies [31,32] showed the association of long sleep duration with obesity, the participants with long sleep duration ($\geq$9.0 h/day) were low (8.0%) in this study. Finally, the menopausal status in this study was divided into two categories. However, more detailed menopausal conditions should be considered in future studies. For example, the 3 to 5 years preceding menopause could be taken into consideration because other physiological changes may occur during the menopausal transition period.

5. Conclusions

In conclusion, the results using representative subject data of Korean women from KNHANE, demonstrated that menopausal status is related to the differences in obesity-related variables and consumption of CHO-rich foods. Indeed, short sleep duration was associated with increased levels of obesity-related variables and increased consumption of CHO-rich foods in premenopausal women, but not in postmenopausal women. These findings suggest that the increased risk for being obese and the consumption of dietary CHO-rich foods that are associated with short sleep duration are likely to be modulated after menopause in Korean women.

Acknowledgments: This research was supported by the Basic Science Research Program through the National Research Foundation of Korea (NRF) funded by the Ministry of Science (NRF-2016R1C1B1010094). The first author was a recipient of the Center for Women in Science, Engineering and Technology (WISET) Grant funded by the Ministry of Science, ICT & Future Planning of Korea (MSIP) under the Program for Returners into R&D.

Author Contributions: The authors' responsibilities were as follows: Y.K. and M.D. created the study concept and design; M.D. performed the statistical analysis, conducted the data interpretation, and drafted the manuscript; Y.K. and M.D. reviewed the manuscript; both authors read and approved the final version of the manuscript.

Conflicts of Interest: The authors declare no conflict of interest.

References

1. Bayon, V.; Leger, D.; Gomez-Merino, D.; Vecchierini, M.F.; Chennaoui, M. Sleep debt and obesity. *Ann. Med.* **2014**, *46*, 264–272. [CrossRef] [PubMed]
2. Rahe, C.; Czira, M.E.; Teismann, H.; Berger, K. Associations between poor sleep quality and different measures of obesity. *Sleep Med.* **2015**, *16*, 1225–1228. [CrossRef] [PubMed]

3. Doo, M.; Kim, Y. Association between sleep duration and obesity is modified by dietary macronutrients intake in Korean. *Obes. Res. Clin. Pract.* **2016**, *10*, 424–431. [CrossRef] [PubMed]
4. Mihm, M.; Gangooly, S.; Muttukrishna, S. The normal menstrual cycle in women. *Anim. Reprod. Sci.* **2011**, *124*, 229–236. [CrossRef] [PubMed]
5. Pankaj, T. *Manual of Cytogenetics in Reproductive Biology*; Jp Medical Ltd.: New Delhi, India, 2014.
6. Weber, M.T.; Rubin, L.H.; Maki, P.M. Cognition in perimenopause: The effect of transition stage. *Menopause* **2013**, *20*, 11–17. [CrossRef] [PubMed]
7. Kravitz, H.M.; Joffe, H. Sleep during the perimenopause: A SWAN story. *Obstet. Gynecol. Clin. N. Am.* **2011**, *38*, 567–586. [CrossRef] [PubMed]
8. Tao, M.F.; Sun, D.M.; Shao, H.F.; Li, C.B.; Teng, Y.C. Poor sleep in middle-aged women is not associated with menopause per se. *Braz. J. Med. Biol. Res.* **2016**, *49*, e4718. [CrossRef] [PubMed]
9. Young, T.; Rabago, D.; Zgierska, A.; Austin, D.; Laurel, F. Objective and subjective sleep quality in premenopausal, perimenopausal, and postmenopausal women in the Wisconsin Sleep Cohort Study. *Sleep* **2003**, *26*, 667–672. [PubMed]
10. Kweon, S.; Kim, Y.; Jang, M.J.; Kim, Y.; Kim, K.; Choi, S.; Chun, C.; Khang, Y.H.; Oh, K. Data resource profile: The Korea National Health and Nutrition Examination Survey (KNHANES). *Int. J. Epidemiol.* **2014**, *43*, 69–77. [CrossRef] [PubMed]
11. The Fifth Korean National Health and Nutrition Survey (KNHANES V). Available online: https://knhanes.cdc.go.kr/knhanes/eng/index.do (accessed on 21 November 2016).
12. World Health Organization. *The Asia-Pacific Perspective: Redefining Obesity and Its Treatment*; WHO: Geneva, Switzerland, 2000.
13. Bixler, E. Sleep and society: An epidemiological perspective. *Sleep Med.* **2009**, *10*, S3–S6. [CrossRef] [PubMed]
14. Gallicchio, L.; Kalesan, B. Sleep duration and mortality: A systematic review and meta-analysis. *J. Sleep Res.* **2009**, *18*, 148–158. [CrossRef] [PubMed]
15. The Korean Nutrition Society. *Dietary Reference Intake for Korean*; Hanareum Press: Seoul, Korea, 2010.
16. Colpani, V.; Oppermann, K.; Spritzer, P.M. Association between habitual physical activity and lower cardiovascular risk in premenopausal, perimenopausal, and postmenopausal women: A population-based study. *Menopause* **2013**, *20*, 525–531. [CrossRef] [PubMed]
17. Mauvais-Jarvis, F.; Clegg, D.J.; Hevener, A.L. The role of estrogens in control of energy balance and glucose homeostasis. *Endocr. Rev.* **2013**, *34*, 309–338. [CrossRef] [PubMed]
18. Teede, H.J.; Lombard, C.; Deeks, A.A. Obesity, metabolic complications and the menopause: An opportunity for prevention. *Climacteric* **2010**, *13*, 203–209. [CrossRef] [PubMed]
19. Walecka-Kapica, E.; Klupińska, G.; Chojnacki, J.; Tomaszewska-Warda, K.; Błońska, A.; Chojnacki, C. The effect of melatonin supplementation on the quality of sleep and weight status in postmenopausal women. *Prz Menopauzalny* **2014**, *13*, 334–338. [CrossRef] [PubMed]
20. Okatani, Y.; Morioa, N.; Wakatsuki, A. Changes in nocturnal melatonin secretion in perimenopausal women: Correlation with endogenous estrogen concentrations. *J. Pineal Res.* **2000**, *28*, 111–118. [CrossRef] [PubMed]
21. Stachowiak, G.; Pertyński, T.; Pertyńska-Marczewska, M. Metabolic disorders in menopause. *Prz. Menopauzalny* **2015**, *14*, 59–64. [CrossRef] [PubMed]
22. Bagnoli, V.R.; Fonseca, A.M.; Arie, W.M.; Das Neves, E.M.; Azevedo, R.S.; Sorpreso, I.C.; Soares Júnior, J.M.; Baracat, E.C. Metabolic disorder and obesity in 5027 Brazilian postmenopausal women. *Gynecol. Endocrinol.* **2014**, *30*, 717–720. [CrossRef] [PubMed]
23. Korea Centers for Disease Control and Prevention. *The Report of the Third Korea National Health and Nutrition Examination Survey (KNHANES III) 2005—Nutrition Survey (I)*; Korea Centers for Disease Control and Prevention: Seoul, Korea, 2006.
24. Markwald, R.R.; Melanson, E.L.; Smith, M.R.; Higgins, J.; Perreault, L.; Eckel, R.H.; Wright, K.P., Jr. Impact of insufficient sleep on total daily energy expenditure, food intake, and weight gain. *Proc. Natl. Acad. Sci. USA* **2013**, *110*, 5695–5700. [CrossRef] [PubMed]
25. Haghighatdoost, F.; Karimi, G.; Esmaillzadeh, A.; Azadbakht, L. Sleep deprivation is associated with lower diet quality indices and higher rate of general and central obesity among young female students in Iran. *Nutrition* **2012**, *28*, 1146–1150. [CrossRef] [PubMed]

26. Nedeltcheva, A.V.; Kilkus, J.M.; Imperial, J.; Kasza, K.; Schoeller, D.A.; Penev, P.D. Sleep curtailment is accompanied by increased intake of calories from snacks. *Am. J. Clin. Nutr.* **2009**, *89*, 126–133. [CrossRef] [PubMed]
27. Davis, S.; Mirick, D.K.; Chen, C.; Stanczyk, F.Z. Night shift work and hormone levels in women. *Cancer Epidemiol. Biomark. Prev.* **2012**, *21*, 609–618. [CrossRef] [PubMed]
28. Cagnacci, A.; Paoletti, A.M.; Soldani, R.; Orrù, M.; Maschio, E.; Melis, G.B. Melatonin enhances the luteinizing hormone and follicle-stimulating hormone responses to gonadotropin-releasing hormone in the follicular, but not in the luteal, menstrual phase. *J. Clin. Endocrinol. Metab.* **1995**, *80*, 1095–1099. [PubMed]
29. Sato, M.; Kanikowska, D.; Iwase, S.; Shimizu, Y.; Nishimura, N.; Inukai, Y.; Sato, M.; Sugenoya, J. Seasonal differences in melatonin concentrations and heart rates during sleep in obese subjects in Japan. *Int. J. Biometeorol.* **2013**, *57*, 743–748. [CrossRef] [PubMed]
30. Walters, J.F.; Hampton, S.M.; Ferns, G.A.; Skene, D.J. Effect of menopause on melatonin and alertness rhythms investigated in constant routine conditions. *Chronobiol. Int.* **2005**, *22*, 859–872. [CrossRef] [PubMed]
31. Nagai, M.; Tomata, Y.; Watanabe, T.; Kakizaki, M.; Tsuji, I. Association between sleep duration, weight gain, and obesity for long period. *Sleep Med.* **2013**, *14*, 206–210. [CrossRef] [PubMed]
32. Knutson, K.L. Sleep duration and cardiometabolic risk: A review of the epidemiologic evidence. *Best. Pract. Res. Clin. Endocrinol. Metab.* **2010**, *24*, 731–743. [CrossRef] [PubMed]

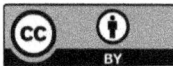

nutrients

MDPI

Article

Serum Amyloid A Production Is Triggered by Sleep Deprivation in Mice and Humans: Is That the Link between Sleep Loss and Associated Comorbidities?

Edson M. de Oliveira [1], Bruna Visniauskas [2], Sergio Tufik [2], Monica L. Andersen [2], Jair R. Chagas [2] and Ana Campa [1,*]

[1] Departamento de Análises Clínicas e Toxicológicas, Universidade de São Paulo, Av. Prof. Lineu Prestes, 580, São Paulo SP 05509-000, Brazil; edson.fbq@gmail.com
[2] Departamento de Psicobiologia, Universidade Federal de São Paulo, Rua Napoleão de Barros, 925, São Paulo SP 04024-002, Brazil; brunavisniauskas@gmail.com (B.V.); sergio.tufik@unifesp.br (S.T.); ml.andersen12@gmail.com (M.L.A.); jchagas1@gmail.com (J.R.C.)
* Correspondence: anacampa@usp.br; Tel.: +55-11-3091-3741; Fax: +55-11-3813-2197

Received: 29 November 2016; Accepted: 16 March 2017; Published: 21 March 2017

Abstract: Serum amyloid A (SAA) was recently associated with metabolic endotoxemia, obesity and insulin resistance. Concurrently, insufficient sleep adversely affects metabolic health and is an independent predisposing factor for obesity and insulin resistance. In this study we investigated whether sleep loss modulates SAA production. The serum SAA concentration increased in C57BL/6 mice subjected to sleep restriction (SR) for 15 days or to paradoxical sleep deprivation (PSD) for 72 h. Sleep restriction also induced the upregulation of *Saa1.1/Saa2.1* mRNA levels in the liver and *Saa3* mRNA levels in adipose tissue. SAA levels returned to the basal range after 24 h in paradoxical sleep rebound (PSR). Metabolic endotoxemia was also a finding in SR. Increased plasma levels of SAA were also observed in healthy human volunteers subjected to two nights of total sleep deprivation (Total SD), returning to basal levels after one night of recovery. The observed increase in SAA levels may be part of the initial biochemical alterations caused by sleep deprivation, with potential to drive deleterious conditions such as metabolic endotoxemia and weight gain.

Keywords: sleep curtailment; sleep loss; obesity; type 2 diabetes; SAA

1. Introduction

Obesity is now reaching pandemic proportions across much of the world and its consequences includes unprecedented health, social and economic issues. Several aggravating factors have been identified and are considered contributors to the current epidemic of obesity. Sleep disorders are among the factors that raised more concerns (for review see [1,2]).

Sleep loss induces metabolic and endocrine alterations, such as decreased glucose tolerance, decreased insulin sensitivity, increased concentrations of cortisol and ghrelin, decreased levels of leptin, and increased hunger and appetite [2]. Although these metabolic and endocrine alterations are frequently used to support a causal relationship between sleep loss and obesity/insulin resistance, it is still missing the identification of a triggering factor for weight gain in sleep disorders.

The difficulty of translating findings directly from animal models to humans and the challenge of finding an experimental model that leads to weight gain are some of the elements that prevent new discoveries regarding the mechanisms involved in weight gain led by sleep loss. Recently, using the multiple platform sleep restriction (SR) experimental model, we were able to link a past history of sleep restriction to subsequent complications arising from a high-fat diet [3].

Several possible causes linking reduced sleep and obesity, such as neuroendocrine changes, increased food intake, decreased energy expenditure and circadian disruption, share an inflammatory status as a common factor. Here, we focused in a specific inflammatory protein that has progressively gained recognition for its role in the obesity process, the acute phase protein serum amyloid A (SAA). Recently, we used SAA-targeted antisense oligonucleotide (ASO$_{SAA}$) on a high-fat diet-induced obesity model and identified SAA as an additional trigger driving endotoxemia, weight gain and insulin signaling impairment [4].

SAA production is upregulated in the liver and adipose tissue in the acute inflammatory process and it has been considered to have a role in the activation of immune cells triggering inflammatory responses [5]. Moreover, SAA has growth factor–like activity, such as increasing the proliferation of different cell types, including preadipocytes [6,7]. SAA is also able to bind to members of the Toll-like receptors (TLRs) family that are involved in the inflammatory process and metabolic control in obesity [8,9]. Here, we addressed if the production of SAA is one of the biochemical factors present in sleep restriction.

2. Materials and Methods

Animals. Male C57BL/6 mouse (three months of age) from CEDEME Universidade Federal de São Paulo (UNIFESP), housed in a room maintained at 20 ± 2 °C in 12:12 h light/dark cycle, chow diet (Nuvilab CR-1, Colombo, Brazil) and water *ad libitum*, were submitted to sleep restriction (SR) or paradoxical sleep deprivation (PSD) protocols. For each experimental group, six to 12 animals were used. The experimental protocol was approved by the Ethical Committee of UNIFESP (approval No. 0474/09). The euthanasia occurred immediately after each last experimental period by anesthesia overdose (i.p. administration of a combination of ketamine (100 mg/kg) and xylazine (15 mg/kg)), and ensured by cervical dislocation. During terminal anesthesia, serum samples were collected by cardiac puncture.

Sleep restriction (SR) protocol. The SR method used in this study was an adaptation of the multiple platform method, originally developed for rats [10], and performed as previously described [3,11,12]. The animals were randomly assigned into control group and SR group. The SR group was sleep restricted for 15 days, 21 h daily. After each 21 h period of SR, the mice were allowed to sleep for 3 h (sleep opportunity beginning at 10 a.m.).

Paradoxical sleep deprivation (PSD) and paradoxical sleep rebound (PSR) protocols. For PSD experiments, the animals were randomly assigned into three groups: the control group, the PSD group and the PSR group. PSD animals were sleep deprived for 72 consecutive hours, using the multiple platform method as previously described [3,13–15]. The PSR mice were sleep deprived for 72 consecutive hours followed by 24 h in sleep rebound period. A home cage control group was in the same room for the duration of the experiment, sleeping ad libitum. During the 72 h PSD period mice were placed inside a water tank (41 cm × 34 cm × 17.5 cm), filled up to 1 cm of the upper border and containing 12 circular platforms, 3.5 cm in diameter. Animals could thus move around inside the tank by jumping from one platform to another. When PSD was reached, muscle atonia set in, animals fell into the water and woke up. Food and water were provided ad libitum. Water in the tank was changed daily throughout the study period.

Human sleep deprivation. The experimental protocol was performed as previously described [16,17] with 30 healthy male volunteers ranging from 19 to 29 years. The exclusion criteria included sleep disorders, shift work, extreme morningness-eveningness, neurological or psychiatric diseases, smoking and alcohol or substance abuse, including any medicine able to change sleep patterns. The participants had normal results on Pittsburgh Sleep Quality Index, Epworth Sleepness Scale and Beck Depression Inventory. Briefly, three experimental groups were randomly assigned (10 non-sleep deprived, 10 total sleep deprived, and 10 REM sleep deprived) and the protocol was performed on nine consecutive days: one adaptation night, one baseline night, two nights of total sleep deprivation (Total SD) or four nights of REM sleep deprivation (REM SD), followed by three nights of sleep recovery for both groups. The control group was also maintained in the laboratory during the entire experimental protocol and had regular nights of sleep monitored by polysomnography (uninterrupted sleep showing normal sleep patterns). All subjects remained in the research center throughout the study period respecting a bedtime schedule (from 11 p.m. to 8 a.m.), in accordance with their regular habits (7–9 h sleep per night), and receiving 4 meals per day [17]. Total SD volunteers could read, play games, watch television or ambulate within the building to help them stay awake. Therefore, we cannot exclude circadian interference on SAA levels. The subjects were also abstained from running or any other type of resistance exercise. The investigators were continuously present to monitor wakefulness to ensure that subjects would not fall asleep during the study. REM SD volunteers were awakened when observed desynchronized EEG without spindles or K complexes and the concomitant reduction of the tonic electromyogram amplitude. The volunteers were kept awake for a sufficient time to avoid an immediate relapse into REM sleep while keeping the waking episodes short enough to allow frequent interventions. The study was conducted at the Sleep Laboratory of the Department of Psychobiology at the Universidade Federal de São Paulo (UNIFESP) with the approval of the Ethics Committee of the University (#1163/2016). All participants provided informed consent prior to enrolling in the study. Blood samples were obtained every morning (8 a.m.) during the experimental protocol (baseline, two nights of Total SD, four nights of REM SD and three nights of recovery). Blood samples were centrifuged immediately at 4 °C, and then the plasma were stored at −80 °C until the assays were conducted.

Quantitative real-time PCR. Total RNA from epididymal adipose tissue and liver was isolated using Qiagen RNeasy® Lipid Tissue Mini kit (Qiagen, Hilden, Germany). cDNA was then synthesized from 1 µg of RNA using the High Capacity cDNA Reverse Transcription (Life Technologies®, Grand Island, NY, USA). Real-time PCR were performed using SyBr® Green Master Mix (Life Technologies®, Grand Island, NY, USA) for *Saa1.1/2.1* (F-5′-AGA CAA ATA CTT CCA TGC TCG G-3′ and R-5′-CAT CAC TGA TTT TCT CAG CAG C-3′). Real-time PCR for *Saa3* was performed using the TaqMan® assay (Applied Biosystems®, Grand Island, NJ, USA), catalogue number Mm00441203_m1–*Saa3* and β-actin (*Actb*), number 4552933E, as an endogenous housekeeping gene control. Relative gene expression was determined using the $2^{-\Delta\Delta Ct}$ method [18].

SAA and endotoxin quantification. Serum/plasma concentrations of SAA were determined using ELISA following the manufacturer's instructions: mouse SAA (Tridelta Development Ltd., Maynooth, Ireland) and human SAA (Invitrogen®, Camarillo, CA, USA). Endotoxin was measured with the limulus amoebocyte lysate (LAL) chromogenic endpoint assay (Lonza, Allendale, NJ, USA).

Immunofluorescence. Using paraffin-embedded sections (5 µm thick) from epididymal adipose tissue, immunofluorescence for SAA was performed using a rabbit anti-mouse SAA (1:200 dilution, kindly produced and provided by De Beer laboratory, University of Kentucky, KY, USA) [19], subsequently incubated with the appropriate secondary fluorescent antibody (Invitrogen®, Camarillo, CA, USA) and the slides mounted using Vectashield set mounting medium with 4,6-diamidino-2-phenylindol-2-HCl (DAPI; Vector Laboratories Inc., Burlingame, CA, USA). An isotype control was used to ensure antibody specificity in each staining. Tissue sections were observed with a Nikon Eclipse 80i microscope (Nikon®, Tokyo, Japan) and digital images were captured with NIS-Element AR software (Nikon®, Tokyo, Japan).

Statistical analysis. Results were presented as mean ± SEM and the number of independent experiments is indicated in each graph. Statistical analysis was performed with Graph Pad Prism4 (Graph Pad Software, Inc., San Diego, CA, USA). When multiple samples were compared with one independent variable, one-way analysis of variance with Newman-Keuls post hoc test was performed. The level of significance was set at $p < 0.05$.

3. Results

Mice subjected to sleep restriction (SR) for 21 h daily during 15 days lost weight (Figure 1A). After seven and 15 days of SR, mice lost approximately 7% and 12% of weight, respectively. SR led to an increase in serum SAA and endotoxin of approximately four times (Figure 1B,C). *Saa1.1/2.1* and *Saa3* are inducible tissue-specific isoforms in the liver and adipose tissue, respectively [5,20,21].

Sleep restriction led to the mRNA expression of tissue-specific isoforms of SAA (Figure 1D–G). In the liver, the isoform *Saa1.1/2.1* was upregulated 10–40 times (Figure 1D) and *Saa3* remained unaltered (Figure 1E). In adipose tissue, whereas no difference in *Saa1.1/2.1* expression was observed (Figure 1F), the isoform *Saa3* was upregulated around seven times (Figure 1G). The data was confirmed by immunostaining the adipose tissue, where SAA production was induced after SR (Figure 1H).

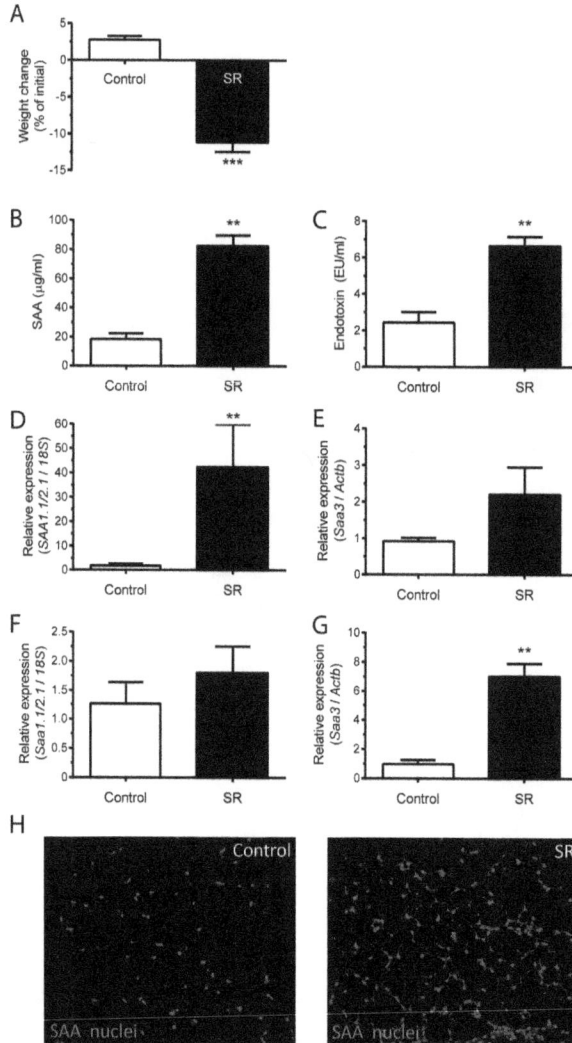

Figure 1. Sleep restriction (SR) causes weight loss and increased SAA production. Mice C57BL/6 were submitted to SR for 21 h daily for 15 days. (**A**) Mice weight change after SR; (**B**) SAA and (**C**) endotoxin concentration in mice serum; Real-time PCR was performed to assess mRNA expression of (**D**) *Saa1.1/2.1* and (**E**) *Saa3* in liver and (**F**) *Saa1.1/2.1* and (**G**) *Saa3* in adipose tissue; (**H**) Control and SR mice adipose tissue stained for SAA. Data are means ± SEM from six to 12 mice per group, with statistical analyses performed by one-way ANOVA followed by Newman-Keuls post hoc test (** $p < 0.01$, *** $p < 0.001$, vs. control).

Paradoxical sleep deprivation (PSD) and paradoxical sleep rebound (PSR) were primarily used to assess the extent, severity and length of the SAA increment induced by sleep loss. Similarly to sleep restriction (SR), mice subjected to paradoxical sleep deprivation (PSD) also showed an increase in serum SAA levels (four times higher than control mice) (Figure 2A). Besides that, PSD mice showed no difference in *Saa1.1/2.1* expression (Figure 2B) in the adipose tissue, with *Saa3* mRNA being upregulated about three times (Figure 2C). Interestingly, PSD regulates SAA production in a stimulus-dependent manner, once it was observed that SAA serum levels and *Saa3* mRNA expression in adipose tissue returned to baseline after the rebound period (Figure 2A,C).

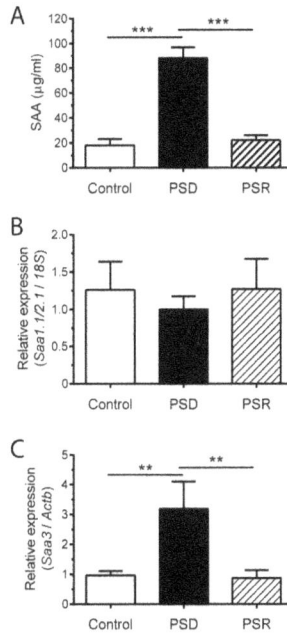

Figure 2. Paradoxical sleep deprivation (PSD) increases SAA levels in a stimulus-dependent manner. C57BL/6 mice were submitted to PSD for 72 uninterrupted hours, followed by a 24 h paradoxical sleep rebound (PSR) period. (**A**) SAA concentration in serum. Real-time PCR was performed to assess mRNA expression of (**B**) *Saa1.1/2.1* and (**C**) *Saa3* in adipose tissue. Data are means ± SEM from six mice per group, with statistical analyses performed by one-way ANOVA followed by Newman-Keuls post hoc test (** $p < 0.01$, *** $p < 0.001$, vs. control).

Finally, it was also possible to measure SAA from plasma derived from healthy human volunteers subjected to two nights of total sleep deprivation (Total SD) or four days in REM sleep deprivation (REM SD) (Figure 3). Although there was no difference regarding the SAA concentration when comparing the control and REM SD groups (Figure 3A), a remarkable four-fold increase in plasma SAA levels was observed after 24 or 48 h of total sleep deprivation (Total SD) (Figure 3B). Interestingly, the SAA levels also returned to basal levels after one night of recovery, showing that Total SD regulates SAA production in humans (Figure 3B).

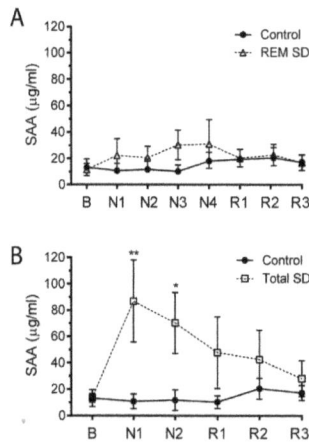

Figure 3. Total sleep deprivation increases plasma SAA in human. Thirty healthy male volunteers aged between 19 to 29 years were randomly assigned to one of three experimental groups after providing a written informed consent (10 in a non-sleep-deprived group (Control), 10 in a total sleep-deprived group (Total SD), and 10 in an REM-sleep-deprived group (REM SD)). Exclusion criteria included the following: sleep disorders, obesity and obstructive sleep apnea (OSA). Plasma SAA concentration in (**A**) REM SD and (**B**) Total SD. Data are means ± SEM (* $p < 0.05$, ** $p < 0.01$).

4. Discussion

The purpose of this study was to determine whether sleep restriction is associated with SAA production. We found that sleep restriction led to an increase in the production of SAA in both mice and humans.

In obesity and diabetes, the increment in SAA serum levels reaches no more than a three-fold increase from baseline [5,22]. Considering that, the four-fold elevation in serum SAA observed in sleep restriction (21 h daily for 15 days) and also in paradoxical sleep deprivation (72 consecutive hours) seems a striking result. Moreover, sleep restriction also caused an increment in lipopolysaccharide (LPS) in serum, achieving levels similar to that observed in metabolic endotoxemia, defined as a mild increment of LPS in serum after a short time on a high-fat diet, associated with the onset of diabetes and obesity [23].

Although it was not possible to identify which specific SAA isoform was increased in the mice serum, it is expected to be the hepatic-induced isoforms *Saa1.1/2.1*, once *Saa3* does not contribute to circulating SAA levels [5,21,24]. SAA3 is related to adipose tissue inflammation and its expression regulation may involve a direct induction by the hepatic isoforms *Saa1.1/2.1* [6,25].

The interplay between SAA and LPS has been suggested to play a role in the adipose tissue, making it prone to hypertrophy and consequent weight gain [4]. Both SAA and LPS are able to cause morphologic changes in the adipose tissue, such as promoting preadipocyte proliferation and tissue inflammation [6,26,27]. Despite the direct induction of migration, adhesion and tissue infiltration of monocytes and polymorphonuclear leukocytes [28], SAA induces the release of other chemoattractive cytokines such as MCP-1 and CCL20 [26,29]. Although sleep restriction led momentarily to weight loss, the increase in *Saa3* expression in adipose tissue may be an important factor to trigger obesity and insulin resistance. Our previous study in mice showed that sleep restriction predisposed them to weight gain and insulin resistance, aggravating the harmful effects of a high-fat diet [3].

Sleep restriction and sleep reestablishment seemed to be a prompt regulator for *Saa3* expression in mice adipose tissue. In a stimulus-dependent manner, an increase in *Saa3* expression was observed in PSD, with a rapid return to the baseline expression after 24 h in recovery.

The increment in SAA observed in humans submitted to two nights of total sleep deprivation was similar to that found in mice submitted to sleep restriction. This increment may be due to an increased SAA production or even due to a reduction in SAA clearance. Besides physiological differences between mice and humans, especially related to sleep habits, the increase in serum levels of SAA in response to sleep restriction seems to be similar between the species. However, if paradoxical sleep deprivation in mice was also able to modulate SAA production, no effect was observed when REM sleep deprivation was applied to humans. It is important to highlight that SAA was already described as being altered in obese patients with obstructive sleep apnea syndrome (OSAS) [30], possibly as a consequence of hypoxia/reoxygenation related to sleep apnea [31]. Our findings point out that even in lean and non-OSAS humans, SR is able to increase SAA levels and it may be related to the onset of subclinical inflammation, weight gain and insulin resistance. Moreover, the elevation in circulating non-esterified fatty acid (NEFA) is another event derived from SR [32] and it might be a direct effect of serum amyloid A, once it is able to induce lipolysis [6,26]. Both SAA and NEFA can lead to insulin resistance and play a central role in the development of metabolic diseases [4,32].

In addition to the role of SAA in obesity and insulin resistance, elevated serum levels of SAA is an independent and strong predictor of coronary artery disease and adverse cardiovascular outcome [33]. More recently, clearer evidence of the involvement of SAA in cardiovascular disease (CVD) showed that a brief elevation in SAA levels is sufficient to increase atherosclerosis [34]. Although no measurement of a direct cardiovascular disease risk factor was taken, it should be addressed in future studies.

5. Conclusions

In summary, our data show that sleep deprivation triggers SAA production in healthy and non-obese mice and humans. Interestingly, the transient increment in SAA levels occurred simultaneously to a metabolic endotoxemia. These results support the continued investigation of the role of SAA in metabolic diseases and also suggest that increased levels of SAA may be part of the signaling linking sleep loss to its associated comorbidities, such as obesity and type 2 diabetes.

Acknowledgments: The authors thank all the financial support and also thank Alexandre Froes Marchi and Thais Palumbo Ascar from the Departamento de Análises Clínicas e Toxicológicas, Faculdade de Ciências Farmacêuticas, Universidade de São Paulo, Brazil and Waldemarks Aires Leite from Departamento de Psicobiologia, Universidade Federal de São Paulo, Brazil, for their technical support. This study was supported by Fundação de Amparo à Pesquisa do Estado de São Paulo (FAPESP) (grant number 2011/24052-4 and 2010/18498-7 (doctoral scholarship)), Coordenação de Aperfeiçoamento de Pessoal de Nível Superior (CAPES), Conselho Nacional de Desenvolvimento Científico e Tecnológico (CNPq) (grant number 47310/2010-6) and Associação Fundo de Incentivo a Pesquisa (AFIP).

Author Contributions: E.M.O. contributed to the study conception and design, acquisition, analysis and interpretation of data, and writing of the article. B.V. contributed to the acquisition and interpretation of data. S.T., M.L.A. and J.R.C. contributed to the study conception and design, and also to the final critical revision of the manuscript. A.C. contributed to the study conception and design, analysis and interpretation of data, and writing and editing of the manuscript. All authors approved the final version of the manuscript to be published. A.C. is the guarantor of this work and, as such, has had full access to all data in the study and takes responsibility for both the integrity of the data and the accuracy of the data analysis.

Conflicts of Interest: The authors declare no conflict of interest.

References

1. Knutson, K.L. Does inadequate sleep play a role in vulnerability to obesity? *Am. J. Hum. Biol.* **2012**, *24*, 361–371. [CrossRef] [PubMed]
2. Taheri, S.; Lin, L.; Austin, D.; Young, T.; Mignot, E. Short sleep duration is associated with reduced leptin, elevated ghrelin, and increased body mass index. *PLoS Med.* **2004**, *1*, 210–217. [CrossRef] [PubMed]
3. De Oliveira, E.M.; Visniauskas, B.; Sandri, S.; Migliorini, S.; Andersen, M.L.; Tufik, S.; Fock, R.A.; Chagas, J.R.; Campa, A. Late effects of sleep restriction: Potentiating weight gain and insulin resistance arising from a high-fat diet in mice. *Obesity* **2015**, *23*, 391–398. [CrossRef] [PubMed]

4. De Oliveira, E.M.; Ascar, T.P.; Silva, J.C.; Sandri, S.; Migliorini, S.; Fock, R.A.; Campa, A. Serum amyloid A links endotoxaemia to weight gain and insulin resistance in mice. *Diabetologia* **2016**, *59*, 1760–1768. [CrossRef] [PubMed]
5. Eklund, K.K.; Niemi, K.; Kovanen, P.T. Immune functions of Serum Amyloid A. *Crit. Rev. Immunol.* **2012**, *32*, 335–348. [CrossRef] [PubMed]
6. Filippin-Monteiro, F.B.; de Oliveira, E.M.; Sandri, S.; Knebel, F.H.; Albuquerque, R.C.; Campa, A. Serum amyloid A is a growth factor for 3t3-l1 adipocytes, inhibits differentiation and promotes insulin resistance. *Int. J. Obes.* **2012**, *36*, 1032–1039. [CrossRef] [PubMed]
7. Cai, X.P.; Freedman, S.B.; Witting, P.K. Serum amyloid A stimulates cultured endothelial cells to migrate and proliferate: Inhibition by the multikinase inhibitor BIBF1120. *Clin. Exp. Pharm. Physiol.* **2013**, *40*, 662–670. [CrossRef] [PubMed]
8. Sandri, S.; Rodriguez, D.; Gomes, E.; Monteiro, H.P.; Russo, M.; Campa, A. Is serum amyloid A an endogenous TLR4 agonist? *J. Leukoc. Biol.* **2008**, *83*, 1174–1180. [CrossRef] [PubMed]
9. Cheng, N.; He, R.; Tian, J.; Ye, P.P.; Ye, R.D. Cutting edge: TLR2 is a functional receptor for acute-phase serum amyloid a. *J. Immunol.* **2008**, *181*, 22–26. [CrossRef] [PubMed]
10. Machado, R.B.; Suchecki, D.; Tufik, S. Comparison of the sleep pattern throughout a protocol of chronic sleep restriction induced by two methods of paradoxical sleep deprivation. *Brain Res. Bull.* **2006**, *70*, 213–220. [CrossRef] [PubMed]
11. Kahan, V.; Ribeiro, D.A.; Egydio, F.; Barros, L.A.; Tomimori, J.; Tufik, S.; Andersen, M.L. Is lack of sleep capable of inducing dna damage in aged skin? *Skin Pharm. Physiol.* **2014**, *27*, 127–131. [CrossRef] [PubMed]
12. Maia, L.O.; Dias, W.; Carvalho, L.S.; Jesus, L.R.; Paiva, G.D.; Araujo, P.; Costa, M.F.O.; Andersen, M.L.; Tufik, S.; Mazaro-Costa, R. Association of methamidophos and sleep loss on reproductive toxicity of male mice. *Environ. Toxicol. Pharm.* **2011**, *32*, 155–161. [CrossRef] [PubMed]
13. Machado, R.B.; Hipolide, D.C.; Benedito-Silva, A.A.; Tufik, S. Sleep deprivation induced by the modified multiple platform technique: Quantification of sleep loss and recovery. *Brain Res.* **2004**, *1004*, 45–51. [CrossRef] [PubMed]
14. Guariniello, L.D.; Vicari, P.; Lee, K.S.; De Oliveira, A.C.; Tufik, S. Bone marrow and peripheral white blood cells number is affected by sleep deprivation in a murine experimental model. *J. Cell. Physiol.* **2012**, *227*, 361–366. [CrossRef] [PubMed]
15. Zager, A.; Andersen, M.L.; Ruiz, F.S.; Antunes, I.B.; Tufik, S. Effects of acute and chronic sleep loss on immune modulation of rats. *Am. J. Physiol. Regul. Integr. Comp. Physiol.* **2007**, *293*, R504–R509. [CrossRef] [PubMed]
16. Ruiz, F.S.; Andersen, M.L.; Martins, R.C.S.; Zager, A.; Lopes, J.D.; Tufik, S. Immune alterations after selective rapid eye movement or total sleep deprivation in healthy male volunteers. *Innate Immun.* **2012**, *18*, 44–54. [CrossRef] [PubMed]
17. Martins, R.C.S.; Andersen, M.L.; Garbuio, S.A.; Bittencourt, L.R.; Guindalini, C.; Shih, M.C.; Hoexter, M.Q.; Bressan, R.A.; Castiglioni, M.L.V.; Tufik, S. Dopamine transporter regulation during four nights of rem sleep deprivation followed by recovery—An in vivo molecular imaging study in humans. *Sleep* **2010**, *33*, 243–251. [PubMed]
18. Livak, K.J.; Schmittgen, T.D. Analysis of relative gene expression data using real-time quantitative PCR and the 2(-Delta Delta C(T)) Method. *Methods* **2001**, *25*, 402–408. [CrossRef] [PubMed]
19. De Beer, M.C.; Wroblewski, J.M.; Noffsinger, V.P.; Rateri, D.L.; Howatt, D.A.; Balakrishnan, A.; Ji, A.L.; Shridas, P.; Thompson, J.C.; van der Westhuyzen, D.R.; et al. Deficiency of endogenous acute phase serum amyloid a does not affect atherosclerotic lesions in apolipoprotein e-deficient mice. *Arterioscler. Thromb. Vasc. Biol.* **2014**, *34*, 255–261. [CrossRef] [PubMed]
20. Sommer, G.; Weise, S.; Kralisch, S.; Scherer, P.E.; Lossner, U.; Bluher, M.; Stumvoll, M.; Fasshauer, M. The adipokine SAA3 is induced by interleukin-1 beta in mouse adipocytes. *J. Cell. Biochem.* **2008**, *104*, 2241–2247. [CrossRef] [PubMed]
21. Uhlar, C.M.; Whitehead, A.S. Serum amyloid A, the major vertebrate acute-phase reactant. *Eur. J. Biochem.* **1999**, *265*, 501–523. [CrossRef] [PubMed]
22. Hatanaka, E.; Monteagudo, P.T.; Marrocos, M.S.M.; Campa, A. Interaction between serum amyloid A and leukocytes—A possible role in the progression of vascular complications in diabetes. *Immunol. Lett.* **2007**, *108*, 160–166. [CrossRef] [PubMed]

23. Cani, P.D.; Amar, J.; Iglesias, M.A.; Poggi, M.; Knauf, C.; Bastelica, D.; Neyrinck, A.M.; Fava, F.; Tuohy, K.M.; Chabo, C.; et al. Metabolic endotoxemia initiates obesity and insulin resistance. *Diabetes* **2007**, *56*, 1761–1772. [CrossRef] [PubMed]

24. Chiba, T.; Han, C.Y.; Vaisar, T.; Shimokado, K.; Kargi, A.; Chen, M.H.; Wang, S.; McDonald, T.O.; O'Brien, K.D.; Heinecke, J.W.; et al. Serum amyloid A3 does not contribute to circulating SAA levels. *J. Lipid Res.* **2009**, *50*, 1353–1362. [CrossRef] [PubMed]

25. Den Hartigh, L.J.; Wang, S.R.; Goodspeed, L.; Ding, Y.L.; Averill, M.; Subramanian, S.; Wietecha, T.; O'Brien, K.D.; Chait, A. Deletion of serum amyloid A3 improves high fat high sucrose diet-induced adipose tissue inflammation and hyperlipidemia in female mice. *PLoS ONE* **2014**, *9*. [CrossRef] [PubMed]

26. Faty, A.; Ferre, P.; Commans, S. The acute phase protein serum amyloid A induces lipolysis and inflammation in human adipocytes through distinct pathways. *PLoS ONE* **2012**, *7*, e34031. [CrossRef] [PubMed]

27. Luche, E.; Cousin, B.; Garidou, L.; Serino, M.; Waget, A.; Barreau, C.; André, M.; Valet, P.; Courtney, M.; Casteilla, L.; et al. Metabolic endotoxemia directly increases the proliferation of adipocyte precursors at the onset of metabolic diseases through a cd14-dependent mechanism. *Mol. Metab.* **2013**, *2*, 281–291. [CrossRef] [PubMed]

28. Badolato, R.; Wang, J.M.; Murphy, W.J.; Lloyd, A.R.; Michiel, D.F.; Bausserman, L.L.; Kelvin, D.J.; Oppenheim, J.J. Serum amyloid-A is a chemoattractant—Induction of migration, adhesion, and tissue infiltration of monocytes and polymorphonuclear leukocytes. *J. Exp. Med.* **1994**, *180*, 203–209. [CrossRef] [PubMed]

29. Sandri, S.; Hatanaka, E.; Franco, A.G.; Pedrosa, A.M.C.; Monteiro, H.P.; Campa, A. Serum amyloid A induces ccl20 secretion in mononuclear cells through mapk (p38 and ERK1/2) signaling pathways. *Immunol. Lett.* **2008**, *121*, 22–26. [CrossRef] [PubMed]

30. Svatikova, A.; Wolk, R.; Shamsuzzaman, A.S.; Kara, T.; Olson, E.J.; Somers, V.K. Serum amyloid A in obstructive sleep apnea. *Circulation* **2003**, *108*, 1451–1454. [CrossRef] [PubMed]

31. De Oliveira, E.M.; Sandri, S.; Knebel, F.H.; Iglesias Contesini, C.G.; Campa, A.; Filippin-Monteiro, F.B. Hypoxia increases serum amyloid A3 (SAA3) in differentiated 3t3-l1 adipocytes. *Inflammation* **2013**, *36*, 1107–1110. [CrossRef] [PubMed]

32. Broussard, J.L.; Chapotot, F.; Abraham, V.; Day, A.; Delebecque, F.; Whitmore, H.R.; Tasali, E. Sleep restriction increases free fatty acids in healthy men. *Diabetologia* **2015**, *58*, 791–798. [CrossRef] [PubMed]

33. Johnson, B.D.; Kip, K.E.; Marroquin, O.C.; Ridker, P.M.; Kelsey, S.F.; Shaw, L.J.; Pepine, C.J.; Sharaf, B.; Merz, C.N.B.; Sopko, G.; et al. Serum amyloid A as a predictor of coronary artery disease and cardiovascular outcome in women—The national heart, lung, and blood institute-sponsored women's ischemia syndrome evaluation (wise). *Circulation* **2004**, *109*, 726–732. [CrossRef] [PubMed]

34. Thompson, J.C.; Jayne, C.; Thompson, J.; Wilson, P.G.; Yoder, M.H.; Webb, N.; Tannock, L.R. A brief elevation of serum amyloid a is sufficient to increase atherosclerosis. *J. Lipid Res.* **2015**, *56*, 286–293. [CrossRef] [PubMed]

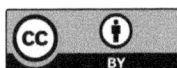

![nutrients logo]

nutrients

MDPI

Article

Sleep Duration and Chronic Fatigue Are Differently Associated with the Dietary Profile of Shift Workers

Georgina Heath [1,*], Alison Coates [2], Charli Sargent [3] and Jillian Dorrian [1]

[1] Centre for Sleep Research, University of South Australia, Adelaide 5000, Australia; jill.dorrian@unisa.edu.au
[2] Alliance for Research in Exercise, University of South Australia, Nutrition and Activity, Adelaide 5000, Australia; alison.coates@unisa.edu.au
[3] Appleton Institute for Behavioural Science, Central Queensland University, Wayville 5034, Australia; charli.sargent@cqu.edu.au
*   Correspondence: Georgina.heath@unisa.edu.au; Tel.: +61-8-8302-9973

Received: 14 October 2016; Accepted: 23 November 2016; Published: 30 November 2016

Abstract: Shift work has been associated with dietary changes. This study examined factors associated with the dietary profiles of shift workers from several industries (n = 118, 57 male; age = 43.4 ± 9.9 years) employed on permanent mornings, nights, or rotating 8-h or 12-h shifts. The dietary profile was assessed using a Food Frequency Questionnaire. Shift-related (e.g., sleep duration and fatigue), work-related (e.g., industry), and demographic factors (e.g., BMI) were measured using a modified version of the Standard Shift work Index. Mean daily energy intake was 8628 ± 3161 kJ. As a percentage of daily energy intake, all workers reported lower than recommended levels of carbohydrate (CHO, 45%–65%). Protein was within recommended levels (15%–25%). Permanent night workers were the only group to report higher than recommended fat intake (20%–35%). However, all workers reported higher than recommended levels of saturated fat (>10%) with those on permanent nights reporting significantly higher levels than other groups (Mean = 15.5% ± 3.1%, $p < 0.05$). Shorter sleep durations and decreased fatigue were associated with higher CHO intake ($p \leq 0.05$) whereas increased fatigue and longer sleep durations were associated with higher intake of fat ($p \leq 0.05$). Findings demonstrate sleep duration, fatigue, and shift schedule are associated with the dietary profile of shift workers.

Keywords: shift work; shift schedule; sleep duration; fatigue; diet; energy intake; macronutrient distribution; dietary profile

1. Introduction

The prevalence of shift work has increased over the past few decades [1]. Shift work has been associated with a number of negative consequences, including circadian disruption, sleep restriction [2,3], and high levels of fatigue [4], leading to detrimental effects for the safety and performance of shift workers [5–8]. The impact of shift work on long-term health is also of concern and numerous studies have linked shift work with several serious health disorders, including cardiovascular disease, metabolic syndrome, type 2 diabetes, gastrointestinal disease, and some forms of cancer [9–12]. Poor diet has been identified as a risk factor for chronic health conditions [13] and, as such, interest in examining the dietary profiles of shift workers has increased.

A recent systematic review and meta-analysis investigating the energy intake of shift workers compared to day workers concluded that there were no differences in total energy intake over a 24-h period between the two groups [14]. In contrast, a subsequent study adjusting for confounding factors, such as age and BMI, found that shift workers reported a higher energy intake compared to day workers [15]. Although this study did not find any differences in the quality of the diet, several previous studies have suggested that shift work might alter macronutrient distribution and food consumption patterns, such as an increased intake of snacks on night shift. Several studies have investigated the dietary profiles of shift workers. Studies have found shift workers report an increased fat intake [16–18], a higher percentage of saturated fat in the diet [16,19], and an increased intake of carbohydrates [17] when compared to day workers. However, findings have been mixed, with variations in methods used to capture dietary intake (e.g., food frequency questionnaires versus food diaries) [20,21], country/culture (e.g., Brazil versus Japan) [19,20], industry (e.g., airline employees versus steel company workers) [18,19], and type of shift work studied (e.g., permanent versus rotating shifts) [16,21]. These differences by shift work type are important, since each shift schedule differentially affects lifestyle factors, such as sleep duration and fatigue [2,5,22,23], which have, themselves, been associated with dietary changes [24–29]. As highlighted in a recent review examining lifestyle habits and health risks in shift workers [30], it is important to measure lifestyle factors associated with shift work as these may at least partially explain the extent to which diet is altered.

Indeed, as a consequence of circadian disruption and/or inadequate rest opportunities between shifts, studies have demonstrated that shift workers obtain less sleep than day workers [2,22,23,31]. Laboratory studies restricting the sleep of their participants have found alterations in macronutrient intake. For example, an increase in carbohydrate intake was observed in a study that restricted participants' sleep opportunity to 5 h for five nights [25]. Other studies (all restricting sleep to 4 h per night) showed an increased consumption of fat following sleep restriction [26–29]. Contrasting findings in these studies could be explained by varied options, timing, and delivery of food. For example, buffet meals were provided at set times in some studies [26], while other studies have offered participants the option to snack ad libitum from a list of set snack choices [25,27]. Additionally, one study allowed participants to purchase foods of their choice at any time [29]. Differences in participant demographics have also been noted across studies, including BMI (e.g., within healthy weight range versus overweight participants) [25,28]; sex (e.g., males only versus mixed sex studies) [26,28], and duration of sleep restriction exposure, ranging from one night [26] to five nights [25,28]. In addition to these laboratory studies, a review of recent epidemiological studies concluded that sleep restriction was associated with an increase in fat consumption [32]. Overall, the findings of these studies suggest reduced sleep duration may result in changes to fat, and potentially carbohydrates, in the diet. However, the additional influence of other factors is yet to be explored.

In addition to sleep restriction, shift workers commonly report experiencing high levels of sleepiness and fatigue [5]. Night shift workers participating in a qualitative study reported increasing their intake of sugar and sweet snacks as a strategy for dealing with decreased alertness due to the circadian disruption associated with the night shift [24]. The term fatigue is sometimes used interchangeably with sleepiness, however, it may be most usefully examined as a separate construct resulting from difficult work, extended duty, and personal circumstance [33], as opposed to the simple desire for sleep. In this context, the term chronic fatigue is often used. To our knowledge no studies have examined whether chronic fatigue is associated with macronutrient intake.

Other work related factors, such the number of years an individual has been employed in shift work, have also been found to influence dietary profile. For example, a longitudinal study found that individuals who were employed in shift work for the full 10 years of the study had higher energy intakes compared to day workers who remained on day shifts for the duration of the study, day workers who changed to shift work during the study, and shift workers who reverted back to day shifts [34]. Similarly, a previous longitudinal study found that participants reported an increase in energy intake since beginning employment in shift work [35]. Very few studies investigating the diet of shift workers have reported the years their participants have been employed on a shift work schedule, however, the findings from these two studies suggest this should be investigated further as long-term shift work may be associated with increased energy intake.

In addition to the above factors that relate specifically to shift work, various other work-related and demographic factors have been found to alter the diet. For example, the industry an individual works in may influence their dietary profile due to the availability of food at the workplace (e.g., canteen facilities) [18] and norms for eating may alter between workplaces [36]. Furthermore, demographic variables, such as age, sex, BMI, number of dependents, and marital and socioeconomic status, have also been found to influence dietary intake and composition [36–40] and, therefore, these factors should also be considered when examining dietary profiles.

Although there have been an increasing number of studies examining the diet of shift workers, very few have investigated factors other than shift schedule to determine if they are associated with dietary profile. Identifying these factors will improve our understanding of the mechanisms that may contribute to health disorders seen in shift work populations and may help in the planning and development of health promotion strategies. Therefore, the aim of the current study was to determine if shift-related factors such as sleep duration, fatigue and years employed in shift work are associated with alterations in dietary profile. As other work-related and demographic factors have been found to alter dietary intake and composition, these will also be examined to determine if they are associated with the dietary profiles of shift workers.

2. Materials and Methods

This cross-sectional study conducted was over two years (2010–2012) and was designed to investigate factors associated with the dietary profiles in shift workers. Ethical approval for this study was obtained from the University of South Australia Human Research Ethics Committee (Ethics Protocol: P008/10). In addition, where required, ethics approval was obtained from the human research ethics committees relevant to the specific organisations.

2.1. Participants

The study recruited 131 participants from six organisations. Participants came from four industries: printing, postal, nursing, and oil and gas. Participants were included in the study if they worked on a shift work schedule in one of these industries at one of these organisations. Participants were excluded from the study if they were under 18 years of age.

2.2. Procedure

Participants were recruited in two different ways depending on the organisation. Three of the six organisations allowed the research team to conduct information sessions in scheduled breaks at the workplace. The remaining three organisations preferred the research team to discuss the study with a manager who then explained the study to employees at workplace meetings. Following the information sessions, interested volunteers were asked to complete a series of questionnaires to capture information about dietary patterns, shift schedule, sleep, etc. As the questionnaire was anonymous a consent form was not required. Return of the questionnaire indicated consent to participate in the study. Questionnaires were returned via post to the Centre for Sleep Research at the University of South Australia and checked for completeness.

2.3. Measures

Dietary profiles were assessed using a semi-quantitative self-administered food frequency questionnaire (FFQ) designed by the Cancer Council Victoria [41]. The FFQ has been validated relative to weighed food records [42,43]. The daily macronutrient and alcohol intakes for each participant were calculated as a percentage of daily energy intake in kilojoules using the following values for each macronutrient: 17 kJ/g for carbohydrate and protein, 29 kJ/g for alcohol, and 37 kJ/g for fat.

Participants reported their sleep duration in hours on a modified version of the Standard Shift work Index (SSI) [44]. The Standard Shift work Index is a questionnaire that has been specifically designed to capture the details of shift workers. It is particularly appropriate for measuring demographic details in shift workers as it contains questions that take the schedules of shift workers into consideration. For example, the questionnaire asks participants to complete detailed information around the times they normally fall asleep and wake up at specific points within their shift system (e.g., before shifts, between shifts, and after the shift). This questionnaire has been used in many studies investigating the behaviour of shift workers worldwide [45]. Section 2 of the SSI (Sleep and Fatigue) was used to determine the amount of sleep each participant typically obtained between each working day for every type of shift they worked (e.g., morning, night and afternoon). Rotating shift workers reported the amount of sleep they typically obtained between each shift type. As rotating shift workers undertook a variety of shifts, average sleep duration between working days was calculated. Therefore, sleep duration was operationalized as the average sleep duration (in hours) a participant reported obtaining between working days.

Chronic fatigue was measured using a scale provided in the modified version of the SSI. The SSI defines chronic fatigue as general tiredness and lack of energy on work and rest days regardless of sleep obtained or work hours [44]. The Chronic Fatigue Scale is a five-point Likert type scale with 10 items. Responses can range from 'not at all' to 'very much so'. Five items in the scale are related to general feelings of tiredness or lack of energy. The remaining five items relate to feelings of vigour and energy, and are reversed scored. The Chronic Fatigue Scale has been found to have a reliability coefficient of 0.91 for internal consistency [46]. Scores on the Chronic Fatigue Scale can range from 10 to 50 with higher scores representing a greater level of chronic fatigue. Chronic fatigue was operationalized as the participant's score on the Chronic Fatigue Scale as a continuous variable.

Shift schedule, shift work history, total hours worked, and industry were reported on the modified version of the SSI [44]. These questions were open ended and asked participants to report their shift schedule, the number of years they have been employed in shift work, typical weekly working hours (including overtime) and the industry they are currently employed in. It was identified that shift workers were employed in one of four different shift schedules: permanent morning (e.g., 07:00–15:30), permanent night (e.g., 21:00–07:30), 8-h rotating (e.g., rotating between morning, afternoon, and night shift), and 12-h rotating (rotating between morning and night shifts). Participants were employed in one of four industries (printing, postal services, nursing, or oil and gas). The responses from completed questionnaires determined shift schedule (permanent morning, permanent night, 8-h rotating, or 12-h rotating); shift work history (the number of years employed in shift work); total hours worked (the number of hours reported working per week); and industry (printing, postal services, nursing or oil and gas). All of these industries were located in the metropolitan area of South Australia, except for oil and gas, which was located in Victoria.

Self-reported data were also collected for age, body mass, and height (from which body mass index (BMI) was derived). The number of dependents living at home, educational level, and marital status were also included in this study, as previous research has suggested that these variables can affect eating behaviour [38]. Participants reported their demographic details on the modified version of the SSI.

2.4. Data Processing and Statistical Analysis

Data were checked for missing values and screened for normality. There were no clear patterns in missing data between participants or variables. Less than 5% of data were missing for all variables except for shift work history (11% missing) and BMI (7% missing). Reported energy intake for one participant was >3 Standard Deviation (SD) above the mean and was, therefore, considered an outlier [47] and this value was removed. Marital status was categorised into 'married' and 'not married' (divorced, widowed, or single) in order to have cell sizes that were sufficient for the analysis. Dependents were categorised into 'yes' (dependent <18 years) or 'no'. Education was categorised into four categories: post-graduate, undergraduate, vocational, and secondary.

In order to examine differences in demographic, sleep, fatigue, work hours, and diet variables across different shift types (morning, night, 8-h rotating, 12-h rotating), univariate analysis of variance (ANOVA) was conducted. F-values and degrees of freedom were reported (F_{df}). Significant F-ratios ($p < 0.05$) were further investigated with pairwise post-hoc testing to identify which shifts were different from each other.

In order to identify associations between sleep, fatigue, work hours, and diet, controlling for other variables, linear regression was conducted. Prior to conducting the regressions, to investigate univariate associations and check for multicollinearity (variables that are too highly correlated), Pearson correlations were calculated for all continuous sleep, fatigue, work, diet, and demographic variables. Magnitudes of correlations were interpreted as trivial <0.1; $0.1 \leq$ small < 0.3; $0.3 \leq$ moderate < 0.5; and large >0.5 [48]. Correlations between all variables and energy intake were trivial. Percentage of fat showed small correlations with chronic fatigue levels ($r = 0.26$) and BMI ($r = 0.27$). Sleep duration showed a small correlation with BMI ($r = -0.21$) and the total hours worked per week ($r = -0.22$). Age showed a small correlation with BMI ($r = 0.22$) and a large correlation with years worked in shift work ($r = 0.58$). The correlation between sleep duration and chronic fatigue was trivial ($r = -0.06$). No sources of multicollinearity were identified.

Subsequent regression analyses for total energy, carbohydrate, protein, fat, saturated fat, and alcohol intake (dependent variables) were conducted using purposeful selection of covariates, as outlined by Hosmer, Lemeshow, and May [49]. This is an alternative to traditional stepwise approaches, which is of particular benefit when the goals of regression analysis are more than simply prediction. In traditional approaches, variables are most commonly retained in a model based on clinical and/or statistical significance. In contrast, the purposeful approach is designed to capture not only significant variables, but also those that are confounders (i.e., they influence the relationship between other variables and the dependent variable) [50]. First, (BMI, sex (ref = male), age, marital status, dependents, education, industry (ref = oil and gas), shift work history, hours worked per week, chronic fatigue score, shift schedule (ref = morning shift), and sleep duration) were entered into the model. Second, covariates that were not significant were removed from the model, leaving a preliminary main effects model. Third, each non-significant covariate was individually re-added to the preliminary main effects model. During this step, any covariates that were significant altered the significance of the other variables, or changed the parameter estimates by more than 20% were retained. Therefore, final models, presented in the results section, include all variables that have a significant effect on the dependent variable, or on the relationship between other independent variables and the dependent variable (referred to as control variables). Parameter estimates, their standard error (SE), significance level (*p*), and 95% confidence intervals (CI) are presented, as well as the R^2 change (ΔR^2) for each independent variable.

3. Results

3.1. Participants

Eight participants were excluded due to incomplete dietary questionnaires. One participant was excluded, as the industry reported on their questionnaire did not match any of the other industry categories. A further four participants were excluded as the work hours they reported (e.g., working between 9 a.m. and 5 p.m.) classified them as day workers rather than shift workers. Therefore, the final sample consisted of 118 participants (68% male) aged between 18 and 62 years (43.4 ± 9.9 years). The average sleep duration between shifts in this sample was 7.0 h. Shift workers on a 12-h rotating shift schedule obtained significantly less sleep than those employed on any of the other shift schedules (see Table 1). Although those on 8-h rotating shift and permanent night shift reported slightly higher levels of fatigue than morning and 12-h rotating shift workers, there was no significant difference in fatigue found between shift types (see Table 1). The average working hours per week for participants was 39.8 ± 11.6 h. On average, shift workers in the present study had been employed in shift work for 14.7 ± 10.0 years (see Table 1). Dietary intake for each shift type is reported in Table 2. All shift workers reported lower than recommended levels (45%–65%) of carbohydrates as a percentage of daily energy intake. Intake of protein as a percentage of energy intake was within recommended levels (15%–25%) for all shift workers. Night shift workers were the only group to report a higher than recommended percentage (20%–35%) of total fat intake. However, all shift workers reported higher than recommended levels of saturated fat (>10%) as a percentage of daily energy intake. The only significant difference by shift schedule in these simple univariate comparisons was for the percentage of saturated fat, with night shift workers consuming the highest proportion.

Table 1. Demographic characteristics of the study population for morning, night, 8-h rotating (8-h R) and 12-h rotating (12-h R) shift workers. The final column shows the F-ratio and degrees of freedom (*df* = 3113) from the univariate ANOVA.

	Morning *n* = 33	Night *n* = 27	8-h R *n* = 29	12-h R *n* = 29	F_{3113}
Demographics					
Age (years)	44.8 (9.9)	42.7 (9.9)	41.2 (11.7)	44.17 (7.9)	0.58
Female (%)	21.2	37.0	65.5	3.6	
BMI (kg/m^2)	25.8 (2.8)	26.8 (5.1)	27.5 (5.5)	28.3 (4.0)	1.68
Married (%)	81.8	74.1	85.7	93.1	
Education					
Postgrad (%)	12.5	7.4	32.1	17.2	
Undergrad (%)	21.9	14.8	32.1	3.4	
Vocational (%)	21.9	7.4	14.3	44.8	
Secondary (%)	43.8	70.4	21.4	34.5	
Sleep/Fatigue					
Sleep duration (h)	7.5 (1.0)	7.0 (1.1)	7.4 (0.9)	6.3 (1.0)	8.42 *,a
Chronic Fatigue (10–50)	25.9 (5.9)	28.1(8.4)	28.0 (7.8)	25.1 (7.7)	1.42
Work					
Work hours (h)	40.4 (16.1)	35.9 (9.6)	38.9 (10.0)	44.0 (7.2)	2.44
Shift work (years)	18.7 (11.5)	9.0 (5.9)	13.5 (10.5)	18.5 (8.8)	6.37 *,b
Industry					
Printing (%)	18.2	14.8	20.7	0	
Postal (%)	63.6	77.8	0	0	
Nursing (%)	15.2	7.4	75.9	0	
Oil and Gas (%)	3	0	3.4	100	

Mean (standard deviation) unless indicated otherwise; * significant at $p < 0.05$; R = rotating; BMI = body mass index; [a] 12-h R sleep duration was significantly shorter compared to all other shift types; [b] 12-h R spent significantly longer years in shift work compared to night and 8-R shift workers.

Table 2. Energy (kJ/1000) and macronutrients (% of energy intake) for morning, night, 8-h rotating (8-h R), and 12-h rotating (12-h R) shift workers. The final column shows the F-ratio and degrees of freedom (*df* = 3113) from the univariate ANOVA.

		Morning *n* = 33	Night *n* = 27	8-h R *n* = 29	12-h R *n* = 29	F_{3113}
Energy (kJ/1000)		7954 (2979)	8816 (3616)	8530 (3080)	9318 (2852)	1.0
CHO	%	40.7 (6.8)	41.8 (6.1)	41.3 (6.8)	38.7 (6.9)	1.1
	g	196.5 (81.2)	211.2 (86.5)	208.5 (87.3)	213.3 (78.8)	
Protein	%	19.0 (2.6)	19.2 (3.7)	20.7 (3.2)	19.6 (3.6)	1.3
	g	89.4 (34.3)	99.9 (43.4)	101.9 (37.6)	105.5 (33.0)	
Fat	%	33.0 (6.0)	35.9 (5.0)	34.3 (5.3)	34.5 (4.0)	1.4
	g	71.0 (28.8)	85.8 (38.9)	79.9 (34.1)	87.2 (30.5)	
SFA	%	12.9 (2.7)	15.5 (3.1)	13.8 (2.8)	14.1 (2.4)	4.2 *,a
	g	30.0 (13.2)	37.3 (16.9)	32.0 (15.1)	33.2 (12.9)	
Alcohol	%	8.8 (9.24)	5.5 (6.79)	6.5 (5.52)	10.1 (8.88)	2.0
	g	17.7 (17.28)	14.1 (21.18)	12.3 (10.53)	24.8 (23.04)	

Mean (standard deviation); * significant $p < 0.05$; kJ = kilojoules; g = grams; %, percent of total daily energy intake; SFA = saturated fat; CHO = carbohydrate; [a] Night shift workers reported a significantly higher percentage of saturated fat compared to morning and 8-R shift workers. It is recommended that the daily energy intake of adults contain between 45% and 65% carbohydrates, 15% and 25% protein, 20% and 35% fat in order to maintain health [13].

3.2. Daily Energy Intake

Sex, age, and total hours worked were significantly related to daily energy intake, controlling for sleep duration (Table 3). Specifically, females and younger participants consumed less energy (kJ) than males and older participants. Participants who worked fewer hours had a higher energy intake. Overall, the model accounted for 16% of the variance of energy intake in the diet.

Table 3. Regression analysis models (energy intake and macronutrient and alcohol intake as a percentage of daily energy intake). Factors include in final models were identified using purposeful selection [37], and are presented in model entry order (BMI, sex (ref = male), age, marital status, dependents, education, industry (ref = oil and gas), shift work history, hours worked per week, chronic fatigue score, shift schedule (ref = morning shift), and sleep duration).

Independent Variable	Parameter Estimate	SE	p	95% LLCI	95% ULCI	ΔR^2
Energy Intake (kJ)						
Sleep duration	−185.80	256.26	0.47	−693.93	322.32	0.01
Female (ref = male)	−2164.12	611.96	<0.01	−3377.54	−756.12	0.07
Age (years)	−69.94	28.04	0.01	−125.55	−14.33	0.04
Hours worked (h)	−60.03	23.78	0.01	−107.19	−12.86	0.05
Carbohydrate Intake (%)						
Chronic fatigue	−0.19	0.08	0.02	−0.37	−0.02	0.04
Shift schedule						
Night (ref = morning)	−1.21	1.89	0.52	−4.97	2.55	
8-h R	−8.33	1.74	0.63	−4.28	2.61	
12-h R	−5.26	1.88	<0.01	−9.00	−1.15	0.03
Sleep duration	−1.59	0.64	0.01	−2.86	0.32	0.05
Protein Intake (%)						
Female (ref = male)	1.33	1.16	0.04	0.02	2.63	0.03
Fat Intake (%)						
Female(ref = male)	1.94	1.66	0.10	−0.37	4.26	0.01
Shift schedule						
Night (ref = morning)	1.48	1.41	0.29	−1.32	4.29	
8-h R	−0.90	1.38	0.51	−3.65	1.85	
12-h R	1.86	1.39	0.18	−0.91	4.64	0.03
BMI (kg/m^2)	0.28	0.10	0.01	0.07	0.49	0.11
Chronic fatigue (10–50)	0.15	0.06	0.01	0.03	0.28	0.06
Sleep Duration (h)	1.04	0.47	0.03	0.10	1.99	0.01
Saturated Fat Intake (%)						
Age	−0.05	0.02	0.05	−0.10	0.00	<0.01
Married (ref = not married)	1.19	0.74	0.11	−0.27	2.67	<0.01
Industry						
Postal (ref = oil and gas)	−3.48	2.64	0.19	−8.75	1.77	
Printing	−3.10	2.61	0.23	−8.29	2.09	
Nursing	−1.13	2.50	0.65	−6.11	3.85	0.01
Hours worked (h)	0.03	0.02	0.16	−0.01	0.08	<0.01
Chronic Fatigue	0.05	0.03	0.14	−0.01	0.11	0.04
BMI (kg/m^2)	0.15	0.05	<0.01	0.03	0.26	0.10
Night (ref = morning)	2.76	0.76	<0.01	1.12	4.27	
8-h R	−0.95	0.99	0.34	−2.93	1.03	
12-h R	−2.28	2.69	0.39	−7.63	3.06	0.11
Sleep duration (h)	0.54	0.25	0.04	0.02	1.05	0.05
Alcohol (%)						
Married (ref = not married)	2.44	1.98	0.22	−1.49	6.37	<0.01
Shift work history (years)	−0.03	0.07	0.64	−0.18	−0.11	0.02
Female (ref = male)	−4.38	1.92	0.02	−8.20	−0.56	0.06
Industry						
Postal (ref = oil and gas)	−4.33	1.92	0.02	−8.14	0.51	
Printing	−1.45	2.49	0.56	−6.41	3.50	
Nursing	−2.11	2.37	0.37	−6.83	2.59	0.02
Hours worked (h)	−0.18	0.07	0.01	0.33	−0.04	0.06

ref = reference category; R = rotating; SE = standard error; LLCI = lower limit confidence interval; ULCI = upper limit confidence interval; ΔR^2 = R^2 change; kJ = kilojoules; % = percent of total daily energy intake; kg = kilograms; m^2 = meters squared.

3.3. Carbohydrate as a Percentage of Daily Energy Intake

Chronic fatigue, shift schedule, and sleep duration were significantly related to carbohydrate intake (Table 3). Figure 1 (upper panel) shows that as sleep duration and chronic fatigue decreased, the percentage of carbohydrates in the diet increased. Shift workers on a 12-h rotating shift schedule consumed less carbohydrates than morning shift workers (reference category). The model explained 12% of the variance of carbohydrate intake in the diet.

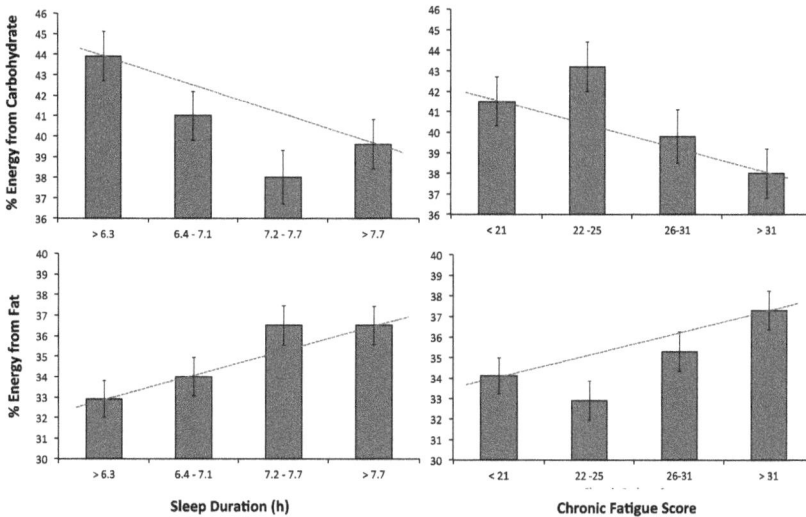

Figure 1. Relationship between sleep duration (**left panels**) and chronic fatigue (**right panels**) grouped into quartiles, for carbohydrate (**upper**) and fat (**lower**) as a percentage of total energy intake. Figures represent estimated marginal means from regression models and standard error bars. Dotted lines through the means of the first and last quartiles are presented as a visual aid—as sleep duration and chronic fatigue score increase, the percent of energy from carbohydrates decreases and the percent of energy from fat increases.

3.4. Protein as a Percentage of Daily Energy Intake

Protein in the daily diet was significantly related to sex (Table 3) such that females consumed a higher percentage of protein in the diet. Sex accounted for 3% of the variance in protein intake.

3.5. Fat as a Percentage of Daily Energy Intake

BMI, chronic fatigue and sleep duration were significantly related to fat, controlling for sex and shift schedule (Table 3). Figure 1 (lower panel) illustrates that as sleep duration and chronic fatigue increased, participants consumed a higher percentage of fat in the diet. The model explained 19% of the variance in fat intake.

3.6. Saturated Fat as a Percentage of Daily Energy Intake

BMI and shift schedule were significantly related to saturated fat, controlling for age, marital status, industry, work hours, and chronic fatigue (Table 3). As BMI increased, the percentage of saturated fat in the diet increased. Compared to morning shift workers (reference category), night shift workers had a higher saturated fat intake (means and SD in Table 2). Overall, the model explained 30% of the variance in saturated fat intake.

3.7. Alcohol as a Percentage of Daily Energy Intake

Alcohol intake was significantly related to sex, industry, and hours worked per week when controlling for marital status and shift work history (Table 3). In particular, males consumed a higher percentage of alcohol when compared to females. Postal workers had a lower percentage of alcohol intake as a percentage of daily energy intake compared to oil and gas workers (reference category). Working fewer hours per week indicated a higher percentage of alcohol in the daily diet. The model accounted for 16% of the variance in alcohol intake.

4. Discussion

The aim of this study was to identify factors associated with the dietary profile of shift workers. Results showed that factors related to shift work were not associated with total energy intake, but were associated with reported macronutrient profiles. Shorter sleep durations and lower levels of fatigue were associated with an increased percentage of carbohydrate in the diet. In contrast, higher levels of fatigue and longer sleep durations were associated with an increased percentage of fat. These findings suggest a trade-off between carbohydrate and fat depending on sleep duration and fatigue levels. Permanent night shift workers reported a higher proportion of saturated fat, and morning shift workers reported a higher proportion of carbohydrate in their diet.

The finding that total energy intake was not different across different shift work schedules supports some previous field studies [21,51,52]. However, results in past literature are mixed. For example, a group of shift working nurses who were working the night shift reported consuming more energy since beginning shift work. These nurses also reported obtaining more sleep than day or afternoon shift working nurses [53]. Interestingly, this study used broad questions focusing on the within-participant changes in sleep duration and energy intake since starting shift work. The current study, using a cross-sectional design, investigated only a single point-in-time snapshot. It would be interesting to further interrogate how sleep and diet may change concurrently within individual workers across time in shift work. Laboratory studies finding that sleep restriction increases energy intake have typically examined severe (5 h or less) sleep restriction [25,26,29]. Shift workers in the current study (apart from 12-h rotating shift workers) reported obtaining recommended levels of sleep on average (7–9 h). Therefore, sleep restriction may need to be severe (e.g., 5 h or less) to result in changes in energy intake.

Indeed, the results of the current study support the importance of measuring and controlling for sleep durations and chronic fatigue when considering diet. The proportion of carbohydrates in the diet for morning shift workers was not different when compared with night or 8-h rotating workers, and significantly higher than for 12-h rotating workers. In contrast, a previous study which examined dietary profiles of garbage collectors on three different shift schedules (morning, afternoon, and night shifts) found that morning shift workers reported the lowest intake of carbohydrates [52]. Whilst sleep duration was reported, and the regression models included a number of covariates, sleep duration was not among them. The current study showed the effect of sleep duration on carbohydrate intake was small–moderate ($r = 0.22$), this finding is similar to the small-moderate effect size of sleep restriction on carbohydrate found in a laboratory study ($r = 0.16$) [25]. Further, in a previous qualitative study, shift workers reported consumption of sweet foods as a strategy for coping with circadian disruption on the night shift [24]. Carbohydrates are often consumed by individuals due to the perception that they increase alertness and energy levels [54,55]. Consistent with this, findings from the current study indicated that increased carbohydrate consumption was associated with shorter sleep durations, perhaps reflecting a strategy to combat sleepiness. The results from the current study also suggest that sleep and chronic fatigue may have contrasting influences on diet. The correlation between the two constructs was trivial, and while reduced sleep was associated with increased carbohydrate consumption, chronic fatigue was associated with increased fat intake (effect size: small–moderate; $r = 0.24$). These findings highlight the importance of differentiating and measuring both constructs when investigating factors associated with dietary intake.

In addition to sleep and fatigue, shift schedule was associated with dietary profile. Shift schedule had small–moderate effect on fat intake in the current study ($r = 0.17$) and a moderate–large effect on saturated fat intake ($r = 0.33$). This is similar to a previous study that found night shift work had a moderate–large effect on saturated fat intake ($r = 0.42$) when night shift workers were compared to day workers. In the current study, night shift workers reported the highest levels of saturated fat. These findings could be a result of food options available to night shift workers, for example, limited access to canteen facilities and reliance on vending machines [56]. It would be useful to consider food purchase and preparation options in future studies investigating the dietary profiles of shift workers. Moreover, all shift workers in the current study consumed higher than recommended levels of saturated fat (recommended level: <10% per day) [57] and consumed more saturated fat than reported by the Australian population in a recent Australian Health Survey (Australian population: fat = 31%, SFA = 12%) [58]. This is in line with previous research showing that, for example, shift workers consume fried food more regularly that day workers [59], consume more butter [60], and report eating more saturated fat than day workers [61]. In contrast, shift workers in the current study reported consuming a slightly lower percentage of carbohydrate, yet a slightly higher percentage of protein than that reported by the Australian population (Australian population: CHO = 45%, protein = 18%) [58].

There is evidence to suggest that shift work may influence patterns of alcohol intake [62]. Shift workers may use alcohol as a sleep aid [63,64] and some studies have found that working the night shift is associated with increased alcohol consumption [52,65]. In contrast to these findings, the current study did not find that shift schedule was associated with alcohol intake. When compared to the findings of the Australian Health Survey, all shift workers in the current study reported consuming a lower percentage of alcohol on average (Australian population = 13%) [58]. However, the reported percentage of alcohol intake for all shift workers in the current study was higher than recommended by Australian guidelines that suggest percentage of daily alcohol intake should form less than 5% of daily energy intake [57]. In the current study industry had a small–moderate effect on alcohol intake ($r = 0.14$) [48], specifically oil and gas workers consumed more alcohol as a percentage of their total energy intake. These findings concur with previous studies demonstrating the industry an individual is employed is associated with alcohol intake [66,67]. Whilst motivation for drinking alcohol was not investigated in the current study, it may have been that oil and gas workers were consuming alcohol to aid their sleep. Alternatively, other work-related factors may explain the differences between the industries. For example, lower demands at work have been associated with reduced odds of risky drinking levels [62]. Whilst investigating these factors was not a focus of the current study they may be useful to include when comparing differences in alcohol consumption between industries.

Findings from previous research suggest that alterations to the diet may be more likely with increasing shift work exposure [33,34]. However, whilst the current study included shift workers who had been employed for lengthy durations (>9 years on average), shift work history was not found to be associated with dietary profile. It has been postulated that shift workers who develop health disorders whilst working shift work revert back to day work (known as the 'healthy worker effect') [68]. Many health disorders are associated with unhealthy eating behaviours, therefore, it is possible that shift workers with unhealthy eating behaviours reverted back to day work and were not included in the current study. Longitudinal studies that follow not only shift workers who remain in shift work, but also those who revert back to day work, would help gain an understanding of how dietary profile changes due to the years employed in shift work.

Whilst the current study provided a general overview of the dietary profiles of shift workers there were some limitations to the study that could be addressed in future research. This study did not include a sample of day workers. Day workers may also experience sleep restriction and fatigue. Indeed, a recent study found that 26.4% of day workers reported never or rarely obtaining recommended levels of sleep and 27.6% reported experiencing frequent fatigue [69]. Therefore, future studies should also examine the influence of sleep and fatigue on dietary profile in day work populations. The current study was a cross-sectional design. This type of design can be advantageous as it allows for a snapshot of shift workers diets from a variety of industries. As mentioned above, to allow for further exploration of these factors in the future, it would be useful to employ a longitudinal design in future studies. A longitudinal design would be particularly useful when investigating rotating shift workers. For example, shift workers on a rotating schedule may have been experiencing

Nutrients **2016**, *8*, 771

different durations of sleep depending on the shift they were working (e.g., night versus afternoon shift). Therefore, capturing an overall estimate of their sleep duration misses the variability in sleep duration and timing, and how this may influence eating patterns. The generalizability of findings should also be taken into consideration. Whilst, the study included shift workers from a variety of industries there was only a small sample from each shift type. Moreover, the shift schedules tended to reflect the industry the individual was employed in and other related factors such as gender and age. For example, all 12-h rotating shift workers were employed in the oil and gas industry. This makes it difficult to separate the influence of shift schedule, industry and other demographic factors.

Studies investigating dietary habits are often subject to limitations. In particular, underreporting is common [70,71]. Additionally, participants choosing to take part in studies involving dietary intake may have an interest in nutrition and health [72]. The current study employed a FFQ to measure usual food intake of the previous 12 months. This method has advantages; for example, it puts less burden on participants compared to collecting diet history via interviews. However, accuracy may be reduced as it is difficult to remember food intake over longer periods of time [73]. Despite issues with accuracy the FFQ used in the current study has been validated relative to weighed food records [42,43]. Furthermore, this method cannot be used to investigate day-to-day variation [74], however, future studies could measure food intake using a food diary to determine how dietary profile differs on a daily basis when individuals are working on different shift types.

There has been limited research investigating factors associated with dietary profile in shift workers. Findings from this study indicate that it is not simply the shift schedule, but also other factors associated with shift work (e.g., sleep duration and chronic fatigue) that contribute to alterations in the dietary profile of shift workers. In particular, sleep duration and fatigue appear to have opposing effects on the diet. It is important to understand the psychological and physiological factors associated with shift work that influence the dietary profile as this can assist with the planning of health promotion strategies.

Acknowledgments: We would like to thank all participants and industry representatives who helped make this research possible. G.H. was funded with an Australian Post Graduate Award; otherwise; this research received no specific grant from any funding agency, commercial or not-for-profit sectors.

Author Contributions: G.H. developed the project, carried out the study, collected data, undertook analysis and prepared the first draft of the manuscript. C.S. and J.D. assisted in developing the project, A.C. and J.D. assisted with analysis, A.C., C.S. and J.D. assisted in revising the manuscript as well as supervising the study.

Conflicts of Interest: The authors declare no conflict of interest.

Abbreviations

The following abbreviations are used in this manuscript:

BMI	Body mass index
CHO	Carbohydrate
FFQ	Food frequency questionnaire
SSI	Standard shift work index
ANOVA	Analysis of variance
kJ	Kilojoules
SFA	Saturated fat
R	Rotating
g	Grams
SE	Standard error
LLCI	Lower limit confidence interval
ULCI	Upper limit confidence interval
Cum	Cumulative
kg	Kilograms
m^2	Meters squared

References

1. Australian Bureau of Statistics. Working Time Arrangements, Australia, November 2012. Available online: http://www.abs.gov.au/ausstats/abs@.nsf/mf/6342.0 (accessed on 18 November 2016).
2. Akerstedt, T. Shift work and disturbed sleep/wakefulness. *Occup. Med.* **2003**, *53*, 89–94. [CrossRef]
3. Costa, G. Shift work and occupational medicine: An overview. *Occup. Med.* **2003**, *53*, 83–88. [CrossRef]
4. Paley, M.J.; Tepas, D.I. Fatigue and the shiftworker: Firefighters working on a rotating shift schedule. *J. Hum. Factors Ergon. Soc.* **1994**, *36*, 269–284.
5. Åkerstedt, T.; Wright, K.P. Sleep loss and fatigue in shift work and shift work disorder. *Sleep Med. Clin.* **2009**, *4*, 257–271. [CrossRef] [PubMed]
6. Arendt, J. Shift work: Coping with the biological clock. *Occup. Med.* **2010**, *60*, 10–20. [CrossRef] [PubMed]
7. Dorrian, J.; Tolley, C.; Lamond, N.; van den Heuvel, C.; Pincombe, J.; Rogers, A.E.; Drew, D. Sleep and errors in a group of australian hospital nurses at work and during the commute. *Appl. Ergon.* **2008**, *39*, 605–613. [CrossRef] [PubMed]
8. Rajaratnam, S.M.; Arendt, J. Health in a 24-h society. *Lancet* **2001**, *358*, 999–1005. [CrossRef]
9. Karlsson, B.; Knutsson, A.; Lindahl, B. Is there an association between shift work and having a metabolic syndrome? Results from a population based study of 27,485 people. *J. Occup. Environ. Med.* **2001**, *58*, 747–752. [CrossRef]
10. Knutsson, A.; Bøggild, H. Gastrointestinal disorders among shift workers. *Scand. J. Work Environ. Health* **2010**, *36*, 85–95. [CrossRef] [PubMed]
11. Puttonen, S.; Härmä, M.; Hublin, C. Shift work and cardiovascular disease—Pathways from circadian stress to morbidity. *Scand. J. Work Environ. Health* **2010**, *36*, 96–108. [CrossRef] [PubMed]
12. Costa, G.; Haus, E.; Stevens, R. Shift work and cancer—Considerations on rationale, mechanisms, and epidemiology. *Scand. J. Work Environ. Health* **2010**, *36*, 163–179. [CrossRef] [PubMed]
13. World Health Organization. Global Strategy on Diet Physical Activity and Health 2015. Available online: http://www.who.int/dietphysicalactivity/diet/en/ (accessed on 18 November 2016).
14. Bonham, M.P.; Bonnell, E.K.; Huggins, C.E. Energy intake of shift workers compared to fixed day workers: A systematic review and meta-analysis. *Chronobiol. Int.* **2016**, *33*, 1086–1100. [CrossRef] [PubMed]
15. Hulsegge, G.; Boer, J.; van der Beek, A.; Verschuren, W.; Sluijs, I.; Vermeulen, R.; Proper, K. Shift workers have a similar diet quality but higher energy intake than day workers. *Scand. J. Work Environ. Health* **2016**, *42*, 459–468. [CrossRef] [PubMed]
16. Padilha, H.G.; Crispim, C.A.; Zimberg, I.Z.; Folkard, S.; Tufik, S.; de Mello, M.T. Metabolic responses on the early shift. *Chronobiol. Int.* **2010**, *27*, 1080–1092. [CrossRef] [PubMed]
17. Schiavo-Cardozo, D.; Lima, M.M.; Pareja, J.C.; Geloneze, B. Appetite-regulating hormones from the upper gut: Disrupted control of xenin and ghrelin in night workers. *Clin. Endocrinol.* **2013**, *79*, 807–811. [CrossRef] [PubMed]
18. Hemiö, K.; Puttonen, S.; Viitasalo, K.; Härmä, M.; Peltonen, M.; Lindström, J. Food and nutrient intake among workers with different shift systems. *J. Occup. Environ. Med.* **2015**, *72*, 513–520. [CrossRef] [PubMed]
19. Morikawa, Y.; Miura, K.; Sasaki, S.; Yoshita, K.; Yoneyama, S.; Sakurai, M.; Ishizaki, M.; Kido, T.; Naruse, Y.; Suwazono, Y. Evaluation of the effects of shift work on nutrient intake: A cross-sectional study. *J. Occup. Health* **2008**, *50*, 270–278. [CrossRef] [PubMed]
20. Balieiro, L.C.T.; Rossato, L.T.; Waterhouse, J.; Paim, S.L.; Mota, M.C.; Crispim, C.A. Nutritional status and eating habits of bus drivers during the day and night. *Chronobiol. Int.* **2014**, *31*, 1123–1129. [CrossRef] [PubMed]
21. Esquirol, Y.; Bongard, V.; Mabile, L.; Jonnier, B.; Soulat, J.-M.; Perret, B. Shift work and metabolic syndrome: Respective impacts of job strain, physical activity, and dietary rhythms. *Chronobiol. Int.* **2009**, *26*, 544–559. [CrossRef] [PubMed]
22. Pilcher, J.J.; Lambert, B.J.; Huffcutt, A.I. Differential effects of permanent and rotating shifts on self-report sleep length: A meta-analytic review. *Sleep* **2000**, *23*, 155–163. [PubMed]
23. Ingre, M.; Kecklund, G.; Åkerstedt, T.; Söderström, M.; Kecklund, L. Sleep length as a function of morning shift-start time in irregular shift schedules for train drivers: Self-rated health and individual differences. *Chronobiol. Int.* **2008**, *25*, 349–358. [CrossRef] [PubMed]

24. Persson, M.; Martensson, J. Situations influencing habits in diet and exercise among nurses working night shift. *J. Nurs. Manag.* **2006**, *14*, 414–423. [CrossRef] [PubMed]

25. Markwald, R.R.; Melanson, E.L.; Smith, M.R.; Higgins, J.; Perreault, L.; Eckel, R.H.; Wright, K.P. Impact of insufficient sleep on total daily energy expenditure, food intake, and weight gain. *Proc. Natl. Acad. Sci. USA* **2013**, *110*, 5695–5700. [CrossRef] [PubMed]

26. Brondel, L.; Romer, M.A.; Nougues, P.M.; Touyarou, P.; Davenne, D. Acute partial sleep deprivation increases food intake in healthy men. *Am. J. Clin. Nutr.* **2010**, *91*, 1550–1559. [CrossRef] [PubMed]

27. Schmid, S.M.; Hallschmid, M.; Jauch-Chara, K.; Wilms, B.; Benedict, C.; Lehnert, H.; Born, J.; Schultes, B. Short-term sleep loss decreases physical activity under free-living conditions but does not increase food intake under time-deprived laboratory conditions in healthy men. *Am. J. Clin. Nutr.* **2009**, *90*, 1476–1482. [CrossRef] [PubMed]

28. Spaeth, A.M.; Dinges, D.F.; Goel, N. Sex and race differences in caloric intake during sleep restriction in healthy adults. *Am. J. Clin. Nutr.* **2014**, *100*, 559–566. [CrossRef] [PubMed]

29. St-Onge, M.-P.; Roberts, A.L.; Chen, J.; Kelleman, M.; O'Keeffe, M.; RoyChoudhury, A.; Jones, P.J. Short sleep duration increases energy intakes but does not change energy expenditure in normal-weight individuals. *Am. J. Clin. Nutr.* **2011**, *94*, 410–416. [CrossRef] [PubMed]

30. Nea, F.M.; Kearney, J.; Livingstone, M.B.E.; Pourshahidi, L.K.; Corish, C.A. Dietary and lifestyle habits and the associated health risks in shift workers. *Nutr. Res. Rev.* **2015**, *28*, 143–166. [CrossRef] [PubMed]

31. Ursin, R.; Bjorvatn, B.; Holsten, F. Sleep duration, subjective sleep need, and sleep habits of 40-to 45-year-olds in the hordaland health study. *Sleep* **2005**, *28*, 1260. [PubMed]

32. Dashti, H.S.; Scheer, F.A.; Jacques, P.F.; Lamon-Fava, S.; Ordovás, J.M. Short sleep duration and dietary intake: Epidemiologic evidence, mechanisms, and health implications. *Adv. Nutr. Res.* **2015**, *6*, 648–659. [CrossRef] [PubMed]

33. Boivin, D.B.; Tremblay, G.M.; James, F.O. Working on atypical schedules. *Sleep Med.* **2007**, *8*, 578–589. [CrossRef] [PubMed]

34. Morikawa, Y.; Nakagawa, H.; Miura, K.; Soyama, Y.; Ishizaki, M.; Kido, T.; Naruse, Y.; Suwazono, Y.; Nogawa, K. Effect of shift work on body mass index and metabolic parameters. *Scand. J. Work Environ. Health* **2007**, *33*, 45–50. [CrossRef] [PubMed]

35. Knutson, A.; Andersson, H.; Berglund, U. Serum lipoproteins in day and shift workers: A prospective study. *Br. J. Ind. Med.* **1990**, *47*, 132–134. [CrossRef] [PubMed]

36. Devine, C.M.; Olson, C.M. Women's perceptions about the way social roles promote or constrain personal nutritional care. *Women Health* **1992**, *19*, 79–95. [CrossRef] [PubMed]

37. Devine, C.M.; Wolfe, W.S.; Frongillo, E.A., Jr.; Bisogni, C.A. Life-course events and experiences: Association with fruit and vegetable consumption in 3 ethnic groups. *J. Am. Diet. Assoc.* **1999**, *99*, 309–314. [CrossRef]

38. Rolls, B.J.; Fedoroff, I.C.; Guthrie, J.F. Gender differences in eating behavior and body weight regulation. *Health Psychol.* **1991**, *10*, 133. [CrossRef] [PubMed]

39. Lissner, L.; Heitmann, B.L. Dietary fat and obesity: Evidence from epidemiology. *Eur. J. Clin. Nutr.* **1995**, *49*, 79. [PubMed]

40. Murphy, S.P.; Rose, D.; Hudes, M.; Viteri, F.E. Demographic and economic factors associated with dietary quality for adults in the 1987–88 nationwide food consumption survey. *J. Am. Diet. Assoc.* **1992**, *92*, 1352–1357. [PubMed]

41. The Cancer Council Victoria. *Dietary Questionnaire for Epidemiological Studies*, version 2; The Cancer Council Victoria: Melbourne, Australia, 1996.

42. Xinying, P.X.; Noakes, M.; Keogh, J. Can a food frequency questionnaire be used to capture dietary intake data in a 4 week clinical intervention trial? *Asia Pac. J. Clin. Nutr.* **2004**, *13*, 318–323. [PubMed]

43. Hodge, A.; Patterson, A.J.; Brown, W.J.; Ireland, P.; Giles, G. The anti cancer council of victoria ffq: Relative validity of nutrient intakes compared with weighed food records in young to middle-aged women in a study of iron supplementation. *Aust. N. Z. J. Public Health* **2000**, *24*, 576–583. [CrossRef] [PubMed]

44. Barton, J.; Folkard, S.; Smith, L.; Spelten, E.; Totterdell, P. Standard shiftwork index manual. *J. Appl. Psychol.* **1993**, *60*, 159–170.

45. Spelten, E.; Barton, J.; Folkard, S. Have we underestimated shiftworkers' problems? Evidence from a 'reminiscence' study. *Ergonomics* **1993**, *36*, 307–312. [CrossRef] [PubMed]

46. Smith, C.; Gibby, R.; Zickar, M.; Crossley, C.; Robie, C.; Folkard, S.; Tuker, P.; Barton, J. Measurement properties of the shiftwork survey and standard shiftwork index. *J. Hum. Ergol.* **2001**, *30*, 191–196.

47. Field, A.P. *Discovering Statistics Using ibm spss Statistics: And Sex and Drugs and Rock 'n' Roll*, 4th ed.; Sage: Los Angeles, CA, USA, 2013.

48. Cohen, J. Set correlation and contingency tables. *Appl. Psychol. Meas.* **1988**, *12*, 425–434. [CrossRef]

49. Hosmer, D.; Lemeshow, S.; May, S. *Applied Survival Analysis*; John Wiley & Sons: Hoboken, NJ, USA, 2008.

50. Bursac, Z.; Gauss, C.H.; Williams, D.K.; Hosmer, D.W. Purposeful selection of variables in logistic regression. *Source Code Biol. Med.* **2008**, *3*. [CrossRef] [PubMed]

51. Pasqua, I.; Moreno, C. The nutritional status and eating habits of shift workers: A chronobiological approach. *Chronobiol. Int.* **2004**, *21*, 949–960. [CrossRef] [PubMed]

52. De Assis, M.A.A.; Kupek, E.; Nahas, M.V.C.; Bellisle, F. Food intake and circadian rhythms in shift workers with a high workload. *Appetite* **2003**, *40*, 175–183. [CrossRef]

53. Geliebter, A.; Gluck, M.E.; Tanowitz, M.; Aronoff, N.J.; Zammit, G.K. Work-shift period and weight change. *Nutrition* **2000**, *16*, 27–29. [CrossRef]

54. Wurtman, R.J.; Wurtman, J.J. Carbohydrates and depression. *Sci. Am.* **1989**, *260*, 68–75. [CrossRef] [PubMed]

55. Thayer, R. Energy, tiredness, and tension effects of a sugar snack versus moderate exercise. *J. Personal. Soc. Psychol.* **1987**, *52*, 119–125. [CrossRef]

56. Stewart, A.J.; Wahlqvist, M.L. Effect of shiftwork on canteen food purchase. *J. Occup. Environ. Med.* **1985**, *27*, 552–554. [CrossRef]

57. Australian Government National Health and Medical Research Council Nutrient Reference Values for Australia and New Zealand. Available online: https://www.nrv.gov.au/ (accessed on 18 November 2016).

58. Australian Bureau of Statistics Australian Health Survey: Nutrition First Results-Food and Nutrients. Available online: http://www.abs.gov.au/ausstats/abs@.nsf/Lookup/4364.0.55.009main+features12011-12 (accessed on 18 November 2016).

59. Harada, H.; Suwazono, Y.; Sakata, K.; Okubo, Y.; Oishi, M.; Uetani, M.; Kobayashi, E.; Nogawa, K. Three-shift system increases job-related stress in japanese workers. *J. Occup. Health* **2005**, *47*, 397–404. [CrossRef] [PubMed]

60. Puttonen, S.; Kivimäki, M.; Elovainio, M.; Pulkki-Råback, L.; Hintsanen, M.; Vahtera, J.; Telama, R.; Juonala, M.; Viikari, J.S.; Raitakari, O.T. Shift work in young adults and carotid artery intima–media thickness: The cardiovascular risk in young finns study. *Atherosclerosis* **2009**, *205*, 608–613. [CrossRef] [PubMed]

61. Di Lorenzo, L.; De Pergola, G.; Zocchetti, C.; L'Abbate, N.; Basso, A.; Pannacciulli, N.; Cignarelli, M.; Giorgino, R.; Soleo, L. Effect of shift work on body mass index: Results of a study performed in 319 glucose-tolerant men working in a southern Italian industry. *Int. J. Obes.* **2003**, *27*, 1353–1358. [CrossRef] [PubMed]

62. Dorrian, J.; Skinner, N. Alcohol consumption patterns of shiftworkers compared with dayworkers. *Chronobiol. Int.* **2012**, *29*, 610–618. [CrossRef] [PubMed]

63. Dorrian, J.; Paterson, J.; Dawson, D.; Pincombe, J.; Grech, C.; Rogers, A.E. Sleep, stress and compensatory behaviors in Australian nurses and midwives. *Rev. Saude Publica* **2011**, *45*, 922–930. [CrossRef] [PubMed]

64. Gold, D.R.; Rogacz, S.; Bock, N.; Tosteson, T.D.; Baum, T.M.; Speizer, F.E.; Czeisler, C.A. Rotating shift work, sleep, and accidents related to sleepiness in hospital nurses. *Am. J. Public Health* **1992**, *82*, 1011–1014. [CrossRef] [PubMed]

65. Härmä, M.; Tenkanen, L.; Sjöblom, T.; Alikoski, T.; Heinsalmi, P. Combined effects of shift work and life-style on the prevalence of insomnia, sleep deprivation and daytime sleepiness. *Scand. J. Work Environ. Health* **1998**, *24*, 300–307. [CrossRef] [PubMed]

66. Howland, J.; Mangione, T.W.; Kuhlthau, K.; Bell, N.; Heeren, T.; Lee, M.; Levine, S. Work-site variation in managerial drinking. *Addiction* **1996**, *91*, 1007–1017. [CrossRef] [PubMed]

67. Larsen, S. Alcohol use in the service industry. *Addiction* **1994**, *89*, 733–741. [CrossRef] [PubMed]

68. Wen, C.; Tsai, S.; Gibson, R. Anatomy of the healthy worker effect: A critical review. *JOM-J. Occup. Med.* **1983**, *25*, 283–289.

69. Skinner, N.; Dorrian, J. A work-life perspective on sleep and fatigue—Looking beyond shift workers. *Ind. Health* **2015**, *53*, 417. [CrossRef] [PubMed]

70. Goris, A.H.; Westerterp-Plantenga, M.S.; Westerterp, K.R. Undereating and underrecording of habitual food intake in obese men: Selective underreporting of fat intake. *Am. J. Clin. Nutr.* **2000**, *71*, 1130–1134.

71. Taren, D.; Tobar, M.; Hill, A.; Howell, W.; Shisslak, C.; Bell, I.; Ritenbaugh, C. The association of energy intake bias with psychological scores of women. *Eur. J. Clin. Nutr.* **1999**, *53*, 570–578. [CrossRef] [PubMed]
72. Rebro, S.M.; Patterson, R.E.; Kristal, A.R.; Cheney, C.L. The effect of keeping food records on eating patterns. *J. Am. Diet. Assoc.* **1998**, *98*, 1163–1165. [CrossRef]
73. Erdman, J.W., Jr.; MacDonald, I.A.; Zeisel, S.H. *Present Knowledge in Nutrition*; John Wiley & Sons: Hoboken, NJ, USA, 2012.
74. Thomson, T.; Subar, A. Dietary assessment methdology. In *Nutrtion in the Prevention and Treatment of Disease*; Coulston, A., Rock, C., Mondsen, E., Eds.; Academic Press: London, UK, 2001; pp. 3–30.

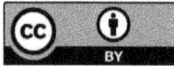

nutrients

MDPI

Article

Influences on Dietary Choices during Day versus Night Shift in Shift Workers: A Mixed Methods Study

Emily K. Bonnell [1,†], Catherine E. Huggins [1,†], Chris T. Huggins [2], Tracy A. McCaffrey [1], Claire Palermo [1] and Maxine P. Bonham [1,*]

[1] Department of Nutrition, Dietetics and Food, Level 1, 264 Ferntree Gully Road, Monash University, Melbourne, Notting Hill VIC 3168, Australia; emilykbonnell@gmail.com (E.K.B.); Catherine.huggins@monash.edu (C.E.H.); tracy.mccaffrey@monash.edu (T.A.M.); claire.palermo@monash.edu (C.P.)
[2] Department of Community Emergency Health and Paramedic Practice, Monash University, Frankston VIC 3199, Australia; chris.huggins@monash.edu
* Correspondence: Maxine.bonham@monash.edu; Tel.: +61-3-9902-4272
† These two authors are the joint first authors.

Received: 12 December 2016; Accepted: 20 February 2017; Published: 26 February 2017

Abstract: Shift work is associated with diet-related chronic conditions such as obesity and cardiovascular disease. This study aimed to explore factors influencing food choice and dietary intake in shift workers. A fixed mixed method study design was undertaken on a convenience sample of firefighters who continually work a rotating roster. Six focus groups ($n = 41$) were conducted to establish factors affecting dietary intake whilst at work. Dietary intake was assessed using repeated 24 h dietary recalls ($n = 19$). Interviews were audio recorded, transcribed verbatim, and interpreted using thematic analysis. Dietary data were entered into FoodWorks and analysed using Wilcoxon signed-rank test; $p < 0.05$ was considered significant. Thematic analysis highlighted four key themes influencing dietary intake: shift schedule; attitudes and decisions of co-workers; time and accessibility; and knowledge of the relationship between food and health. Participants reported consuming more discretionary foods and limited availability of healthy food choices on night shift. Energy intakes (kJ/day) did not differ between days that included a day or night shift but greater energy density (ED_{energy}, kJ/g/day) of the diet was observed on night shift compared with day shift. This study has identified a number of dietary-specific shift-related factors that may contribute to an increase in unhealthy behaviours in a shift-working population. Given the increased risk of developing chronic diseases, organisational change to support workers in this environment is warranted.

Keywords: nutrition; shift work; communicative disease; qualitative methodology

1. Introduction

Compared to day workers, shift workers are at a higher risk of many diet-related chronic conditions, including obesity [1,2], cardiovascular disease (CVD) [3,4], and type 2 diabetes [5,6]. Across the world, the proportion of the workforce who engage in shift work varies, ranging from around 10% in Brazil to 16% in Australia, 24% in Czech Republic, and greater than 50% in Jamaica [7].

Shift work that includes overnight shifts disrupts the circadian biological clock governing the body's internal regulation of sleep and wake times, which in turn affects energy metabolism and may promote weight gain [8]. During nighttime sleep, the body is in a fasting state promoting release of stored glucose and relative insulin resistance (compared with day) to permit preferential usage of glucose by the central nervous system rather than for muscle energy [9,10]. Eating during nocturnal hours, when the body is programmed to be asleep, disrupts the metabolic milieu [11]. Acute experimental studies have found that a meal eaten at night generates an exaggerated glucose and lipid response compared with the same meal eaten during the day [12]. Long-term excursions in glucose and lipids are risk factors for cardiovascular disease [13].

Eating at work during night shift is, therefore, a modern-day risk factor for cardiovascular disease.

Although shift workers have a propensity for snacking at night [14] and making poor food choices [15], these habits do not appear to be at the expense of an increased energy intake. A recent systematic review and meta-analyses reporting on a total of 12 studies with 10,367 day workers and 4726 shift workers concluded no difference in energy intake between shift workers and their daytime counterparts [16]. These findings suggest that meal timing and food choice at night, rather than energy intake per se, is a key contributor to the increased risk of CVD observed in shift workers and imply that shift workers eat a substantial proportion of their meals during a time of suboptimal glucose and lipid tolerance. Recommending complete avoidance of food at night is unrealistic for many shift workers. Thus, the development of strategies to minimise the metabolic disturbance to food intake at night are required. These strategies will rely, in part, on an understanding of dietary practices of shift workers. Physiological, psychosocial, environmental, and organisational influences were identified as the main themes affecting food choices in a qualitative study of Australian paramedics (an essential shift work profession), however, shift-specific factors (i.e., night shift vs. day shift) were not explored [17]. Understanding shift-specific factors is important to permit development of dietary advice that is practical and feasible for shift workers.

Using a fixed mixed methods approach, the aim of this study was to: (1) explore, in rotating shift workers, factors influencing dietary intake on day shift and on night shift; (2) assess the types of foods and drinks consumed and the timing of each eating occasion on work days. A mixed method approach was taken to facilitate a more complete understanding of food choices and the factors affecting these choices.

2. Materials and Methods

2.1. Design

A fixed mixed method study design was undertaken (i.e., the decision to undertake both qualitative and quantitative methods was made before the research is started), with concurrent data collection methods [18]. Focus groups were conducted to establish the factors affecting dietary intake of rotational shift workers whilst at work and quantitative assessment of their dietary intake using 24 h dietary recalls. Ethics approval for this study was granted by Monash University Human Research Ethics Committee (CF14/1491-2014000703) and signed informed consent was obtained from all participants.

2.2. Sampling

A convenience-based sample of firefighters from Melbourne provided a population of rotating shift workers for the study. Potential participants were a mixture of recruit firefighters (<1 year) or experienced firefighters. All participants were provided with information about the aims of the research study by the researcher face to face at the beginning of a 2-day mandatory training course and then were invited to participate in the focus group and/or dietary assessment after the completion of their training. This sample followed a 10/14 rotating shift schedule: two consecutive 10 h day shifts followed by two consecutive 14 h night shifts, then four rostered days off. Recruitment continued until the female researcher (EB) determined that further discussions would not disclose new information [19].

2.3. Data Collection

Participants were required to self-report their age, height, and weight (current weight and weight on starting shift work). Body mass index (BMI) was calculated from body height and weight in kg/m^2.

Focus groups were held at the training facility of the employer and facilitated by the same student researcher (EB) using a list of semi-structured open questions (Table 1) developed by the research team.

EB is also an accredited practising dietitian with research training in qualitative methods. The approach was pragmatic, aiming to elicit information that would support understanding of data collected from quantitative methods. Participants were prompted to discuss factors that influenced their food choices at work and each focus group lasted between 40 min and 1 h. Each group was audio-recorded and transcribed verbatim by the student researcher (EB) with confidentiality maintained. Transcripts were completed within the week following each focus group to allow a determination to be made whether data saturation had been reached and thus whether recruitment of new focus groups should be halted. Transcripts were not returned to participants for comment.

Table 1. Questions used to guide semi-structured focus group discussions.

Question	Information Sought
Can you run me through what you would eat and drink at work on a day shift?	Usual dietary intake during a day shift
Where does your food come from on a day shift? For example, do you bring it from home, buy it at work . . . ?	Source of food during a day shift
What influences these food choices on day shift? Do you ever find that you eat on a day shift for reasons other than hunger? If yes, what are these reasons? Why do eat at the times that you do?	Factors influencing food choices during a day shift
Can you now run me through what you would eat and drink at work on a night shift?	Usual dietary intake during a night shift
On a night shift, where does your food come from?	Source of food during a night shift
What influences the types of foods that you eat on night shift? Thinking about a night shift, what are the reasons for you choosing to eat when you do? Say you have just come back from a call at 2 a.m., will you have something to eat or go straight to bed?	Factors influencing food choices during a night shift
Recruit firefighters (<1 year): Since starting shift work, have there been any notable changes in what influences your food choices? *Experienced firefighters*: Have you noticed any dietary changes over your years of working with the Metropolitan Fire Brigade?	Long-term effects of shift work on dietary intake

Dietary intakes were assessed using an adapted version of the United States Department of Agriculture (USDA) multiple-pass 24 h recall method [20]. Two recalls covered 24 h periods during which an entire night shift was worked (for example, midday Thursday to midday Friday, encompassing the 1700–0700 h night shift) and two covered equivalent 24 h periods encompassing the entire day shift (0700–1700 h). As food intake can vary from day to day, the paired repetition of 24 h recalls allowed the capture of food intake on different days of the week. All dietary recalls were conducted over the telephone by the same researcher (EB). Participants were provided with an adapted copy of the 4000 for Health food model booklet on enrolment into the study [21], which provided visual examples of meal portions and mug and cup sizes, to assist them to describe the quantity of food and beverages consumed.

2.4. Data Analysis

Data from the dietary intake and focus groups were analysed concurrently to look for congruence and difference. Quantitative data were used to assist in the interpretation of qualitative data and to verify its accuracy.

A manual thematic analysis was undertaken using qualitative description [22] with simple depiction of the factors influencing shift workers' food intake. Transcript data were initially analysed by the first author (EB). The texts were coded and then grouping codes were used to identify common ideas and themes. Two focus groups were independently analysed (by CP) using the same approach. The themes identified independently were then discussed by both authors and agreement sought on final themes. Descriptors with illustrative quotes were selected to aid interpretation. Representative quotes are presented from each focus group rather than individually.

Only participants who completed two or more dietary recalls (at least one day shift and one night shift) were included in the dietary analysis. Dietary data were entered into FoodWorks (Xyris Software, Brisbane, Australia). Energy, macronutrient, and fibre intakes were calculated based on food composition data available from Nutrient Tables (NUTTAB) 2011 (Food Standards Australia and New Zealand) and Australian Food, Supplement and Nutrient Database (AUSNUT) 2013 (Food Standards Australia and New Zealand). Energy density (ED, kJ/g/day) was calculated in three ways [23]: ED of all food and beverages (EDall); ED of solid foods only (EDsolid), and ED of all solid foods plus soups, milk as food, milk as a drink, and beverages containing >21 kJ/100 g (EDenergy). Eating occasions during each 24 h recall were described using participants' definitions (e.g., breakfast, lunch, dinner, snack and beverage, or beverage only). Lunch and dinner meals were further classified into three categories: cooked meals, takeaway meals, and easy-to-prepare meals (sandwiches, rolls, wraps, salads, or heat-and-serve dishes (e.g., microwave rice) based on examples provided in the focus groups. Snacks were classified into food groups based on the Australian dietary guidelines [24].

Descriptive statistics were calculated using Statistical Packages for the Social Sciences (SPSS; IBM SPSS Statistics for Windows, Version 23.0. Armonk, NY, USA; IBM Corp.). Data were tested for normality using the Shapiro–Wilk test, and reported as median (25th and 75th percentiles). Wilcoxon signed-rank test was used to compare dietary intake between 24 h periods where a day shift was worked compared to a night shift. Differences in dietary intake during hours at work were also compared (i.e., day shift (10 h) versus night shift (14 h)) using the Wilcoxon signed-rank test. Significance was reported as $p < 0.05$.

3. Results

3.1. Participation

Fifty-five potential participants attended the mandatory training program during the data collection period. Forty-one took part in six focus groups (*n* = 8, *n* = 7, *n* = 7, *n* = 4, *n* = 12, and *n* = 3 participants, respectively) and participant characteristics are presented in Table 2. Recruit firefighters and experienced firefighters were in different focus groups due to the scheduling of the training. The median (25th, 75th percentile) years working rotating shift work was 6 (0.58, 29). A total of 29 people consented to participate in the dietary intake collection, all but one of whom participated in the focus groups. Fifteen participants completed four dietary recalls and four competed two or more, and thus 19 were included in the dietary analysis. The other 10 participants were excluded as follows: *n* = 9 could not be contacted during the study period (on annual leave, incorrect contact details, unresponsive to contact attempts) and *n* = 1 only completed one dietary recall. Participants represented 27 of the 47 fire stations across metropolitan Melbourne.

Table 2. Characteristics of study participants.

	Focus Group *n* = 41	Dietary Recall [c] *n* = 19
Age (years)	36 (30, 52) [a]	36 (29, 51)
Body mass index (BMI) (kg/m^2)	26 (24.7, 27.8) [a]	24.7 (23.4, 26.5)
Self-reported weight gain since starting shift work (kg)	24 (58.5) [a]	9 (47.4)
Male gender (%) [b]	40 (97.6)	18 (94.7)
Proportion aged: (%) [b]		
<25 years	2 (4.9)	1 (5.3)
25–34 years	16 (39)	8 (42.1)
35–44 years	6 (14.6)	3 (15.8)
>45 years	17 (41.5)	7 (36.8)

[a] Median (25th, 75th percentiles); [b] % of total group; [c] *n* = 18 also completed the focus groups.

3.2. Factors Affecting Dietary Intake

Four key themes related to factors influencing dietary intake emerged from the focus groups (Table 3) and include shift schedule; attitudes and decisions of co-workers; time and accessibility; and knowledge of the relationship between food and health. Each theme was connected to the workplace and included social (attitudes and choices of others), cultural (demands of daily tasks), and physical factors (environmental) that affect decision making around food choices. Dietary data that support the emergent themes are presented at the end of each relevant Theme, with differences between night shift and days shift emphasised where evident.

Table 3. Themes identified from focus groups of rotating shift workers.

Themes	Descriptors
1. Shift schedule influences types of meals and snacks consumed at work.	Meals prepared at work: "Communal cook-ups" Meals bought during shift: Takeaway choices Meals brought to work from home Meals provided by the organisation Snacks during work hours
2. Dietary intake is affected (both positively and negatively) by the dietary choices and attitudes of co-workers.	Impact of others' dietary choices Impact of co-workers' attitudes toward food and health
3. Food choices during a shift are dependent on time availability and ease of access.	Non-hungry eating Impact of workplace protocol, structure and location Demands of the day's tasks
4. Firefighters endeavour to make healthy food choices due to growing awareness of health within the brigade.	Preparing balanced meals together Cooking facilities Greater interest in health

3.2.1. Theme 1: Shift Schedule Influences Types of Meals and Snacks Consumed at Work

Participants reported that irrespective of shift, the main meal consumed at work might include: communal meals cooked at the workplace, takeaway food purchased during shifts, or food brought from home. Lunch intake differed from dinner. Four of the six focus groups reported that for lunch they would choose an easy-to-prepare meal, such as meat and salad rolls or wraps, roast rolls, and schnitzel rolls. Their communal evening meals generally took much more time to prepareand they placed much higher value on these dinner meals:

> "You pride yourself on what you cook for dinner so yeah. Lot more effort goes into dinner."

—Focus group 5

For takeaway foods, participants stated that they would more often choose foods considered to be healthy when they were on day shift than when they were on night shift. They also consumed takeaway foods more often on night shift. This was partly due to the presence of established routines at particular fire stations where takeaway meals were consumed every second night shift (Focus groups 2–4), every Friday night (Focus groups 1, 2, 4, 6), or over a weekend shift (Focus group 6).

> "Night shift: fish and chips or takeaway. Day shift I generally try and keep that clean and go to the supermarket."

—Focus group 3

Lack of time for preparing food to take to work was highlighted as an important reason for purchasing takeaway food during night shift. Some firefighters worked other jobs on their days off and/or during the day before beginning their night shift. Others had family commitments (young families) that prevented them preparing their own food:

> "At work sometimes it is hard for me to bring stuff in if I'm on the nightshift sometimes because of what I've been doing, looking after the kids during the day or whatever. So it's convenient to just get takeaway when you're at work."

—Focus group 4

Participants noted that other meals provided to them by their brigade when they were on call were usually unhealthy regardless of shift schedule:

> "I think one disadvantage with this organisation is when we go to fire duties the organisation sends out high fat foods. They send out pizza, pies, soft drinks and stuff like that."
>
> —Focus group 3

The majority of work snacks were brought from home. Irrespective of shift schedule, these were mainly fruit, nuts, and yoghurt. Some participants said that they were more likely to eat chocolates and ice cream, supplied at the workplace, after dinner (on a night shift) than when they were on a day shift; other groups indicated no difference. However, workers indicated that they would eat chocolates and sweet biscuits after an extended night call because nothing else was available.

> "You'd start eating a packet of biscuits coz that's the only thing around at the station to eat, yeah so that's the worst part . . . night shifts where you do go on call, you come back and . . . you don't plan on eating as such but you (have) got to basically or you starve."
>
> —Focus group 2

A deductive examination of the dietary data for the frequency of main meal types (Figure 1A) and snacks (Figure 1B) consumed at work supports the findings of the focus groups. On night shift, compared with day shift, a greater proportion of discretionary snack foods were consumed comprising mostly of chocolates, ice creams, and sweet pastries (Figure 1B).

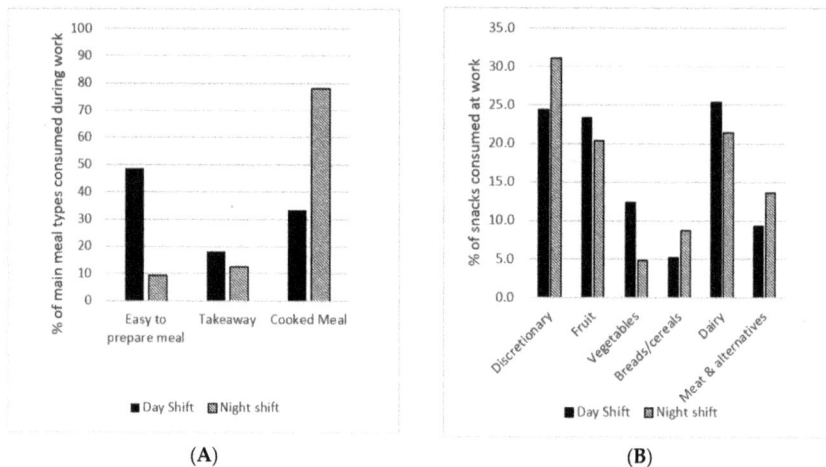

(A) (B)

Figure 1. Comparison of main meal and food groups consumed by rotating shift workers (*n* = 19) comparing dietary intake from day shift and night shift: (**A**) Categories of main meals were identified during focus groups. Easy-to-prepare meals included sandwiches, rolls, wraps, or salads, or heat-and-serve dishes (e.g., microwave rice); (**B**) snacks were categorised according to the Australian Guide to Healthy Eating food groups (*n* = 296 snack foods consumed over 70 snacking occasions).

Energy intakes (kJ/day) were not different between day or night shift (Table 4). A significantly higher percentage energy from sugar was observed during the 24 h period that included a night shift compared with the 24 h period that included a day shift ($p = 0.036$). There were fewer eating occasions, and a greater overall energy density (ED_{energy}, kJ/g/day) of the diet during a 24 h period that included a night shift compared with a day shift period ($p < 0.05$, Table 4).

Table 4. Median dietary intake of shift workers (*n* = 19) using 24 h dietary recalls.

	Total Daily Intake 24 h Period Includes Day Shift		Total Daily Intake 24 h Period Includes Night Shift		*p* Value *	Dietary Intake at Work (Day Shift 10 h)		Dietary Intake at Work (Night Shift 14 h)		*p* Value *
Energy (kJ/day)	11,491	(9986, 13,452)	10,350	(8519, 12,939)	0.295	6403	(4609, 7808)	5693	(4072, 6900)	0.171
Protein %EI	23.2	(19.5, 28)	21.4	(19.8, 24.2)	0.053	21.1	(19.4, 27.2)	23.1	(21.7, 25.2)	0.968
Total fat %EI	32.4	(27.6, 38.4)	33.0	(29, 36.8)	0.904	31.5	(28.8, 40.6)	29.2	(22.1, 36.7)	0.295
Saturated fat %EI	12.3	(9.7, 14.1)	12.5	(10.5, 13.5)	0.936	11.9	(10.4, 12.4)	11.9	(7.5, 14.2)	0.841
Carbohydrate %EI	38.9	(34.2, 44)	43.8	(36.5, 45.7)	0.117	43.6	(30.4, 46.4)	43.2	(36.5, 49.5)	0.277
Sugar %EI	15.5	(11.3, 19.7)	16.8	(14.2, 19.6)	0.036	17.8	(12.1, 19.2)	15.0	(10.9, 18.4)	0.494
Number of foods consumed	27.5	(21.5, 30)	25.0	(20, 30)	0.029	16.0	(12, 18)	11.5	(8, 15)	0.001
ED_{all} (kJ/g/day)	6.62	(6.16, 7.12)	7.36	(6.06, 8.14)	0.077	6.85	(5.69, 7.97)	6.61	(5.64, 7.55)	0.546
ED_{solid} (kJ/g/day)	6.56	(6.11, 6.8)	6.40	(6.04, 7.99)	0.117	8.68	(6.77, 9.55)	8.95	(7.14, 10.02)	0.421
ED_{energy} (kJ/g/day)	5.52	(4.72, 5.83)	5.73	(5.08, 6.88)	0.044	7.81	(6.45, 9.34)	7.37	(6.65, 9.55)	0.904

* Calculated using Wilcoxon signed-rank test. Significance level *p* < 0.05. All values are median (25th, 75th percentiles) %EI—percentage of total energy intake; ED_{all}—all food and beverages; ED_{solid}—solid foods only; ED_{energy}—all solid foods, soups, milk as food, soups, milk as a drink and beverages containing > 21 kJ/100 g.

3.2.2. Theme 2: Dietary Intake Is Affected by the Dietary Choices and Attitudes of Co-Workers

Social influence was reported as a major factor influencing dietary choices at work and in some cases, carried over to impact choices made at home.

"Most things that we do we generally do with someone else … it's a pretty social job so you're generally … sitting around (with) other people so you do a lot of stuff together."

—Focus group 5

Selection of meals purchased or cooked communally at lunch and dinner tended to be a majority decision, with group consensus valued over individual preference. This could have both a positive and negative impact on dietary intake.

"You don't want to be the odd one out, so if everyone wants to get salad rolls you're hardly gonna (sic) say well no I want Maccas (McDonalds) or I want pizza, but then if like 2 or 3 guys go 'ohh let's get pizza tonight boys' you don't want to be the guy who goes nah I'd rather have a salad roll so … it's a group decision."

—Focus group 5

"Couple of guys you know you'll say 'alright we'll have a salad tonight' and they'll just laugh at you kind of thing. So you gotta (sic), if you're gonna (sic) cook for the station you gotta (sic) cook for everyone."

—Focus group 2

The choice to purchase takeaway food on shift was influenced by others. Participants explained that the crew must accompany one another to purchase food in case they are called out during this time. The temptation then arises to purchase what others are getting, neglecting an often-healthier choice brought from home.

"If we go out and someone else has to buy lunch and I like what they're getting, I'll forget what I took into work and I'll say 'I'll have some of that!' That's how I have more takeaway."

—Focus group 1

The strongest predictor of whether meals were cooked communally was the presence of somebody interested in food and cooking, which tended to encourage others to cook as well. If this person then left the station, motivation within the crew faded:

> "We had a guy come from ah from out of town … and he enjoyed cooking, so for that whole month that he was with us he was cooking meals, motivated the guys and that lasted probably two or three months (afterwards) and then ended up going to get takeaway food that was ah around the back of the station."

—Focus group 5

These participants also initially felt peer pressure to become involved in communal cook-ups:

> "If you're at a station where they do cook together there's a pretty big culture around it so you don't want to be a splitter and not eat with them so yeah, you tend to have bigger meals and maybe not as healthy because you don't want to not eat with them."

—Focus group 2

3.2.3. Theme 3: Food Choices Are Dependent on the Availability of Time and Ease of Accessibility

Accessibility to food was reported to influence food choices. Convenience and temptation were highlighted as major reasons for non-hungry eating at work. During two focus groups, it was reported that eating was a way to combat boredom on quiet work days. The majority of non-hungry eating occasions involved discretionary items freely available at the workplace.

> "It's always a battle because they're there (chocolates). We never have that stuff at home so … the opportunity is there, which is quite tempting."

—Focus group 6

The type of takeaway bought on shift was reported to be largely dependent on the location of the station and whether convenience food stores were close by. Participants described challenges obtaining food when they were "moved up"—that is, when a crew shifts to cover another station that is out on an extended call. Workers described snacking on chocolates and ice creams available at the station because they either did not have an opportunity to prepare a meal or they had left it behind at their home station. The drive back to their home station or during shifts with repeated call-outs were identified as situations where they might stop to purchase something quick, easy, and often of poor nutritional quality, depending on the length and timing of the move-up or call-outs.

> "When you get a move up because you don't know how long (it) is going to be … it's getting past 3 o'clock (a.m.) … you're getting hungry and you're like, 'Oh crap, I will have that Magnum (ice-cream bar)' … and you do go and buy something crap because it's been that long since you've had anything to eat."

—Focus group 3

> "We had a heap of calls in a row, we had a fire, a couple of false alarms and something else and by the time we got back to the station it was about 9.30 (p.m.) and I think (colleague) and myself both had about three goes at cooking our dinner and mine ended up in the bin … we walked up to McDonalds on the corner."

—Focus group 4

Participants varied in the foods they chose when tired after a busy shift. One group noted that the day after a busy night shift they were more likely to choose takeaway foods or easy-to-prepare meals, because they were too tired to put effort into cooking:

"After I've finished a night shift I'll often, like first two days after, I'll just go and get Subway for lunch or something coz I can't' be bothered putting the same effort into preparing my food as when I feel fully ah, revitalised."

—Focus group 5

Meals might be delayed by calls or in some instances missed all together. For example, breakfast following night shift might be missed entirely if the end of shift was delayed, as this was not designated as a mealtime. As each shift is unpredictable, the participants explained that they prepare for calls and busy shifts by eating when the opportunity arises, with the expectation that this could be their only chance to eat during the rest of the shift.

"You (might) get delayed in the morning and you don't get breakfast. You get a call. The next thing you know by the time you get home it's half past 10 or 11 o'clock in the morning and the last time you ate was at 6.30 the night before."

—Focus group 3

"Even though you're not hungry, you will eat because you know you could have a bad night."

—Focus group 3

3.2.4. Theme 4: Firefighters Endeavour to Make Healthy Food Choices Due to Growing Awareness of Health

Participants, who were experienced in the workplace, described a move towards a healthier lifestyle and healthier food choices in more recent years. They reported that in the past, communal "cook-ups" had involved cooking with large amounts of added fat and salt and few vegetables. Today, despite large portion sizes, all groups believed their "cook-ups" were more balanced meals. Moreover, the workers today said they were more likely to bring in home-cooked meals or ingredients to cook with at work, while previously an energy-dense takeaway meal was eaten at the start of shifts. Factors contributing to this culture change included: improved cooking facilities at the stations, generational change with greater interest in health, fitness and cooking, regular work-health checks, improved health education, growing public awareness of men's health issues, and improved awareness of potential health concerns in the ageing workforce.

The majority of participants, who were recruit firefighters, reported that they were more likely to prepare a balanced meal during shifts compared to their previous jobs, attributing this to the kitchen facilities, time available, and the social influence of others eating well.

"[My diet has] improved a little bit from my last job, just because there is a kitchen and you can cook and prepare your own food."

—Focus group 2

Similarly, the presence of passionate health and fitness advocators within a station encouraged others to choose healthy foods at work, which occasionally carried over to home-life. As one participant explained:

"We actually have a very passionate personal trainer at our station . . . to the point where when he's on shift people tend to eat healthier just because they don't want to have to have that confrontation where they have to explain what they're eating to him."

—Focus group 5

4. Discussion

This mixed methods study found that shift schedule influenced food choices. It also highlighted that there are opportunities to modify the workplace environment to support healthier food choices of those working both at night and during the day and influence positive health behaviours by using a group/work culture approach. These findings are important for developing strategies in the workplace that will encourage behaviour change to promote healthy eating for those who work shifts. This is important given the data that suggest negative metabolic consequences of working night shift [3,5].

Food choices are key modifiable determinants of chronic diseases such as cardiovascular disease and type 2 diabetes. This study showed that amongst shift workers, the meal consumed during a day shift differed from the meal consumed on night shift, but there were no differences in overall energy intake (kJ/day), which is consistent with findings of a recent systematic review and meta-analysis [16]. The foods chosen at lunch were bread-based products, whereas the meals consumed at night were hot "home-cooked" style meals with a higher energy density (ED_{energy} kJ/g). Following this type of meal structure appeared important to the participants, and the opportunity to prepare a cooked meal and share with colleagues was associated with emotions of pride (Focus group 5). Even when shifts occurred at the weekend, this brought about different food choices than during the week, consistent with the usual variation displayed by those who work a standard working week pattern [25].

Snacking behaviour was different when on night shift compared with day shift. Both the focus groups and dietary data suggest that snacks were more likely to comprise discretionary foods at night. These foods are generally higher in energy, sugar, and fat and may be adverse for metabolic control at night. Habit and lack of healthy alternatives in the workplace were discussed in the focus groups as reasons for discretionary snack choices at night. A previous study of U.S. firefighters also described the availability of unhealthy snacks at their fire stations as a barrier to healthy eating at work, however, it was not indicated whether this was influenced by shift schedule [26]. Other studies have found that increased snacking is related to a change in food preferences at night and the use of sugar and/or caffeine to improve alertness [14,15,27]. A recent narrative review summarising studies that have examined dietary behaviours of shift workers supports the findings of our study that eating frequency, quality of diet, and energy distribution are impacted by shift work [28]. Workplaces should make a concerted effort to ensure that the snacks and food items supplied at work (both night and day) are nutritious.

It has been established that the health behaviours of a group influence the behaviour of an individual [29] and workplace environment is recognised as a strong predictor of individual dietary behaviours [30]. Participants in this study demonstrated a collegial approach to food selection, preparation, and consumption. This may be more evident in this working group due to the type of work activities they engage in, which require exceptional teamwork to prevent potentially devastating consequences. These participants have a group culture not only towards the duties they perform at work, but also to eating and, at times, sleeping as a group. Previous studies of employees working within a team have found that co-workers have an impact on individual health choices. Nurses have reported craving discretionary items after seeing their colleagues eating them, a finding mirrored in the present study [31]. Another study found that the attitude towards fitness among highly ranked firefighters had a strong influence on their crew's physical activity and fitness [32]. The PHLAME (Promoting Healthy Lifestyles: Alternative Models' Effects) Firefighters study demonstrated that group support for nutritious eating can result in group commitment towards health promoting behaviour [33]. This evidence supports the finding of the present study that co-worker attitudes and dietary choices can have both a positive and negative effect on health. The theoretical domains framework (TDF) is a single framework used to inform intervention design and fits within the Behaviour Change Wheel which enables characterisation of the target behaviour in terms of Capability, Opportunity, and Motivation (COM-B). To support translation of our outcomes into strategies promoting dietary change in shift workers, we have mapped these key findings to behaviour system COM-B [34] and theoretical domains framework change theory [35] (Table 5).

Table 5. Theoretical behaviour change components (COM-B) to address when implementing dietary changes for rotating shift workers.

COM-B Components		TDF Domain	Examples of Outcomes
Capability	Psychological	Knowledge Skills	Training/education in meal preparation and how to prepare for unexpected shift durations or tiredness
Opportunity	Physical Social	Environmental context and Resources Social influences	Provide meal preparation environments Ensure employer supplied meals and snacks are healthy Group commitment to healthy food environment
Motivation	Reflective	Social/Professional role and Identity Beliefs about consequences Optimism	Co-workers choices and attitudes affect dietary choices Knowledge of food choices and health outcomes—and that these health outcomes may differ with shift work Proud of having a well prepared dinner

COM-B: Capability, Opportunity, and Motivation (the COM-B system in the Behaviour change wheel), TDF: Theoretical Domain Framework.

In a recent report that explored eating patterns and related lifestyle behaviours in shift workers in Ireland, personal (intrinsic) factors that influenced (dietary) behaviour included motivation to change, nutritional knowledge, and organisational and planning skills [36]. A study in paramedics (*n* = 15) in Australia identified a number of physiological factors that impacted food choice including fatigue, hunger, and physical health [17]. Similar to the current study, data from these two studies were collected through focus groups; however, in our focus groups, personal factors that impacted food choice did not emerge as a Theme in the data.

Strengths of the study include the mixed methods approach, which allows stronger conclusions to be drawn from this study through the affirmation of qualitative and quantitative findings [37]. Furthermore, the repeated use of a multiple-pass method to collect dietary data allowed for the more accurate reporting of dietary intake, although the small sample for the dietary assessment component could be considered a limitation. As participants opted into the study, a risk of sampling bias was introduced. Lastly, firefighters are a unique group of shift workers and, consequently, some of the findings of this study may not be generalizable to the broader Australian shift working population, but may have applicability to related occupations such as other emergency services, law enforcement, and hospital emergency departments that share similar unpredictable work demands and work closely in teams.

5. Conclusions

This study identified a number of factors that may contribute to an increase in unhealthy dietary behaviours in a shift-working population, including an increase in discretionary foods and lack of availability of healthy food choices at night. As shift workers are at an increased risk of developing obesity [1,2,38,39] and cardiovascular disease [3,4] compared to the non-shift-working population, these findings provide important data to inform workplace health policy to support improving the health of these at risk and vulnerable employees.

Acknowledgments: Thanks to the participants from the Melbourne Metropolitan Fire Brigade for taking part in this project.

Author Contributions: M.P.B., C.E.H., C.T.H. conceived and designed the experiments; E.K.B. performed the experiments; E.K.B., C.P., T.A.M. and C.E.H. analysed the data; E.K.B., M.P.B., C.E.H. wrote the paper.

Conflicts of Interest: The authors declare no conflict of interest.

References

1. Amani, R.; Gill, T. Shiftworking, nutrition and obesity: Implications for workforce health—A systematic review. *Asia Pac. J. Clin. Nutr.* **2013**, *22*, 505–515. [CrossRef] [PubMed]
2. Antunes, L.C.; Levandovski, R.; Dantas, G.; Caumo, W.; Hidalgo, M. Obesity and shift work: Chronobiological aspects. *Nutr. Res. Rev.* **2010**, *23*, 155–168. [CrossRef] [PubMed]

3.   Brown, D.; Feskanich, D.; Sánchez, B.; Rexrode, K.; Schernhammer, E.; Lisabeth, L. Rotating night shift work and the risk of ischemic stroke. *Am. J. Epidemiol.* **2009**, *169*, 1370–1377. [CrossRef] [PubMed]

4.   Tüchsen, F.; Hannerz, H.; Burr, H. A 12 year prospective study of circulatory disease among Danish shift workers. *Occup. Environ. Med.* **2006**, *63*, 451–455. [CrossRef] [PubMed]

5.   Gan, Y.; Yang, C.; Tong, X.; Sun, H.; Cong, Y.; Yin, X.; Li, L.; Cao, S.; Dong, X.; Gong, Y.; et al. Shift work and diabetes mellitus: A meta-analysis of observational studies. *Occup. Environ. Med.* **2015**, *72*, 72–78. [CrossRef] [PubMed]

6.   Kecklund, G.; Axelsson, J. Health consequences of shift work and insufficient sleep. *BMJ* **2016**, *355*, i5210. [CrossRef] [PubMed]

7.   Lee, S.; McCann, D.; Messenger, J.C. *Working Time around the World: Trends in Working Hours, Laws and Policies in a Global Comparative Perspective*; Routledge: Geneva, Switzerland, 2007.

8.   Ekmekcioglu, C.; Touitou, Y. Chronobiological aspects of food intake and metabolism and their relevance on energy balance and weight regulation. *Obes. Rev.* **2011**, *12*, 14–25. [CrossRef] [PubMed]

9.   Lowden, A.; Moreno, C.; Holmbäck, U.; Lennernäs, M.; Tucker, P. Eating and shift work—Effects on habits, metabolism, and performance. *Scand. J. Work Environ. Health* **2010**, *36*, 150–162. [CrossRef] [PubMed]

10. Nagaya, T.; Yoshida, H.; Takahashi, H.; Kawai, M. Markers of insulin resistance in day and shift workers aged 30–59 years. *Int. Arch. Occup. Environ. Health* **2002**, *75*, 562–568. [CrossRef] [PubMed]

11. Morgan, L.; Arendt, J.; Owens, D.; Folkard, S.; Hampton, S.; Deacon, S.; English, J.; Ribeiro, D.; Taylor, K. Effects of the endogenous clock and sleep time on melatonin, insulin, glucose and lipid metabolism. *J. Endocrinol.* **1998**, *157*, 443–451. [CrossRef] [PubMed]

12. Lund, J.; Arendt, J.; Hampton, S.M.; English, J.; Morgan, L.M. Postprandial hormone and metabolic responses amongst shift workers in Antarctica. *J. Endocrinol.* **2001**, *171*, 557–564. [CrossRef] [PubMed]

13. Onat, A.; Sari, I.; Yazici, M.; Can, G.; Hergenç, G.; Avci, G. Plasma triglycerides, an independent predictor of cardiovascular disease in men: A prospective study based on a population with prevalent metabolic syndrome. *Int. J. Cardiol.* **2006**, *108*, 89–95. [CrossRef] [PubMed]

14. De Assis, M.A.A.; Kupek, E.; Nahas, M.V.; Bellisle, F. Food intake and circadian rhythms in shift workers with a high workload. *Appetite* **2003**, *40*, 175–183. [CrossRef]

15. Lasfargues, G.; Vol, S.; Cacès, E.; Le Clésiau, H.; Lecomte, P.; Tichet, J. Relations among night work, dietary habits, biological measures, and health status. *Int. J. Behav. Med.* **1996**, *3*, 123–134. [CrossRef] [PubMed]

16. Bonham, M.P.; Bonnell, E.K.; Huggins, C.E. Energy intake of shift workers compared to fixed day workers: A systematic review and meta-analysis. *Chronobiol. Int.* **2016**, *33*, 1086–1100. [CrossRef] [PubMed]

17. Anstey, S.; Tweedie, J.; Lord, B. Qualitative study of Queensland paramedics' perceived influences on their food and meal choices during shift work. *Nutr. Diet.* **2015**, *73*, 43–49. [CrossRef]

18. Creswell, J.; Clark, V. *Designing and Conducting Mixed Methods Research*, 2nd ed.; SAGE Publications: London, UK, 2007.

19. Patton, M. *Qualitative Research and Evaluation Methods. Integrating Theory and Practice*, 4th ed.; SAGE Publications: Thousand Oaks, CA, USA, 2015.

20. Raper, N.; Perloff, B.; Ingwersen, L.; Steinfeldt, L.; Anand, J. An overview of USDA's dietary intake data system. *J. Food Compos. Anal.* **2004**, *17*, 545–555. [CrossRef]

21. Baker IDI. *4000 for Health Food Model Booklet*, 1st ed.Victorian Government Department of Human Services: Melbourne, Australia, 2009.

22. Sandelowski, M. Whatever happened to qualitative description? *Res. Nurs. Health* **2000**, *23*, 334–340. [CrossRef]

23. McCaffrey, T.A.; Rennie, K.L.; Kerr, M.A.; Wallace, J.M.; Hannon-Fletcher, M.P.; Coward, W.A.; Jebb, S.A.; Livingstone, M.B.E. Energy density of the diet and change in body fatness from childhood to adolescence; is there a relation? *Am. J. Clin. Nutr.* **2008**, *87*, 1230–1237. [PubMed]

24. Australian Dietary Guidelines. Available online: https://www.nhmrc.gov.au/guidelines-publications/n55 (accessed on 22 February 2017).

25. An, R. Weekend-weekday differences in diet among, U.S. adults, 2003–2012. *Ann. Epidemiol.* **2016**, *26*, 57–65. [CrossRef] [PubMed]

26. Geibe, J.R.; Holder, J.; Peeples, L.; Kinney, A.M.; Burress, J.W.; Kales, S.N. Predictors of On-Duty Coronary Events in Male Firefighters in the United States. *Am. J. Cardiol.* **2008**, *101*, 585–589. [CrossRef] [PubMed]

27. Waterhouse, J.; Buckley, P.; Edwards, B.; Reilly, T. Measurement of, and Some Reasons for, Differences in Eating Habits between Night and Day Workers. *Chronobiol. Int.* **2003**, *20*, 1075–1092. [CrossRef] [PubMed]

28. Nea, F.M.; Kearney, J.; Livingstone, M.B.; Pourshahidi, L.K.; Corish, C.A. Dietary and lifestyle habits and the associated health risks in shift workers. *Nutr. Res. Rev.* **2015**, *28*, 143–166. [CrossRef] [PubMed]

29. Pettinger, C.; Holdsworth, M.; Gerber, M. Psycho-social influences on food choice in Southern France and Central England. *Appetite* **2004**, *42*, 307–316. [CrossRef] [PubMed]

30. Shimotsu, S.T.; French, S.A.; Gerlach, A.F.; Hannan, P.J. Worksite environment physical activity and healthy food choices: Measurement of the worksite food and physical activity environment at four metropolitan bus garages. *Int. J. Behav. Nutr. Phys. Act.* **2007**, *4*, 17. [CrossRef] [PubMed]

31. Persson, M.; Mårtensson, J. Situations influencing habits in diet and exercise among nurses working night shift. *J. Nurs. Manag.* **2006**, *14*, 414–423. [CrossRef] [PubMed]

32. Staley, J.A.; Weiner, B. Firefighter fitness, coronary heart disease, and sudden cardiac death risk. *Am. J. Health Behav.* **2011**, *35*, 603–617. [CrossRef] [PubMed]

33. Ranby, K.W.; MacKinnon, D.P.; Fairchild, A.J.; Elliot, D.L.; Kuehl, K.S.; Goldberg, L. The PHLAME (Promoting Healthy Lifestyles: Alternative Models' Effects) Firefighter Study: Testing Mediating Mechanisms. *J. Occup. Health Psychol.* **2011**, *16*, 501–513. [CrossRef] [PubMed]

34. Michie, S.; van Stralen, M.M.; West, R. The behaviour change wheel: A new method for characterising and designing behaviour change interventions. *Implement. Sci.* **2011**, *6*, 42. [CrossRef] [PubMed]

35. Cane, J.; O'Connor, D.; Michie, S. Validation of the theoretical domains framework for use in behaviour change and implementation research. *Implement. Sci.* **2012**, *7*, 37. [CrossRef] [PubMed]

36. Managing Food on Shift Work. Available online: http://www.safefood.eu/Publications/Research-reports/Managing-food-on-shift-work.aspx (accessed on 22 February 2017).

37. Johnson, R.B.; Onwuegbuzie, A.J. Mixed Methods Research: A Research Paradigm Whose Time Has Come. *Educ. Res.* **2004**, *33*, 14–26. [CrossRef]

38. Barbadoro, P.; Santarelli, L.; Croce, N.; Bracci, M.; Vincitorio, D.; Prospero, E.; Minelli, A. Rotating shift-work as an independent risk factor for overweight Italian workers: A cross-sectional study. *PLoS ONE* **2013**, *8*, e63289. [CrossRef]

39. Eberly, R.; Feldman, H. Obesity and shift work in the general population. *IJAHSP* **2010**, *8*, 10.

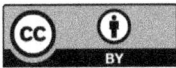

nutrients

MDPI

Article

Shift in Food Intake and Changes in Metabolic Regulation and Gene Expression during Simulated Night-Shift Work: A Rat Model

Andrea Rørvik Marti [1,*], Peter Meerlo [2], Janne Grønli [1,3,4], Sjoerd Johan van Hasselt [2], Jelena Mrdalj [1,5], Ståle Pallesen [6,7], Torhild Thue Pedersen [1], Tone Elise Gjøterud Henriksen [7,8] and Silje Skrede [9]

[1] Department of Biological and Medical Psychology, University of Bergen, Bergen 5009, Norway; janne.gronli@uib.no (J.G.); jelena.mrdalj@uib.no (J.M.); torhildp@hotmail.com (T.T.P.)
[2] Groningen Institute for Evolutionary Life Sciences, University of Groningen, 9700 CC Groningen, The Netherlands; p.meerlo@rug.nl (P.M.); sjoerdvanhasselt@live.nl (S.J.v.H.)
[3] College of Medical Sciences, Washington State University, Spokane, WA 99210, USA
[4] Sleep and Performance Research Center, Washington State University, Spokane, WA 99210, USA
[5] Norwegian Competence Center for Sleep Disorders, Haukeland University Hospital, Bergen 5021, Norway
[6] Department of Psychosocial Science, University of Bergen, Bergen 5015, Norway; staale.pallesen@uib.no
[7] Section of Psychiatry, Department of Clinical Medicine, Faculty of Medicine and Dentistry, University of Bergen, Bergen 5021, Norway; tone.elise.gjotterud@helse-fonna.no
[8] Division of Mental Health Care, Valen Hospital, Fonna Local Health Authority, Valen 5451, Norway
[9] Dr. Einar Martens Research Group for Biological Psychiatry, Center for Medical Genetics and Molecular Medicine, Haukeland Univeristy Hospital, 5021 Bergen, Norway; silje.skrede@uib.no
* Correspondence: andrea.marti@uib.no; Tel: +47-55-58-65-50

Received: 30 August 2016; Accepted: 28 October 2016; Published: 8 November 2016

Abstract: Night-shift work is linked to a shift in food intake toward the normal sleeping period, and to metabolic disturbance. We applied a rat model of night-shift work to assess the immediate effects of such a shift in food intake on metabolism. Male Wistar rats were subjected to 8 h of forced activity during their rest (ZT2-10) or active (ZT14-22) phase. Food intake, body weight, and body temperature were monitored across four work days and eight recovery days. Food intake gradually shifted toward rest-work hours, stabilizing on work day three. A subgroup of animals was euthanized after the third work session for analysis of metabolic gene expression in the liver by real-time polymerase chain reaction (PCR). Results show that work in the rest phase shifted food intake to rest-work hours. Moreover, liver genes related to energy storage and insulin metabolism were upregulated, and genes related to energy breakdown were downregulated compared to non-working time-matched controls. Both working groups lost weight during the protocol and regained weight during recovery, but animals that worked in the rest phase did not fully recover, even after eight days of recovery. In conclusion, three to four days of work in the rest phase is sufficient to induce disruption of several metabolic parameters, which requires more than eight days for full recovery.

Keywords: shift work; night work; animal model; metabolism; circadian rhythmicity; gene expression; body temperature; body weight; food intake

1. Introduction

Working shifts is common in modern societies [1], despite the fact that chronic night-shift work is linked to an increased risk for a wide variety of diseases, including metabolic disorders such as obesity and diabetes [2–8].

The regulation of daily rhythmicity in physiology and behaviour is closely intertwined with the regulation of metabolism. The circadian clock in the suprachiasmatic nuclei (SCN) of the hypothalamus influence other hypothalamic regions and peripheral tissues involved in regulation of feeding behaviour, metabolism, energy storage, and energy breakdown [9].

An important function of the endogenous circadian system is that it allows for anticipation of meals, and thereby facilitates efficiency in metabolic regulation [10]. The activity of organs involved in food processing and energy metabolism—including the digestive tract [11], liver [12,13], and pancreas [14]—shows clear circadian rhythmicity. Food intake is thought to be one of the primary zeitgebers (time-givers) for the coordination and timing of these rhythms [15].

Night-shift workers are exposed to conflicting zeitgebers, imposed by changes in food intake and activity patterns, as well as nocturnal light exposure [16–18]. Consequently, during night-shift work, endogenous circadian rhythms become desynchronized, as conflicting signals are sent to different tissues and organs. Often, the desynchronization is prolonged, as entrainment of rhythms in different tissues occurs at different rates [10].

The effects of working at night are immediate, and although humans may partially adapt to the night-shift, many physiological systems fail to adjust [19]. In Norway and Europe generally, night workers commonly work three to four night shifts in a row. Data from a simulated night-shift study in humans indicate that the metabolic effects are most pronounced during the initial two days, followed by compensatory mechanisms triggered by negative metabolic effects [20]. Ribeiro and colleagues induced a 9 h phase delay in a human simulated shift work study. Controlling energy and macronutrient intake, they showed that plasma levels of free fatty acids and triglycerides were reduced postprandially, indicative of poor metabolic regulation, but that this reduction was partially normalized on the third day following the phase delay [20].

Animal models of shift work may provide important clues to the mechanisms by which shift work causes metabolic disruption. Although several animal models indicate marked metabolic changes due to rest-work [21], only models involving relatively extreme rest-work schedules have been applied so far. The early metabolic effects of simulated night-shift work have yet to be investigated in animal models.

In the present study, we utilized a rat model of shift work to investigate the early effects of simulated night work on metabolism. We hypothesized that a shift in feeding rhythm during work hours occurs during a four-day rest-work schedule, as a sign of metabolic compensation. Specifically, we proposed that compensatory mechanisms triggered by negative metabolic effects would be displayed in liver gene expression due to a shift in the timing of food intake.

2. Materials and Methods

2.1. Ethical Approval

This project was approved by the Norwegian Animal Research Authority (permit number: 2012463) and performed according to Norwegian laws and regulations, and The European Convention for the Protection of Vertebrate Animals used for Experimental and Other Scientific Purposes.

2.2. Animals and Housing

Adult male rats ($n = 40$, Wistar, NTac:WH, Taconic, Silkeborg, Denmark) weighing approximately 300 g at arrival, were group housed in individually ventilated cages (IVC, Tecniplast, Buggugitate, Italy, 75 air changes/h) type IV ($480 \times 375 \times 210$ mm, 1500 cm^2). After surgery and during the experiment, animals were single housed (IVC cage type III, $425 \times 266 \times 185$ mm, 800 cm^2). The study was performed under a 12 h light/12 h dark (LD) cycle (lights on at 06:00, zeitgeber time 0; ZT0). Lights were gradually dimmed on and off over a period of 1 h, and were fully on at 07:00 and fully off at 19:00. Food (rat and mouse No. 1, Special Diets Services, Witham, Essex, UK) and water were provided ad libitum throughout the experiment.

2.3. Study Design

To assess changes in food timing, rats were randomly assigned to one of two treatment groups, either rest-work (RW, $n = 24$) or active-work (AW, $n = 16$). The experiment first consisted of four days of undisturbed baseline, followed by a four-day work period. A subset of animals was monitored during eight days of undisturbed recovery (RW $n = 14$, AW $n = 11$). See Figure 1 for a graphical overview of the study design. A shift in feeding rhythm of RW animals was observed during work session three. For assessment of changes in metabolic gene expression in the liver during this shift, another experiment was conducted in a subset of animals (RW $n = 10$, AW $n = 10$) after five weeks of recovery from the initial four-day shift-work period. Since the animals were still young adults [22], we consider it unlikely that ageing affected the results of this second experiment. The animals were randomly assigned to three consecutive days of either AW or RW as described above, euthanized after the third work session, and compared to time-matched non-working controls ($n = 5$, each condition).

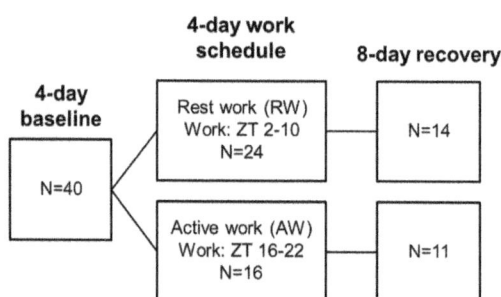

Figure 1. Overview of the study design. Animals were monitored for four baseline days, and a four-day work schedule during which animals were exposed to either rest-work or active work. The work schedule was followed by eight days of recovery. After at least five weeks of recovery, a subset of animals underwent a three-day work schedule (not shown) before euthanasia and tissue harvest from experimental animals and undisturbed time-matched controls.

2.4. Simulated Shift Work Procedure

To mimic human shift work and compare this with normal daytime work, rats were exposed to forced activity for 8 h per day, centred either during the rats' normal active phase (AW; ZT 14-22) or during the rats' normal rest phase (RW; ZT 2-10), as described previously [23]. Forced activity was achieved by placing the rats in automatically rotating wheels (Rat Running Wheel, TSE running wheel system, Bad Homburg, Germany; 24 cm diameter; 3 rpm; 1440 revolutions or 1.086 km of linear distance per 8 h session). Food and water was available ad libitum. Rotating wheels, feeders, and water bottles were cleaned after each work session with a 5% ethanol solution. Between sessions, animals were housed in their home cages.

2.5. Telemetric Recording and Analyses of Body Temperature

Rats were implanted with transmitters (Physiotel, Data Sciences International, St. Paul, MN, USA) for continuous wireless recording of body temperature, as previously described [24]. In brief, animals were anaesthetized with subcutaneous injection of a mixture of fentanyl 0.277 mg/kg, fluanizone 8.8 mg/kg, and midazolam 2.5 mg/kg (Hypnorm, Janssen, Beerse, Belgium; Dormicum, Roche, Basel, Switzerland; Midazolam Actavis, Actavis, Parsippany-Troy Hills, NJ, USA), and the transmitters were placed in subcutaneous pockets in the dorsomedial lumbar region (4ET transmitters) or in the neck region (F40-EET transmitters). Animals were allowed to recover for 14 days before entering the experiment. Body temperature was recorded every 10 s, at 50 Hz sampling rate, and signals were collected with Dataquest ART software (version 4.1, Data Sciences International, St. Paul, MN, USA).

Chronos-Fit software (Heidelberg University, Heidelberg, Germany) [25] was used for linear analyses of body temperature. From the linear analysis, 24 h mean, 12 h rest phase mean (lights on; ZT 12–24), and 12 h active phase mean (lights off; ZT 0–12) were calculated.

2.6. Body Weight and Food Intake Measurements

At baseline, all animals were weighed to assess 24 h and four-day body weight change. Baseline food and water intake were monitored across an 8 h window equal to the length of one work session, and across a 16 h window equal to the time between each work session. During the four-day work period, body weight change, food intake, and water intake were monitored for each 8 h work session and the 16 h between the work sessions. During the eight-day recovery phase, body weight change was monitored every four days.

2.7. Assessment of Metabolic Gene Expression in the Liver

Following the third work session, animals were fasted for 2 h to avoid the immediate effects of food intake on gene expression, anaesthetized with isoflurane, and sacrificed by decapitation. AW were sacrificed at ZT0, before the transition from dark to light phase, and RW at ZT12, before the transition from light to dark phase. A separate group of undisturbed animals never exposed to simulated work were used as time-matched controls, and sacrificed at the same zeitgeber times as experimental animals (AW control: ZT0; and RW control: ZT12). Liver tissue was harvested, flash frozen, and stored at $-80\,^{\circ}$C until analysis. Samples were homogenized using a TissueLyser (Qiagen, Valencia, CA, USA). RNA extraction was performed using a 6100 Nucleic acid PrepStation (Applied Biosystems, Foster City, CA, USA). A total of 20 ng RNA was transcribed to cDNA using the High Capacity RNA-to-cDNA kit (Applied Biosystems). Real-time polymerase chain reaction (PCR) was run on the Applied Biosystems 7900 Real-Time PCR System, with each sample run in triplicate. Relative gene expression levels were determined using the comparative ΔCt method, using β-actin (Actb) and ribosomal protein lateral stalk subunit P0 (Rplp0) as endogenous controls. Sequence names, main function, accession numbers, and primer sequences are shown in Table 1.

2.8. Statistical Analyses

Statistical analyses were conducted using STATA (release 14; StataCorp LP, College Station, TX, USA). Baseline food intake and body weight were compared between groups using student's t-test (two-tailed). For all other statistical analyses of food intake, body weight, and body temperature, we used mixed model analysis using restricted maximum likelihood estimation with the unstructured covariance between random effects. Where significant effects were observed, pairwise comparisons of groups at each time point were performed as well as comparing each day to baseline. Difference in gene expression (fold change) between groups was evaluated using student's t-test (two-tailed). Statistical significance was accepted at $p < 0.05$.

Nutrients **2016**, 8, 712

Table 1. Sequence names, accession numbers, and primer sequences for genes examined for hepatic transcriptional levels.

Gene	Main Function	Accession Number	Forward Primer	Reverse Primer
Fatty acid synthase (*Fasn*)	Fatty acid synthesis	NM_017332	CCATCATCCCCTTGATGAAGA	GTTGATGTCGATGCCTGTGAG
Stearoyl-CoA 9-desaturase; Stearoyl-CoA desaturase 1 (*Scd1*)	Fatty acid desaturation	NM_139192	TCAATCTCGGGAGAACATCC	CATGCAGTCGATGAAGAACG
Diacylglycerol O-acyltransferase 1 (*Dgat1*)	Triglyceride synthesis	NM_053437	AATGCTGCGGAAAAACTACG	TTGCTGGTAACAGTGCTTGC
Diacylglycerol O-acyltransferase 2 (*Dgat2*)	Triglyceride synthesis	NM_001012345	AATCTGTGTGCCGCCAG	TCCCTGCAGCACACAGCTTTG
Glycerol-3-phosphate acyltransferase 1, mitochondrial (*Gpam*)	Triglyceride synthesis	NM_017274	AATGCTGCGGAAAAACTACG	TTGCTGGTAACAGTGCTTGC
Sterol regulatory element-binding protein 1c (*Srebf1*)	Key regulator of fatty acid/triglyceride synthesis	NM_001271207	GAACCGCAAAGGCTTTGTAAA	ACCCAGATCAGCTCCATGGC
Hydroxymethylglutaryl-CoA synthase, cytoplasmic (*Hmgcs1*)	Sterol synthesis	NM_017268	CAGCTCTTGGGATGGACGA	GGCGTTTCCTGAGGCATATATAG
Sterol regulatory element-binding protein 2 (*Srebf2*)	Key regulator of sterol synthesis	NM_001033694.1	GCCGCAACCAGCTTTCAA	CCTGCTGCACCTGTGTGTA
Peroxisome proliferator-activated receptor alpha (*Ppara*)	Fatty acid oxidation	NM_013196	AATGCAATCCGTTTTGGAAGA	ACAGGTAAGGATTTCTGCCTTCAG
Peroxisome proliferator-activated receptor gamma (*Pparg*)	Adipocyte differentiation	NM_001145366	CCACAAAAAGAGTAGAAATAAATGTCAGTAC	CAAACCTGATGGCCATTGTGAGA
Insulin receptor substrate 2 (*Irs2*)	Mediation of insulin effects	NM_001168633	GAAGCGGCTAAGTCTCATCG	CTGGCTGACTTGAAGGAAGG
Phosphorylase, glycogen, liver (*Pygl*)	Glycogen breakdown	NM_022268	AAAAGCCTGGAACACAATGG	TCGGTCACTGGAGAACTTCC
Mechanistic target of rapamycin (*Mtor*)	Mediation of cellular metabolic stress response	NM_019906	CATGAGATGTGGCATGAAGG	AAACATGCCTTTGACGTTCC
Carbohydrate responsive element binding protein (ChREBP/Mlxipl)	Triglyceride synthesis in response to carbohydrates	AB074517	CTCTCAGGGAATACACGTCTCC	ATCTTGGTCTTTGGGTCTTCAGG
β-actin (*Actb*)	Endogenous control	NM_031144	TACAGCTTCACCACCACAGC	CTTCTCCAGGGAGGAAGAGG
Rattus norvegicus ribosomal protein lateral stalk subunit P0 (*Rplp0*)	Endogenous control	NM_022402.2	CATTGAAATCCTGACGCGATGT	AGATGTTCAACATGTTCAGCAG

3. Results

3.1. Baseline Parameters

At baseline, the two groups on average had similar body weight and food intake ($p > 0.09$ in all cases). The absolute baseline food intake across 24 h was 23.1 (± 0.53 g) for RW and 21.36 (± 0.70 g) for AW. Eight hours baseline food intake was 4.39 (± 0.37 g) for RW and 8.54 (± 0.70 g) for AW. Moreover, there were no significant differences in body temperature parameters (24 h mean, active phase mean, rest phase mean; $p > 0.10$ in all cases). Baseline day three was used as baseline reference in the subsequent analyses.

3.2. Feeding and Body Temperature Rhythms, during and after One Rest-Work Period

In RW, total 24 h food intake was significantly reduced on all four work days compared to baseline ($p < 0.001$ for all days; Figure 2a), but not compared to AW. RW food intake gradually increased across the first two 8 h work sessions. On day three, food intake stabilized, and was significantly increased in the 8 h work sessions on both days three and four ($p < 0.02$; Figure 2b). Hence, RW shifted the timing of food intake on work day three. This shift was also significant compared to AW food intake during the work session on days three and four ($p < 0.01$, both work sessions; Figure 1b). Between work sessions, food intake was decreased on all work days ($p < 0.001$, all days) compared to baseline.

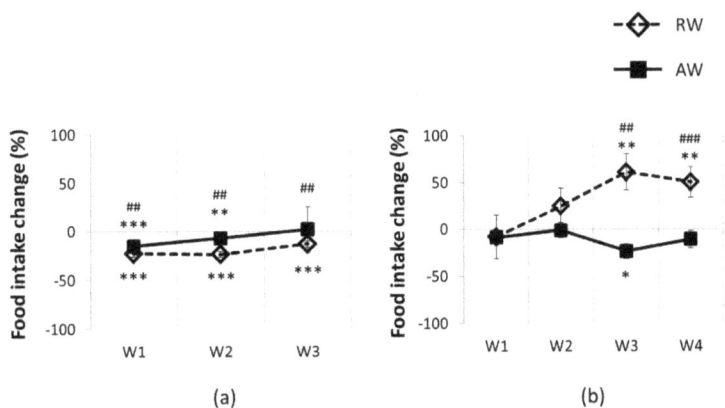

Figure 2. Food intake across one shift work period for active workers (AW) and rest-workers (RW): (**a**) 24 h food intake; (**b**) 8 h food intake (during work session). Data are shown as percentage change relative to baseline. Error bars indicate SEM. W1–4 indicates work days 1 to 4. W4 not included in 24 h food intake due to missing measurements. * $p < 0.05$; ** $p < 0.01$; *** $p < 0.001$, compared to baseline. ## $p < 0.01$; ### $p < 0.001$, between groups.

RW body weight dropped and remained below baseline across the whole four-day rest-work period (Figure 3). The reduced body weight was evident across 24 h, and during the 8 h work sessions. RW gained less weight between the work sessions, both compared to baseline ($p < 0.001$, all work days) and to AW ($p < 0.008$, all work days). The most pronounced body weight loss was observed during work day two, before body weight loss appeared to attenuate (see Figure 3).

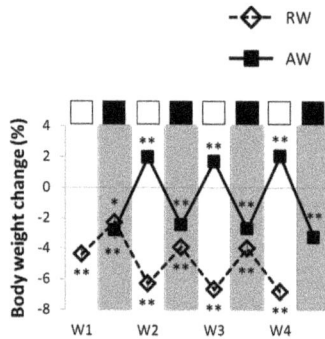

Figure 3. Body weight change during and between work sessions for active workers (AW) and rest-workers (RW). White rectangles indicate work hours for RW. Black rectangles indicate work hours for AW. Data are shown as percentage change relative to baseline. Shaded bars indicate lights off (active phase). Error bars indicate SEM. W1–4 indicates work days 1 to 4. * $p < 0.05$; *** $p < 0.001$, compared to baseline.

In RW, mean 24 h body temperature during the four-day rest-work period did not significantly differ from baseline or AW. However, RW body temperature was elevated during the 12 h rest phase (which now included the 8 h work session; $p < 0.001$ for all four work days), and was reduced during the 12 h active phase on work days two to four ($p < 0.003$ all three work days, Figure 4b). The 12 h body temperature increase from baseline during rest phase was more pronounced in RW than in AW on work days three and four ($p < 0.02$ both), and lower during the 12 h active phase on work day four ($p = 0.02$).

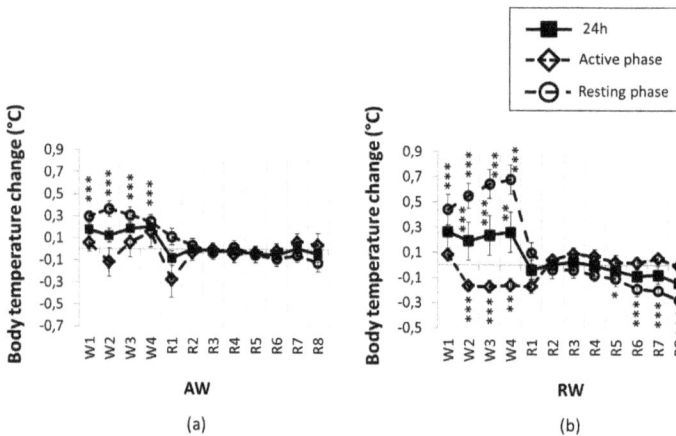

Figure 4. Mean body temperature during one shift work period (W1–4) and recovery (R1–8) for (**a**) active workers (AW) and (**b**) rest-workers (RW). Data are shown as mean percentage change relative to baseline. Error bars indicate SEM. W1–4 indicate work days 1 to 4. ** $p < 0.01$; *** $p < 0.001$, compared to baseline.

In AW, total 24 h food intake was reduced on work days one and two compared to baseline ($p < 0.05$, both days), but not on work days three to four (Figure 2a). During the 8 h work sessions, food intake was only significantly reduced on work day three compared to baseline ($p < 0.001$, Figure 2b). Food intake in the 16 h between work sessions was not significantly different from baseline.

AW body weight was reduced across 24 h ($p < 0.001$, all workdays) and during the 8 h work sessions ($p < 0.001$, all work sessions), but increased more during the 16 h between the work sessions ($p < 0.001$, all workdays) compared to baseline condition (Figure 3).

Mean 24 h body temperature during the four-day work period in AW was slightly elevated (0.17 °C on average), but not significantly different from baseline (Figure 4a). AW mean 12 h body temperature during the active phase (including the 8 h work session) was unaltered compared to baseline. Mean 12 h body temperature during the rest phase between work sessions was increased by 0.31 °C on average compared to baseline ($p < 0.001$, all days).

3.3. The Recovery Period

Rest-workers increased but did not regain the lost body weight during the 8 days recovery phase ($p < 0.001$; Figure 5). Mean body temperature for 24 h and for 12 h active phase was not significantly different from baseline, while mean body temperature during the 12 h rest phase progressively declined in the course of the recovery period, until it was significantly lower than baseline on recovery days five to eight ($p < 0.02$; Figure 4b).

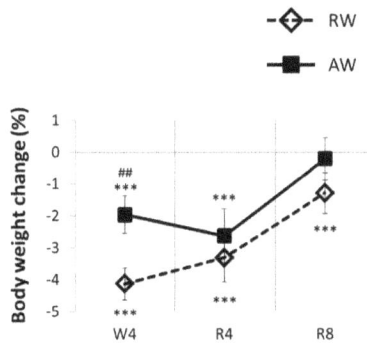

Figure 5. Body weight change during the recovery period for active workers (AW) and rest-workers (RW). Data are shown as percentage change relative to baseline. Error bars indicate SEM. W4 indicates work day. R4–8 indicates recovery days 4 and 8. *** $p < 0.001$, compared to baseline; ## $p < 0.01$, between groups.

Active-workers gradually increased their body weight, and returned to baseline level in the course of the eight-day recovery period (Figure 5). On recovery day four, body weight was still significantly lower than baseline ($p < 0.001$), but not on recovery day eight ($p = 0.20$). Mean values of body temperature in the recovery period did not differ from baseline.

3.4. Metabolic Gene Expression in the Liver at the Shift in Feeding Rhythm of Rest-Workers

In our protocol, AW and RW animals were euthanized on opposite zeitgeber time points, which allowed for comparison to time-matched controls only. Transcriptional alterations in several key genes involved in glucose metabolism, insulin sensitivity, fatty acid synthesis, triglyceride synthesis, cholesterol synthesis, and fatty acid oxidation were present in RW compared to undisturbed, time-matched control animals (Figure 6). mRNA levels for the genes encoding Insulin receptor substrate 2 (*Irs2*), Hydroxymethylglutaryl-CoA synthase, cytoplasmic (*Hmgcs1*), and Glycerol-3-phosphate acyltransferase 1, mitochondrial (*Gpam*) were all upregulated in RW compared to time-matched controls. Less-pronounced upregulation of *Hmgcs1* was present in AW, compared to time-matched controls. Transcriptional levels of Fatty acid synthase (*Fas*) were upregulated four-fold both in RW and in AW, while transcription of Stearoyl-CoA desaturase 1 (*Scd1*) was significantly downregulated in the liver from both groups. Transcription of Peroxisome proliferator-activated receptor alpha (*Ppara*, a major regulator of fatty acid oxidation) was downregulated in RW, but not in AW.

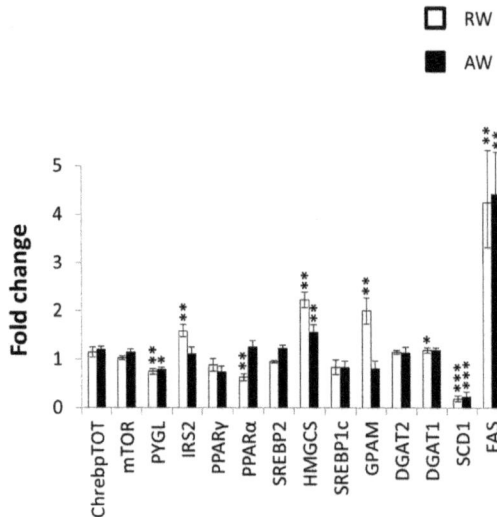

Figure 6. Expression levels of key metabolic genes in the liver from rest-workers (RW) and active workers (AW) following three work sessions, compared to undisturbed rats never exposed to simulated shift work. AW ($n = 10$) were sacrificed at zeitgeber time (ZT)24, and RW ($n = 10$) at ZT12. Undisturbed rats (RW control ($n = 5$) and AW control ($n = 5$) were sacrificed in a time-matched manner (i.e., at the same zeitgeber times as experimental animals). Fold changes for each gene represent the relative difference between shift work rats and controls. A fold change of 1 means no difference compared to controls, while a fold change of 2 means a doubling of transcriptional level, and a fold change of 0.5 a halving of the transcriptional level. * $p < 0.05$; ** $p < 0.01$; *** $p < 0.001$. ChrebpTOT, Carbohydrate-responsive element-binding protein; mTOR, Machanistic target of repemycin; PYGL, Phosphorylase, glycogen, liver; IRS2, Insulin receptor substrate 2; PPAR, Peroxisome proliferator-activated receptor; SREBP, Sterol regulatory element-binding protein; HMGCS, Hydroxymethylglutaryl-CoA synthase; GPAM, Glycerol-3-phosphate acyltransferase 1 mitochondrial; DGAT, Diacylglycerol O-acyltransferase; SCD1, Stearoyl-CoA desaturase 1; FAS, fatty acid synthase.

4. Discussion

The aim of this study was to examine how one period of simulated night-shift work affects metabolism in male rats. Results show that three successive days, each with 8 h of forced activity, led to a shift in the feeding rhythm during the rest-work sessions in rats. Measures of food intake and body weight appear to partially stabilize after three days of rest-work, indicating an adaptation in the regulation of metabolism at this time point.

In this study, both RW and AW exhibited an overall reduction in food intake during the four-day work period. Other studies in animals report inconsistent results regarding food intake during day- and night-shift work. A review of animal models of shift work and effects on metabolism found that effects depended on the species examined (rat or mouse) and the protocol used (manipulate timing of activity, light, food intake, and/or sleep) [21]. In human night workers, a recent meta-analysis reported no change in total calorie intake [26], although there are many other documented changes, such as timing of food intake, number, size, and nutritional content of meals [27].

Our data demonstrated that the metabolic gene expression after three days of work was more affected in RW than in AW. Correspondingly, a previous study concluded that following a long period (five weeks) of forced shift work, synchronization of clock genes (controlled by the SCN) and metabolic genes was lost in the liver of RW rats, primarily due to a shift in food intake towards the rest phase [28]. We found that the gene encoding *Irs2* (which is linked to liver insulin sensitivity and lipid metabolism) was upregulated in RW, in correspondence with reduced total food intake [29–31]. Upregulation of the gene encoding the central cholesterol-producing enzyme *Hmgcs1* could also be related to reduced food intake, with SREBP2 activation triggered by reduced sterol levels in the liver. However, the genes encoding *Fasn*—the rate-limiting enzyme in de novo fatty acid synthesis—and *Gpam*—which catalyses the first acylation step in the synthesis of glycerophospholipids—were also upregulated in RW. Such upregulation would not be expected to accompany decreased food intake [32]. The increased hepatic expression of these genes in RW may be indicative of paradoxical or compensatory fatty acid and triglyceride synthesis in the liver, via as-of-yet undisclosed molecular mechanisms. In addition, the reduced expression of *Ppara*—indicating decreased fatty acid oxidation—is paradoxical. This uncoupling between food intake, body weight, and lipid biosynthesis/oxidation underlines the metabolically-disruptive potential of rest-work.

While these data on liver gene expression clearly suggest effects of rest phase work, the results should be considered with some care, for several reasons. First, liver gene expression was measured at only a single time point after three work days in both the AW and RW groups. Since time of day was controlled for by comparing gene expression of working animals to undisturbed time-matched controls, the results do not reflect effects of zeitgeber time only, but more probably reflect the effects of forced activity. Nevertheless, a more detailed study is required to understand the temporal dynamics of these changes in gene expression, not only in the course of the four-day work period, but also during recovery thereafter. Second, in our current protocol, animals were fasted from 2 h before euthanasia, but this may not fully exclude the possibility that our gene expression data were affected by difference in food intake prior to tissue harvesting. Additionally, for this reason, future studies are required to assess in more detail the complex interactions between food intake, metabolic state, and gene expression in the liver. Moreover, in order to examine the significance of transcriptional alterations, relevant protein levels and metabolites such as glucose, insulin, and lipids should be investigated in future studies.

Very few animal studies report or discuss immediate early metabolic effects of night-shift work. Some studies present day-by-day body weight data visually, and appear to indicate a shift in metabolic (body weight) regulation following 2–3 days of simulated night-shift work, but this shift is generally not acknowledged or discussed [33–35]. Our data demonstrated that AW maintained a normal rhythm of food intake during the work period, consuming most of the food during their usual active phase, whereas RW gradually shifted timing of food intake towards working hours in their normal rest phase, with a stable high food intake reached and maintained at the third work session. A shift in timing of food intake is consistent with previous findings in the laboratory rat [36]. In parallel, human night-shift workers typically consume the majority of their calories during shifts [37]. Interestingly, the shift in food intake occurred between work days two and three in our study—a time window that parallels the shift in metabolism-related processes during simulated night-shift in humans [20,38].

In accordance with the overall reduction in food intake, a net weight loss was observed during the shift work period. Weight loss was more evident in RW than AW, and although body weight increased sharply during the eight-day recovery period, RW did not fully recover body weight to baseline level. Previous studies have reported both weight gain and weight loss during simulated rest-work [34,36]. However, in these studies, rats were exposed to much longer periods of rest-work (4–5 weeks), making it difficult to directly compare our short-term results. Additionally, in the present study, simulated work was achieved with wheels rotating at a faster pace than in previous studies (e.g., [34,36]), which might explain a more negative energy balance. Still, the rats in our study were forced to walk only approximately 1.1 km each work session. Although this physical activity is not considered strenuous, as rats with free access to a running wheel may voluntarily run 6–9 km each day [39], the work sessions may have contributed to weight loss through increased energy expenditure. Such increased energy expenditure might be a direct consequence of the increased physical activity, but it might also partly depend on indirect mechanisms, such as an elevated body temperature. Intriguingly, this presumed increase in energy expenditure was not compensated for by food intake.

While the rats in the RW group consumed more food during the 8 h work sessions than they normally would during the same phase of the day under baseline conditions, they reduced food intake during the 16 h period between sessions (the net result being a reduction in 24-h food intake). Despite this reduction in energy intake between work sessions, body weight increased between sessions, presumably because the lower energy intake was compensated for by parallel reduction in energy expenditure. In agreement with this, RW body temperature was decreased between sessions, perhaps partly as a consequence of increased sleep [23]. This possibly represents a compensatory mechanism aimed at maintaining body weight. A previous study in humans suggests that two to three days of night-shift work is required for such metabolic compensatory mechanisms to take effect [20]. Thus, it may be that the initial days of night-shift work are the most straining on the metabolic system. Measurements of thermogenesis could have shed light on the energy expenditure gap demonstrated by our results, and should be included in future experiments.

Mean body temperature levels in AW rapidly normalized on the first day of recovery. Surprisingly, while RW initially recovered from the aberrant mean body temperature patterns displayed during the work period, they developed progressive hypothermia in the rest phase later on in the recovery phase. On recovery day eight, rest phase mean body temperature was almost 0.3 °C lower than at baseline. Since recordings were ended at recovery day eight, we do not know how many days hypothermia lasted, or how severe it became. The long-term effect on body temperature may be due to either stress, metabolic dysfunction, or a combination of both [40–43]. Based on the unexpected failure of all parameters to return to baseline levels, future studies should aim to prolong recovery time after forced work periods.

The model applied in the present study inherently entails that RW were exposed to light during work sessions, whereas AW were not. Due to the study design, we are precluded from investigating the contribution of light exposure to the metabolic changes. This should be addressed in future studies.

5. Conclusions

Our results indicate that in male rats, 3–4 days of forced work is sufficient to induce disruption to several metabolic parameters, particularly in rats exposed to forced activity during their rest phase. The current findings suggest that the initial days of night-shift work put the most strain on the metabolic system, inducing compensatory effects after 2–3 days, and that neither body weight nor body temperature is fully normalized in eight days of recovery.

Acknowledgments: This research was supported by grants from Faculty of Psychology, University of Bergen (Småforsk), Helse Vest Regional Health Authority (911781) and Norwegian Competence Center for Sleep Disorders. The authors express their thanks to Anne Marie Kinn Rød and Nina Harkestad for their assistance with collecting the data.

Author Contributions: Janne Grønli, Ståle Pallesen, Silje Skrede, Peter Meerlo and Jelena Mrdalj conceived and designed the experiments; Janne Grønli, Jelena Mrdalj, Andrea Rørvik Marti, Torhild Thue Pedersen and Silje Skrede performed the experiments; Janne Grønli, Jelena Marti, Sjoerd Johan van Hasselt and Silje Skrede analysed the data; Andrea Rørvik Marti, Peter Meerlo, Janne Grønli, Sjoerd Johan van Hasselt, Jelena Mrdalj, Ståle Pallesen, Torhild Thue Pedersen, Tone Elise Gjøtterud Henriksen and Silje Skrede wrote the paper.

Conflicts of Interest: The authors declare no conflict of interest. The founding sponsors had no role in the design of the study; in the collection, analyses, or interpretation of data; in the writing of the manuscript, and in the decision to publish the results.

References

1. European Foundation for the Improvement of Living and Working Conditions. *Fourth European Working Conditions Survey*; Eurofound: Luxembourg, 2007.

2. Karlsson, B.; Knutsson, A.; Lindahl, B. Is there an association between shift work and having a metabolic syndrome? Results from a population based study of 27 485 people. *Occup. Environ. Med.* **2001**, *58*, 747–752. [CrossRef] [PubMed]
3. Scheer, F.A.; Hilton, M.F.; Mantzoros, C.S.; Shea, S.A. Adverse metabolic and cardiovascular consequences of circadian misalignment. *Proc. Natl. Acad. Sci. USA* **2009**, *106*, 4453–4458. [CrossRef] [PubMed]
4. Knutsson, A. Health disorders of shift workers. *Occup. Med. (Lond.)* **2003**, *53*, 103–108. [CrossRef] [PubMed]
5. Puttonen, S.; Harma, M.; Hublin, C. Shift work and cardiovascular disease—Pathways from circadian stress to morbidity. *Scand. J. Work. Environ. Health* **2010**, *36*, 96–108. [CrossRef] [PubMed]
6. Van Drongelen, A.; Boot, C.R.; Merkus, S.L.; Smid, T.; van der Beek, A.J. The effects of shift work on body weight change—A systematic review of longitudinal studies. *Scand. J. Work. Environ. Health* **2011**, *37*, 263–275. [CrossRef] [PubMed]
7. Gan, Y.; Yang, C.; Tong, X.; Sun, H.; Cong, Y.; Yin, X.; Li, L.; Cao, S.; Dong, X.; Gong, Y.; et al. Shift work and diabetes mellitus: A meta-analysis of observational studies. *Occup. Environ. Med.* **2015**, *72*, 72–78. [CrossRef] [PubMed]
8. Wang, J.B.; Patterson, R.E.; Ang, A.; Emond, J.A.; Shetty, N.; Arab, L. Timing of energy intake during the day is associated with the risk of obesity in adults. *J. Hum. Nutr. Diet.* **2014**, *27* (Suppl. 2), 255–262. [CrossRef] [PubMed]
9. Hastings, M.; O'Neill, J.S.; Maywood, E.S. Circadian clocks: Regulators of endocrine and metabolic rhythms. *J. Endocrinol.* **2007**, *195*, 187–198. [CrossRef] [PubMed]
10. Dibner, C.; Schibler, U. Circadian timing of metabolism in animal models and humans. *J. Intern. Med.* **2015**, *277*, 513–527. [CrossRef] [PubMed]
11. Konturek, P.C.; Brzozowski, T.; Konturek, S.J. Gut clock: Implication of circadian rhythms in the gastrointestinal tract. *J. Physiol. Pharmacol.* **2011**, *62*, 139–150. [PubMed]
12. Reddy, A.B.; Karp, N.A.; Maywood, E.S.; Sage, E.A.; Deery, M.; O'Neill, J.S.; Wong, G.K.; Chesham, J.; Odell, M.; Lilley, K.S.; et al. Circadian orchestration of the hepatic proteome. *Curr. Biol.* **2006**, *16*, 1107–1115. [CrossRef] [PubMed]
13. Akhtar, R.A.; Reddy, A.B.; Maywood, E.S.; Clayton, J.D.; King, V.M.; Smith, A.G.; Gant, T.W.; Hastings, M.H.; Kyriacou, C.P. Circadian cycling of the mouse liver transcriptome, as revealed by cDNA microarray, is driven by the suprachiasmatic nucleus. *Curr. Biol.* **2002**, *12*, 540–550. [CrossRef]
14. Sadacca, L.A.; Lamia, K.A.; deLemos, A.S.; Blum, B.; Weitz, C.J. An intrinsic circadian clock of the pancreas is required for normal insulin release and glucose homeostasis in mice. *Diabetologia* **2011**, *54*, 120–124. [CrossRef] [PubMed]
15. Damiola, F.; Le Minh, N.; Preitner, N.; Kornmann, B.; Fleury-Olela, F.; Schibler, U. Restricted feeding uncouples circadian oscillators in peripheral tissues from the central pacemaker in the suprachiasmatic nucleus. *Genes Dev.* **2000**, *14*, 2950–2961. [CrossRef] [PubMed]
16. Eastman, C.I.; Stewart, K.T.; Mahoney, M.P.; Liu, L.; Fogg, L.F. Dark goggles and bright light improve circadian rhythm adaptation to night-shift work. *Sleep* **1994**, *17*, 535–543. [PubMed]
17. Crowley, S.J.; Eastman, C.I. Phase advancing human circadian rhythms with morning bright light, afternoon melatonin, and gradually shifted sleep: Can we reduce morning bright-light duration? *Sleep Med.* **2015**, *16*, 288–297. [CrossRef] [PubMed]
18. Wyse, C.A.; Biello, S.M.; Gill, J.M. The bright-nights and dim-days of the urban photoperiod: Implications for circadian rhythmicity, metabolism and obesity. *Ann. Med.* **2014**, *46*, 253–263. [CrossRef] [PubMed]
19. Folkard, S. Do permanent night workers show circadian adjustment? A review based on the endogenous melatonin rhythm. *Chronobiol. Int.* **2008**, *25*, 215–224. [CrossRef] [PubMed]
20. Ribeiro, D.C.; Hampton, S.M.; Morgan, L.; Deacon, S.; Arendt, J. Altered postprandial hormone and metabolic responses in a simulated shift work environment. *J. Endocrinol.* **1998**, *158*, 305–310. [CrossRef] [PubMed]
21. Opperhuizen, A.L.; van Kerkhof, L.W.; Proper, K.I.; Rodenburg, W.; Kalsbeek, A. Rodent models to study the metabolic effects of shiftwork in humans. *Front. Pharmacol.* **2015**, *6*, 50. [CrossRef] [PubMed]
22. Sengupta, P. The laboratory rat: Relating its age with human's. *Int. J. Prev. Med.* **2013**, *4*, 624–630. [PubMed]
23. Gronli, J.; Meerlo, P.; Pedersen, T.; Pallesen, S.; Skrede, S.; Marti, A.R.; Wisor, J.; Murison, R.; Henriksen, T.E.; Rempe, M.; et al. A rodent model of night-shift work induces short-term and enduring sleep and electroencephalographic disturbances. *J. Biol. Rhythms* **2016**, in press.

24. Mrdalj, J.; Pallesen, S.; Milde, A.M.; Jellestad, F.K.; Murison, R.; Ursin, R.; Bjorvatn, B.; Gronli, J. Early and later life stress alter brain activity and sleep in rats. *PLoS ONE* **2013**, *8*, e69923. [CrossRef] [PubMed]
25. Zuther, P.; Gorbey, S.; Lemmer, B. Chronos-Fit 1.05. Available online: http://www.ma.uni-heidelberg.de/inst/phar/lehre/chrono.html (accessed on 1 June 2009).
26. Bonham, M.P.; Bonnell, E.K.; Huggins, C.E. Energy intake of shift workers compared to fixed day workers: A systematic review and meta-analysis. *Chronobiol. Int.* **2016**, *33*, 1086–1100. [CrossRef] [PubMed]
27. Lowden, A.; Moreno, C.; Holmback, U.; Lennernas, M.; Tucker, P. Eating and shift work—Effects on habits, metabolism and performance. *Scand. J. Work. Environ. Health* **2010**, *36*, 150–162. [CrossRef] [PubMed]
28. Salgado-Delgado, R.C.; Saderi, N.; Basualdo Mdel, C.; Guerrero-Vargas, N.N.; Escobar, C.; Buijs, R.M. Shift work or food intake during the rest phase promotes metabolic disruption and desynchrony of liver genes in male rats. *PLoS ONE* **2013**, *8*, e60052. [CrossRef] [PubMed]
29. Awazawa, M.; Ueki, K.; Inabe, K.; Yamauchi, T.; Kubota, N.; Kaneko, K.; Kobayashi, M.; Iwane, A.; Sasako, T.; Okazaki, Y.; et al. Adiponectin enhances insulin sensitivity by increasing hepatic IRS-2 expression via a macrophage-derived IL-6-dependent pathway. *Cell Metab.* **2011**, *13*, 401–412. [CrossRef] [PubMed]
30. Taniguchi, C.M.; Ueki, K.; Kahn, R. Complementary roles of IRS-1 and IRS-2 in the hepatic regulation of metabolism. *J. Clin. Investig.* **2005**, *115*, 718–727. [CrossRef] [PubMed]
31. Dong, X.; Park, S.; Lin, X.; Copps, K.; Yi, X.; White, M.F. Irs1 and Irs2 signaling is essential for hepatic glucose homeostasis and systemic growth. *J. Clin. Investig.* **2006**, *116*, 101–114. [CrossRef] [PubMed]
32. Jensen-Urstad, A.P.; Semenkovich, C.F. Fatty acid synthase and liver triglyceride metabolism: Housekeeper or messenger? *Biochim. Biophys. Acta* **2012**, *1821*, 747–753. [CrossRef] [PubMed]
33. Murphy, H.M.; Wideman, C.H.; Nadzam, G.R. A laboratory animal model of human shift work. *Integr. Physiol. Behav. Sci.* **2003**, *38*, 316–328. [CrossRef] [PubMed]
34. Leenaars, C.H.; Kalsbeek, A.; Hanegraaf, M.A.; Foppen, E.; Joosten, R.N.; Post, G.; Dematteis, M.; Feenstra, M.G.; van Someren, E.J. Unaltered instrumental learning and attenuated body-weight gain in rats during non-rotating simulated shiftwork. *Chronobiol. Int.* **2012**, *29*, 344–355. [CrossRef] [PubMed]
35. Barf, R.P.; Desprez, T.; Meerlo, P.; Scheurink, A.J. Increased food intake and changes in metabolic hormones in response to chronic sleep restriction alternated with short periods of sleep allowance. *Am. J. Physiol. Regul. Integr. Comp. Physiol.* **2012**, *302*, R112–R117. [CrossRef] [PubMed]
36. Salgado-Delgado, R.; Angeles-Castellanos, M.; Buijs, M.R.; Escobar, C. Internal desynchronization in a model of night-work by forced activity in rats. *Neuroscience* **2008**, *154*, 922–931. [CrossRef] [PubMed]
37. De Assis, M.A.; Kupek, E.; Nahas, M.V.; Bellisle, F. Food intake and circadian rhythms in shift workers with a high workload. *Appetite* **2003**, *40*, 175–183. [CrossRef]
38. McHill, A.W.; Melanson, E.L.; Higgins, J.; Connick, E.; Moehlman, T.M.; Stothard, E.R.; Wright, K.P., Jr. Impact of circadian misalignment on energy metabolism during simulated nightshift work. *Proc. Natl. Acad. Sci. USA* **2014**, *111*, 17302–17307. [CrossRef] [PubMed]
39. Rodnick, K.J.; Reaven, G.M.; Haskell, W.L.; Sims, C.R.; Mondon, C.E. Variations in running activity and enzymatic adaptations in voluntary running rats. *J. Appl. Physiol.* **1989**, *66*, 1250–1257. [PubMed]
40. Siyamak, A.Y.; Macdonald, I.A. Sub-acute underfeeding but not acute starvation reduces noradrenaline induced thermogenesis in the conscious rat. *Int. J. Obes. Relat. Metab. Disord.* **1992**, *16*, 113–117. [PubMed]
41. Mrdalj, J.; Lundegaard Mattson, A.; Murison, R.; Konow Jellestad, F.; Milde, A.M.; Pallesen, S.; Ursin, R.; Bjorvatn, B.; Gronli, J. Hypothermia after chronic mild stress exposure in rats with a history of postnatal maternal separations. *Chronobiol. Int.* **2014**, *31*, 252–264. [CrossRef] [PubMed]
42. Harris, R.B.; Zhou, J.; Youngblood, B.D.; Rybkin, I.I.; Smagin, G.N.; Ryan, D.H. Effect of repeated stress on body weight and body composition of rats fed low- and high-fat diets. *Am. J. Physiol.* **1998**, *275 6 Pt 2*, R1928–R1938. [PubMed]
43. Shibli-Rahhal, A.; Van Beek, M.; Schlechte, J.A. Cushing's syndrome. *Clin. Dermatol.* **2006**, *24*, 260–265. [CrossRef] [PubMed]

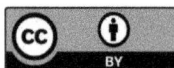

nutrients

MDPI

Article

Relevance of Morning and Evening Energy and Macronutrient Intake during Childhood for Body Composition in Early Adolescence

Tanja Diederichs [1], Sarah Roßbach [1], Christian Herder [2,3], Ute Alexy [1] and Anette E. Buyken [1,*]

[1] IEL-Nutritional Epidemiology, DONALD Study, University of Bonn, Heinstueck 11, 44225 Dortmund, Germany; tdiederi@uni-bonn.de (T.D.); srossbac@uni-bonn.de (S.R.); alexy@uni-bonn.de (U.A.)
[2] Institute for Clinical Diabetology, German Diabetes Center, Leibniz Center for Diabetes Research at Heinrich Heine University Düsseldorf, Auf'm Hennekamp 65, 40225 Düsseldorf, Germany; Christian.Herder@ddz.uni-duesseldorf.de
[3] German Center for Diabetes Research (DZD), Ingolstädter Landstr. 1, 85764 München-Neuherberg, Germany
* Correspondence: buyken@uni-bonn.de; Tel.: +49-231-792102-50; Fax: +49-231-711581

Received: 11 August 2016; Accepted: 7 November 2016; Published: 10 November 2016

Abstract: (1) Background: This study investigated the relevance of morning and evening energy and macronutrient intake during childhood for body composition in early adolescence; (2) Methods: Analyses were based on data from 372 DONALD (DOrtmund Nutritional and Anthropometric Longitudinally Designed study) participants. Explorative life-course plots were performed to examine whether morning or evening energy and macronutrient intake at 3/4 years, 5/6 years, or 7/8 years is critical for fat mass index (FMI [kg/m^2]) and fat free mass index (FFMI [kg/m^2]) in early adolescence (10/11 years). Subsequently, exposures in periods identified as consistently critical were examined in depth using adjusted regression models; (3) Results: Life-course plots identified morning fat and carbohydrate (CHO) intake at 3/4 years and 7/8 years as well as changes in these intakes between 3/4 years and 7/8 years as potentially critical for FMI at 10/11 years. Adjusted regression models corroborated higher FMI values at 10/11 years among those who had consumed less fat ($p = 0.01$) and more CHO ($p = 0.01$) in the morning at 7/8 years as well as among those who had decreased their morning fat intake ($p = 0.02$) and increased their morning CHO intake ($p = 0.05$) between 3/4 years and 7/8 years; (4) Conclusion: During childhood, adherence to a low fat, high CHO intake in the morning may have unfavorable consequences for FMI in early adolescence.

Keywords: childhood; adolescence; morning intake; evening intake; macronutrient intake; fat mass

1. Introduction

Primary school years have recently been identified as a potentially "critical period" for the development and persistence of overweight and obesity [1] in different Western societies [2,3]. Moreover, children with a body mass index (BMI) in the upper normal range before and during primary school were at higher risk for obesity development until the end of primary school compared to those who had a BMI in the lower range [4]. These developments may in part be attributable to the considerable changes in children's daily routine, as entry into institutions like kindergarten and primary school results in an externally determined time window for morning intake and affects the timing and duration of evening intake due to less flexible bed times. These changes in circadian (=approximately 24 h) rhythmicity may entail changes in morning and evening energy and macronutrient intake.

Among adults, severe disruptions of circadian rhythm induced by shiftwork or jetlag are known to increase the risk for obesity, type 2 diabetes, and cardiovascular diseases [5,6]. Similar associations have been suggested for moderate disruptions due to irregular meal times or delayed bed times [7].

Moreover, studies among adults revealed that a number of metabolic processes follow circadian rhythms: levels of hunger are known to increase over the day [8], accompanied by a reduced ability to compensate for higher evening energy intakes [9]; in addition, insulin sensitivity [10] and diet-induced thermogenesis [11] may decrease over the day. It is hence plausible that day-time specific energy or macronutrient intake—in particular, if not in balance with the circadianity of these metabolic processes—may have longer-term effects on body composition. However, evidence of these aspects among children is lacking. This study therefore examined, whether morning or evening energy and macronutrient intake during kindergarten and primary school age is of prospective relevance for body composition in early adolescence (i.e., the end of primary school).

2. Methods

2.1. DONALD Study

The DONALD (DOrtmund Nutritional and Anthropometric Longitudinally Designed) study is an ongoing open cohort study conducted in Dortmund, Germany, which was previously described in detail [9]. Briefly, since recruitment began in 1985, detailed information on diet, growth, development, and metabolism between infancy and early adulthood has been collected from >1550 children. Every year, 35 to 40 healthy infants with no prevalent diseases affecting growth and/or diet are newly recruited and first examined at the ages of three or six months. Each child returns for three more visits in the first year, two in the second, and then once annually until early adulthood. The health status is re-assessed at each visit.

The study was approved by the Ethics Committee of the University of Bonn; all examinations are performed with parental and later the children's written consent.

2.2. Nutritional Data

Nutritional data are assessed by 3-day weighed dietary records on three consecutive days. Participants are free to choose the days of recording. Overall, 37% of the 3–8 years old participants eligible for the present analysis chose to record their intake over three consecutive weekdays only, while 19% documented their intake on two weekdays and one weekend day, and 44% chose one weekday and two weekend days. Parents and/or participants are instructed by dietitians to weigh all foods and beverages consumed by the participant, including leftovers, to the nearest 1 g over three consecutive days with the use of regularly calibrated electronic food scales (initially Soehnle Digita 8000 (Leifheit AG, Nassau, Germany), now WEDO digi 2000 (Werner Dorsch GmbH, Muenster/Dieburg, Germany)). Semi-quantitative measures (e.g., number of spoons) are allowed when exact weighing is not possible. Information on recipes and on the types and brands of food items consumed is also requested. The dietary records are analyzed using the continuously updated in-house nutrient database LEBTAB [10], which includes information from standard nutrient tables, product labels, or recipe simulations based on the listed ingredients and nutrients. Additionally, the time of every eating occasion is recorded.

2.3. Anthropometric Data

Participants are measured at each visit by trained nurses according to standard procedures (WHO 1995), dressed in underwear only and barefoot. From the age of two onward, standing height is measured to the nearest 0.1 cm with a digital stadiometer. Weight is measured to the nearest 0.1 kg with an electronic scale (model 753 E; Seca, Hamburg, Germany). Skinfold thicknesses are measured from the age of six months onward on the right side of the body at the biceps, triceps, subscapular, and suprailiac sites to the nearest 0.1 mm with a Holtain caliper (Holtain Ltd., Crymych, UK). For assurance of quality data, inter- and intra-observer agreement is monitored regularly (average inter- and intra-individual variation coefficients obtained between 2005 and 2015 were 10.0% and

13.0% for biceps, 4.5% and 5.7% for triceps, 5.0% and 7.6% for subscapular, and 7.6% and 9.0% for suprailiacal skinfolds).

Body mass index (BMI, kg/m^2) was calculated, percent body fat (%BF) was estimated for children up to age 8 years from all four skinfolds using the Deurenberg equation [11], and for children above age 8 years, from two skinfolds (triceps, subscapular) using the Slaughter equation [12]. Body fat mass (kg) and fat-free body mass (kg) were calculated ("(%BF × body mass)/100" and "((100 − %BF) × body mass)/100", respectively) and related to the square of height to obtain fat mass index (FMI, kg/m^2) and fat free mass index (FFMI, kg/m^2). Since the distribution of FMI was skewed, log-transformed values were used in analyses.

2.4. Familial Characteristics

On their child's admission to the study and at regular intervals thereafter, parents are interviewed concerning the child's early life data as well as familial and socio-economic characteristics. Additionally, parents are weighed and measured. Information on birth anthropometrics and gestational age are abstracted from a standardized document (Mutterpass) given to all pregnant women in Germany.

2.5. Definition of Morning and Evening

For estimation of morning and evening energy and macronutrient intake, food consumption documented between an age-specific end of the night and 11 a.m. and between 6 p.m. and an age-specific start of the night was used. The cut-points at 11 a.m. in the morning and 6 p.m. in the evening emerged in a preliminary analysis of DONALD data, showing that children and adolescents (2–18 years) consume their first (and second) breakfast until 11 a.m., and that 6 p.m. marks the point in time between afternoon snacks and the main evening meals. The age-specific start and end of the night was estimated using all available consecutive 3-day dietary records from DONALD participants of the respective age. The age-specific start of the night was defined as the time of the day, after which less than 5% of the last eating occasions (≥10 kcal) before midnight were documented; the age-specific end of the night was the time of the day past 5 a.m., after which more than 5% of the first eating occasions (≥10 kcal) were documented.

2.6. Study Sample

The present analysis included term (gestational age 37–42 weeks) singletons with a minimum birth weight of 2500 g. Regarding exposure data, weighed dietary records had to be available from three consecutive days to allow the derivation of the start and end of the night. The outcomes FMI and FFMI were estimated from the latest available anthropometric measurement at age 10 or 11 years.

In an initial explorative analysis, we were interested in the identification of one or more potentially critical time period(s) for later body composition. To this end, life-course plots (see statistical analysis) allow a first data screening. For this analysis, we considered participants who had provided at least one 3-day weighed dietary record in each of the three potentially critical time periods 3/4 years, 5/6 years, and 7/8 years, and anthropometric data at age 10/11 years ($N = 499$). Additionally, data on the age marking the start of the pubertal growth spurt "age at take-off" (ATO) had to be available, resulting in a final sample size of $N = 372$ for the explorative analysis.

For the in-depth analyses, more strict inclusion criteria were used. We only considered participants who had provided two plausible 3-day weighed dietary records and additional covariates (see statistical analysis) for the respective time periods identified by the explorative analysis. A 3-day weighed dietary record was considered plausible when the total recorded energy intake was adequate in relation to the estimated basal metabolic rate (BMR) using modified age-dependent cutoffs from Goldberg et al. [13].

2.7. Statistical Analysis

SAS procedures (SAS version 9.2, SAS Institute, Cary, NC, USA) were used for data analysis. Significance level was set at $p < 0.05$; $p < 0.1$ was considered to indicate a trend. Since there were no interactions between sex and the exposure–outcome associations, data from boys and girls were pooled. The statistical analysis was performed in a two-stage approach, starting with an initial explorative analysis followed by an in-depth analysis.

For the initial explorative analysis, life-course plots [14] were used to simultaneously consider a repeatedly measured exposure (e.g., morning fat intake at 3/4 years, 5/6 years, 7/8 years) in relation to one outcome (e.g., FMI at 10/11 years). Energy intake in the morning and in the evening was expressed as percentage of total daily energy intake (TEI); morning and evening macronutrient intake was expressed as percentages of fat, carbohydrate (CHO), or protein of energy intake before 11 a.m. and after 6 p.m., respectively. For all three potentially critical periods (i.e., 3/4 years, 5/6 years, 7/8 years), exposures were averaged (if two records were available), checked for normal distribution, transformed (if necessary), and standardized (mean = 0, standard deviation = 1) by critical time period. Multivariable linear regression models were calculated with continuous macronutrient intake as independent exposures and FMI or FFMI as outcomes (adjusted for ATO and mean standardized TEI between age 3–8 years). The resulting regression coefficients were plotted against age, and both their own value (representing the strength of the relation at a distinct time point) and their changes (representing the association between outcome and the exposure's change over time) and were evaluated to identify a potentially critical time period of one or more intake variables with respect to body composition in early adolescence.

The in-depth multivariable linear regression analyses focused on the time period(s) and specific intake (morning/evening, energy/macronutrient) identified by the life-course plot approach. Energy-adjusted morning and evening macronutrient intakes were calculated using the residual method [15]. Intakes were entered individually as independent exposures together with ATO into multivariable linear regression models (crude models). Predicted means of FMI or FFMI were presented by tertiles of the respective intake. In a further step, potentially confounding factors were considered as covariates: sex (male/female), FMI- or FFMI at the analysis-specific baseline (i.e., 3/4 years, 5/6 years, or 7/8 years), birth year, appropriateness for gestational age (i.e., whether birth weight and length were appropriate for gestational age yes/no), full breastfeeding ($\geq$4 months yes/no), maternal overweight ($\geq$25 kg/m^2 yes/no), maternal educational status ($\geq$12 years of schooling yes/no) and smoking in the household (yes/no). Only covariates which modified the exposure's regression coefficient in the crude model by $\geq$10% [16] or were independent predictors of the outcome variable [17] were included into a hierarchical approach of covariate selection [18]. The following hierarchy was used: (1) general characteristics (sex and baseline FMI- or FFMI); (2) early life characteristics (birth year, appropriateness for gestational age, full breastfeeding); (3) familial and socio-economic characteristics (maternal overweight, maternal educational status, smoking in the household). To ensure comparability, model building was performed for the strongest exposure–outcome association per time period and outcome. Identified confounders were also used in all other models. Sensitivity analyses using individually constructed models for each exposure–outcome association yielded similar results. Additional sensitivity analyses were performed to address the possibility that observed prospective relations were driven by cross-sectional associations of the respective predictor at age 10/11 years with body composition at age 10/11 years.

3. Results

3.1. Explorative Analysis

Table 1 gives the characteristics of the explorative life-course plot analysis sample (*N* = 372). According to the cut-points of the International Obesity Task Force (IOTF) [19], 16% of the children were overweight at 10/11 years; according to McCarthy [20], 21% had an excessive body fatness.

Table 1. Early life, pubertal, familial-, and socio-economic characteristics, as well as data on the outcome body composition (explorative analysis sample, N = 372).

Variable	Explorative Analysis Sample
Sex (♀ n (%))	182 (48.9)
Early life factors	
Birth year	1992 (1987; 1996)
Appropriate for gestational age (n (%))	285 (76.6)
Fully breastfed (n (%) ≥ 4 months) [1]	223 (60.1)
Puberty marker	
Age at takeoff (ATO, years)	9.7 (8.7; 10.5)
Socio-economic status	
Maternal overweight, ≥25 kg/m^2, (n (%)) [1]	110 (29.7)
Maternal educational status, ≥12 years of schooling, (n (%))	223 (60.0)
Smoking in the household (n (%))	86 (23.1)
Body composition at age 10/11 years (Outcome) [2]	
BMI (kg/m^2)	17.6 (16.1; 19.5)
♀	17.5 (16.0; 19.6)
♂	17.7 (16.2; 19.3)
FMI (kg/m^2)	3.1 (2.3; 4.6)
♀	3.5 (2.5; 4.8)
♂	2.9 (2.0; 4.3)
FFMI (kg/m^2)	14.3 (13.5; 14.9)
♀	14.0 (13.2; 14.6)
♂	14.5 (13.8; 15.2)
Overweight (n (%)) [3]	60 (16.1)
♀	30 (16.5)
♂	30 (15.8)
Excessive body fatness (n (%)) [4]	78 (20.1)
♀	33 (18.1)
♂	45 (23.7)

Values are shown as n (%) for categorized variables and as median (25th; 75th percentile) for continuous variables. BMI—body mass index, FFMI—fat free mass index, FMI—fat mass index, IOTF—international obesity task force, ♀ - girls, ♂ - boys. [1] N = 371; [2] latest available measurement; [3] including overweight and obese participants, according to IOTF, Cole, 2000 [19]; [4] including overweight and obese participants, according to McCarthy, 2006 [20] with body fat estimation after Slaughter, 1988 [12].

Nutritional data of the explorative sample are presented in Table 2 for each potentially critical time period. Morning, evening, and daily fat consumption decreased with age, whereas CHO consumption increased; protein intake was broadly consistent. Regardless of age, children consumed more CHO and less fat or protein in the morning compared to the evening.

Table 2. Dietary characteristics in three potentially critical time periods (explorative analysis sample, N = 372).

Exposure	Time Period 1 (Age 2.5 Years–<4.5 Years)	Time Period 2 (Age 4.5 Years–<6.5 Years)	Time Period 3 (Age 6.5 Years–<8.5 Years)	p for Trend [3]
Daily energy intake (MJ)	4.7 (4.3; 5.3)	5.7 (5.2; 6.3)	6.6 (5.9; 7.3)	<0.001
Daily energy intake (kcal)	1132 (1023; 1254)	1364 (1236; 1501)	1564.8 (1409.3; 1735.9)	<0.001
Fat (E% [1])	37.0 (33.5; 39.7)	36.2 (33.2; 39.1)	35.3 (32.9; 38.2)	0.002
Carbohydrates (E% [1])	50.2 (46.7; 54.2)	51.0 (48.1; 54.4)	52.0 (48.7; 54.7)	0.001
Protein (E% [1])	12.8 (11.6; 13.9)	12.6 (11.3; 13.6)	12.6 (11.6; 13.8)	0.055
Energy intake before 11 a.m. (kcal)	347.0 (295.5; 405.2)	379.0 (309.4; 451.2)	438.9 (369.7; 534.0)	<0.001
Energy intake before 11 a.m. (E% [1])	30.9 (26.7; 34.8)	27.5 (23.7; 32.9)	28.3 (24.3; 33.1)	<0.001
Fat (E% [2])	35.9 (30.9; 40.2)	34.9 (29.9; 39.7)	33.1 (28.9; 37.7)	<0.001
Carbohydrates (E% [2])	50.9 (46.3; 57.0)	52.6 (47.6; 58.1)	54.7 (49.6; 58.7)	<0.001
Protein (E% [2])	12.8 (11.2; 14.6)	12.3 (10.8; 13.9)	12.4 (10.9; 14.1)	0.013
Energy intake after 6 p.m. (kcal)	259.6 (199.2; 315.3)	334.5 (275.1; 403.5)	417.0 (332.4; 490.2)	<0.001
Energy intake after 6 p.m. (E% [1])	22.6 (17.7; 26.9)	24.6 (20.8; 29.0)	26.2 (22.4; 30.2)	<0.001
Fat (E% [2])	40.8 (34.8; 46.5)	39.2 (34.0; 45.0)	37.4 (32.6; 41.8)	<0.001
Carbohydrates (E% [2])	43.7 (37.4; 51.3)	46.4 (40.1; 52.8)	48.4 (43.2; 54.0)	<0.001
Protein (E% [2])	14.2 (12.1; 16.1)	14.0 (12.2; 15.8)	14.0 (12.0; 15.7)	0.361

Values are estimated from one or two 3-day dietary records, shown as median (25th; 75th percentile).
[1] % of daily energy intake; [2] % of energy intake before 11 a.m./after 6 p.m.; [3] differences between time periods using Kruskal–Wallis test.

The explorative life-course plot analysis (adjusted for ATO and TEI) consistently revealed associations of morning fat and morning CHO intake with FMI at 10/11 years (Figure 1A1,B1). Similar, albeit non-significant, associations were seen with FFMI (Figure 1A2,B2). Life-course plots show that a higher fat intake at 3/4 years was related to a higher FMI at 10/11 years ($p = 0.02$) (A1), just as a lower CHO intake was related to a higher FMI ($p = 0.04$) (B1). These trends reversed at 7/8 years (%fat $p = 0.004$, %CHO $p = 0.03$ before 11 a.m.), when a higher fat intake (A1) and a lower CHO intake (B1) before 11 a.m. were related to a lower FMI at 10/11 years. Moreover, the clear switch in signs of the regression coefficients between 3/4 years and 7/8 years suggested an additional relevance of the change in macronutrient intake over this time course (A1, B1) [21]. Morning energy or protein and evening energy or macronutrient intakes at 3/4 years, 5/6 years, or 7/8 years were not associated with FMI or FFMI at 10/11 years (data not shown).

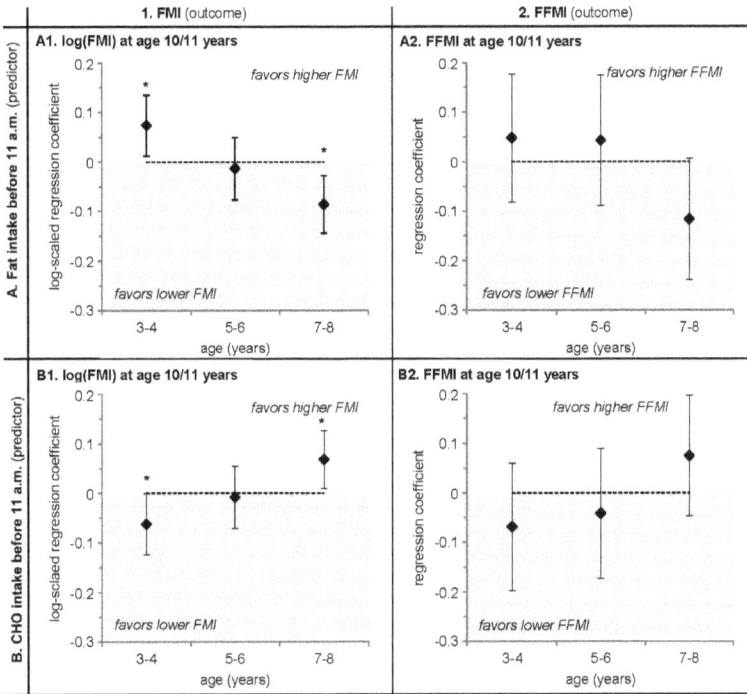

Figure 1. Life-course plots of multivariable linear regression analyses with log-transformed FMI (kg/m^2) and crude FFMI (kg/m^2) in early adolescence at 10/11 years as the outcome and the standardized intake of (**A**) morning fat (% of energy) and (**B**) morning carbohydrate (CHO) (% of energy) as predicting variables. Analyses were adjusted for age at take-off (ATO) and mean standardized daily energy intake (TEI) from 3 to 8 y. Values are regression coefficients (95% CI) from models ran on $N = 372$ participants of the DONALD study. * $p < 0.05$. ATO—age at take-off, CHO—carbohydrates, FFMI—fat free mass index (kg/m^2), FMI—fat mass index (kg/m^2).

3.2. In-Depth Analysis

On the basis of the results of the life-course plots, subsequent in-depth regression analyses (adjusted for ATO and baseline FMI or FFMI, respectively) focused on the prospective relevance of morning fat and CHO intake at 3/4 years and 7/8 years, as well as the change in these intakes between 3/4 years and 7/8 years for FMI at 10/11 years. Characteristics of the in-depth analyses sample ($N = 297$) were very similar to the explorative analysis sample (Supplementary Material Tables S1 and S2).

In these in-depth analyses, morning %CHO and %fat intake at age 3/4 years were not relevant for FMI at age 10/11 years (%fat $p = 0.93$, %CHO $p = 0.80$) (Table 3). By contrast, higher morning %fat intake and lower morning %CHO intake at 7/8 years continued to be predictive of a lower FMI at 10/11 years in multivariable models (%fat $p = 0.01$, %CHO $p = 0.01$). Moreover, a decrease in morning %fat intake and an increase in morning %CHO intake between 3/4 years and 7/8 years was related to a higher FMI at 10/11 years (Δ%fat $p = 0.02$, Δ%CHO $p = 0.05$). Additional adjustment for the corresponding macronutrient intake at age 10/11 years did not change the associations of morning %CHO or %fat intake at age 7/8 years or Δ%fat or Δ%CHO with FMI at 10/11 years (data not shown). For comparative purposes, we also ran multivariable regression models with FFMI as an outcome (Supplementary Material Table S3). However, neither morning %fat nor morning %CHO intake at 3/4 years or 7/8 years nor the change in intakes between 3/4 years and 7/8 years were related to FFMI at 10/11 years.

Table 3. Relation of fat and carbohydrate (CHO) intake before 11 a.m. during different critical time periods throughout childhood to FMI in early adolescence at age 10/11 years (in-depth analysis sample, N = 297).

	Predicted FMI Means in Tertiles of Corresponding Exposures [1] (Fat, CHO, ΔFat, ΔCHO)			%Difference T1–T3 [2]	p for Trend [3]
	Low Intake or Decrease in Intake (T1)	Average Intake or Constant Intake (T2)	High Intake or Increase in Intake (T3)		
At age 3/4 years					
Fat (*%E of breakfast* [4])					
Median intake (25th; 75th)	28.30 (25.24; 30.70)	36.17 (34.65; 37.53)	42.26 (40.08; 45;07)	+49.3%	<0.0001
Model 1 [5]	3.21 (2.90–3.55)	3.33 (3.01–3.68)	3.39 (3.06–3.74)	+5.6%	0.49
Model 2 [6]	3.25 (2.98–3.55)	3.25 (3.09–3.68)	3.30 (3.03–3.60)	+1.5%	0.93
CHO (*%E of breakfast* [4])					
Median intake (25th; 75th)	44.16 (40.53; 46.74)	50.91 (49.64; 52.14)	59.63 (56.95; 62.89)	+35.0%	<0.0001
Model 1 [5]	3.36 (3.04–3.72)	3.39 (3.07–3.75)	3.18 (2.87–3.51)	−5.4%	0.25
Model 2 [6]	3.26 (2.99–3.56)	3.39 (3.11–3.70)	3.27 (2.99–3.57)	−0.3%	0.80
At age 7/8 years					
Fat (*%E of breakfast* [4])					
Median intake (25th; 75th)	27.38 (25.07; 29.37)	33.20 (32.05; 34.58)	40.16 (38.01; 43.40)	+46.7%	<0.0001
Model 1 [5]	3.67 (3.33–4.06)	3.21 (2.90–3.54)	3.07 (2.78–3.39)	−16.4%	0.02
Model 2 [6]	3.48 (3.28–3.69)	3.30 (3.12–3.50)	3.15 (2.97–3.34)	−9.5%	0.01
CHO (*%E of breakfast* [4])					
Median intake (25th; 75th)	45.78 (41.76; 49.30)	54.23 (52.02; 56.45)	60.25 (58.21; 63.06)	+31.6%	<0.0001
Model 1 [5]	3.14 (2.84–3.47)	3.30 (2.99–3.65)	3.49 (3.16–3.85)	+11.1%	0.14
Model 2 [6]	3.15 (2.97–3.33)	3.23 (3.05–3.42)	3.56 (3.36–3.77)	+13.0%	0.01
Change (Δ) between age 3/4 years and age 7/8 years					
ΔFat (*Δ%E of breakfast* [4])					
Median Δ intake (25th; 75th)	−9.02 (−12.54; −6.72)	−1.81 (−3.73; 0.17)	5.14 (2.67; 8.57)	+157.0%	<0.0001
Model 1 [5]	3.60 (3.26–3.98)	3.25 (2.95–3.59)	3.09 (2.80–3.41)	−14.2%	0.01
Model 2 [6]	3.55 (3.26–3.87)	3.25 (2.98–3.54)	3.14 (2.88–3.43)	−11.6%	0.02
ΔCHO (*Δ%E of breakfast* [4])					
Median Δ intake (25th; 75th)	−6.02 (−10.41; −2.8)	2.53 (−0.38; 3.87)	10.28 (8.25; 13.20)	−270.8%	<0.0001
Model 1 [5]	3.13 (2.83–3.46)	3.22 (2.92–3.56)	3.59 (3.25–3.97)	+14.7%	0.02
Model 2 [6]	3.24 (2.97–3.54)	3.20 (2.93–3.49)	3.49 (3.20–3.81)	+7.7%	0.05

CHO—carbohydrates, FMI—fat mass index, - %E—energy percent; Δ, Change in intake between the age of 3/4 years and 7/8 years (Δ = 7/8 years–3/4 years); [1] Model-values are least square means (95% confidence intervals) of the FMI; [2] % difference between median intakes or predicted FMI means in tertile 1 and tertile 3; [3] p-values for differences in median intake or Δ intake are based on Kruskal–Wallis test; p-values for model 1 and model 2 are based on linear regression analyses (fat, CHO, Δ fat, Δ CHO as continuous exposure variables); [4] Residuals used in linear regression models; [5] Model 1 (crude model) adjusted for age at take-off (ATO); [6] Model 2 additionally adjusted for baseline FMI; no other covariates emerged as relevant.

4. Discussion

The present study provides first evidence for a prospective relevance of children's habitual macronutrient intake on a day-time specific level for their fat mass in early adolescence. Our results indicate that a higher FMI in early adolescence (i.e., around the end of primary school) may result if primary school children have a habitual low fat, high CHO intake during the morning, and if children decrease their morning fat intake and increase their morning CHO intake from kindergarten to primary school age.

For the interpretation of our results it is important to note that the analyzed data were collected in healthy free-living children following their habitual dietary habits. Morning CHO intake was moderate to high (age-dependent tertile medians: 44E% to 60E%, Table 3), and morning fat intake was low to moderate (age-dependent tertile medians: 27E% to 42E%, Table 3). Examples for low fat, high CHO breakfasts were ready-to-eat cereal with milk or bread with jam, often combined with juice and/or fruits and/or sweetened milk beverages. In turn, examples of moderate-fat, low-CHO breakfasts were oat(-nuts)-cereal with milk, bread with cheese, or sausage/ham or eggs, often combined with fruits or vegetables. Hence, modest differences in food choices translated into considerable differences in morning macronutrient intakes and subsequent fat mass in early adolescence.

Mechanisms to explain our results are unknown, but the following possible reasons are plausible and should be considered.

Breakfasts with a lower CHO-to-fat ratio compared to a higher one elicit lower overall postprandial blood glucose and insulin responses [22]. This may have consequences for levels of hunger/satiety and subsequent energy intake. In 64 overweight adults, a low CHO, high fat breakfast compared to a high CHO, low fat breakfast resulted in lower levels of hunger and a higher perceived fullness [22]. Data from children and adolescents stem largely from studies analyzing breakfast glycemic index (GI), supporting a short-term role of breakfast GI for subsequent levels of hunger and energy intake at lunch, as a low-GI compared to a high-GI breakfast resulted in lower levels of hunger and energy intake at lunch among normal weight or obese children and adolescents [23,24]. Beyond these acute effect studies, there are no intervention studies analyzing the longer-term impact of modulating breakfast fat/CHO content on body composition development among children. Of note, in our study, additional analyses did not confirm a role of morning dietary GI in the prospective associations of morning carbohydrate intake with adolescent body composition (data not shown). Nonetheless, higher postprandial blood glucose and insulin responses elicited by the high morning carbohydrate intake may be a relevant mechanism for our observation.

The specificity of our findings for morning intakes may also reflect a relevance of circadianity. Postprandial insulin and blood glucose responses follow a diurnal rhythm, at least in adults. Two small studies suggest a decrease in insulin sensitivity throughout the day [25,26], which would imply that a high morning CHO intake would be preferable over a high evening CHO intake. In fact, CHO intake was 6E%–7E% (absolute) higher in the morning than in the evening in our sample (Table 2). However, for our observation of an unfavorable association between higher morning CHO intakes and subsequent fat mass, two physiologically occurring phenomena may play a decisive role. First, pubertal insulin resistance, characterized by a decrease in peripheral insulin sensitivity accompanied by a lower increase in acute insulin response [27], emerges as early as at age 7 years [28]. This may translate into an enhanced vulnerability to high CHO loads among primary school children. Second, the dawn phenomenon, defined as an early morning rise in blood glucose levels and/or insulin requirements without food intake, was observed in patients with diabetes mellitus [29], as well as in healthy individuals [30]. Data for healthy children and adolescents on the dawn phenomenon are scarce and controversial: a difference in insulin levels during the night was neither observed in 31 healthy children and adolescents [31] nor in 10 healthy adolescents [32]. However, for the latter, a significantly higher insulin clearance rate was shown during the dawn period (5–8 a.m.) compared to the night (1–4 a.m.) [32]. Therefore, since insulin clearance rate—a potential characteristic of the dawn phenomenon—seems to rise physiologically in the morning, an additional stimulation by a CHO-rich breakfast may not be beneficial for the development of body composition, and may be specifically disadvantageous throughout puberty, when insulin resistance is known to be elevated [33].

In the context of circadianity, social jetlag must also be considered. The concept of social jetlag describes a misalignment of biological and social time [34]. Due to the natural chronotype delay during childhood and puberty [35] and an increasing sleep pressure as soon as children enter social institutions [36], social jetlag occurs already in young children [37] and increases until the end of adolescence [34]. The thereby disrupted circadian rhythm may interrelate with macronutrient intake and contribute to an adverse development of body composition, as was already shown for obesity development in adults [34]. Interestingly, data of 305 adolescents revealed that 20% of the association between habitual sleep variability and visceral fat was explained by CHO intake [38]. Additionally, the sleep duration of 767 Danish children aged 8–11 years correlated negatively with higher consumption of added sugar and sugar-sweetened beverages [39]. Therefore, a changing sleep pattern potentially induced by social jetlag may result in higher CHO intake—possibly mainly in the morning, when CHO intake was shown to be highest (Table 2).

Besides the morning, the evening is also discussed as potentially relevant for body composition. Chronobiological studies in adults indicate the already mentioned reduction in insulin sensitivity over the day [26], as well as a reduction in diet-induced thermogenesis [40] and an increasing level of hunger [8], accompanied by a reduced ability to compensate for higher evening energy intakes [41]. Interestingly, in our longitudinal analysis, evening macronutrient intakes did not emerge as relevant exposures for subsequent body composition.

Moreover, neither morning nor evening energy intake in childhood was associated with body composition in early adolescence. This may in part be attributable to a better ability of children to compensate for higher day-time specific energy intakes at subsequent meals when compared to adults [41–43]. Alternatively, we may have been unable to discern existing associations due to the fact that one or two 3-day dietary records may not be sufficient to characterize habitual energy intake.

Results of this study must be considered in the light of several limitations. First, FMI and FFMI were estimated from skinfold thicknesses, which have been criticized for being susceptible to measurement error. However, measurements were performed by trained and quality-monitored study personnel, which resulted in comparably low intra- and inter-observer differences [44]. Moreover, percent body fat estimated from skinfold measurements using the equation proposed by Slaughter [12] was shown to be comparable to, for example, body fat estimation by dual-energy X-ray absorptiometry [45]. Given that the variance in FMI explained by morning fat and CHO intake is smaller than the measurement error, it could be argued that our results reflect chance or bias rather than "true effects". However, our findings emerged from a two-stage statistical approach (exploratory and in-depth analyses) and remained largely unaffected by adjustment for potential confounders. Nonetheless, confounding by unmeasured covariates remains a possibility. Second, the DONALD population is characterized by a high socio-economic status [9]; i.e., the extremes in nutritional behavior may be under-represented. However, due to the relatively homogeneous sample, our results may be less vulnerable to residual confounding. The overall strengths of the study are the closely-spaced data, including day-time specific nutritional data for every age during childhood. Due to the early recruitment of the study participants and the annually repeated data collection, 3-day weighed dietary records are documented by participants accustomed to the procedure. Moreover, data on several important potential confounders (early-life characteristics, anthropometric, familial, and socio-economic factors) were available.

5. Conclusions

Our study suggests that a habitual low fat, high CHO intake during the morning among primary school children may contribute to an increase of their FMI in early adolescence. If confirmed by other studies, adherence to current dietary recommendations favoring a low-fat, high-CHO breakfast may fuel rather than abate the current obesity epidemic among children and adolescents. Further studies are needed to address the potential day-time specific underlying mechanisms.

Supplementary Materials: Tables S1–S3 are available online at http://www.mdpi.com/2072-6643/8/11/716/s1. They provide data on the in-depth analysis sample (*N* = 297). Table S1. Early life, pubertal, familial-, and socio-economic characteristics, as well as data on the outcome body composition (in-depth analysis sample, *N* = 297), Table S2. Dietary characteristics for time periods identified as critical (in-depth analysis sample, *N* = 297), Table S3. Relation of morning fat and morning carbohydrate (CHO) intake during different critical time periods throughout childhood to FFMI in early adolescence at age 10/11 years (in-depth analysis sample, *N* = 297).

Acknowledgments: This research project is funded by the German Research Foundation (Bu1807/3-1). The DONALD Study is supported by the Ministry of Science and Research of North Rhine Westphalia, Germany. With respect to the co-authorship of C.H., the following applies: The German Diabetes Center is funded by the German Federal Ministry of Health and the Ministry of Innovation, Science, Research and Technology of the State North Rhine-Westphalia. His participation in this project was supported in part by a grant from the German Federal Ministry of Education and Research to the German Center for Diabetes Research (DZD e.V.). We thank the staff of the DONALD study for carrying out the anthropometric measurements as well as for collecting and coding dietary records and all participants of the study for providing their data.

Author Contributions: T.D. conducted the statistical analysis and wrote the manuscript; A.E.B. supervised the study; A.E.B., U.A., C.H. conceived the project; all authors: made substantial contributions and read and approved the final manuscript.

Conflicts of Interest: Anette E. Buyken is a member of the International Carbohydrate Quality Consortium. All other authors declare no conflicts of interest. The funding sponsors had no role in the design of the study; in the collection, analyses, or interpretation of data; in the writing of the manuscript, and in the decision to publish the results.

References

1. Hughes, A.R.; Sherriff, A.; Lawlor, D.A.; Ness, A.R.; Reilly, J.J. Incidence of obesity during childhood and adolescence in a large contemporary cohort. *Prev. Med.* **2011**, *52*, 300–304. [CrossRef] [PubMed]

2. Fryar, C.D.; Carroll, M.D.; Ogden, C.L. Prevalence of Obesity among Children and Adolescents: United States, Trends 1963–1965 through 2009–2010. 2012. Available online: http://www.cdc.gov/nchs/data/hestat/obesity_child_09_10/obesity_child_09_10.pdf (accessed on 6 November 2015).

3. Kurth, B.-M.; Schaffrath Rosario, A. Die Verbreitung von Übergewicht und Adipositas bei Kindern und Jugendlichen in Deutschland. Ergebnisse des bundesweiten Kinder- und Jugendgesundheitssurveys (KiGGS). *Bundesgesundheitsblatt Gesundheitsforschung Gesundheitsschutz* **2007**, *50*, 736–743. [CrossRef] [PubMed]

4. Nader, P.R.; O'Brien, M.; Houts, R.; Bradley, R.; Belsky, J.; Crosnoe, R.; Friedman, S.; Mei, Z.; Susman, E.J. Identifying risk for obesity in early childhood. *Pediatrics* **2006**, *118*, e594–e601. [CrossRef] [PubMed]

5. Scheer, F.A.J.L.; Hilton, M.F.; Mantzoros, C.S.; Shea, S.A. Adverse metabolic and cardiovascular consequences of circadian misalignment. *Proc. Natl. Acad. Sci. USA* **2009**, *106*, 4453–4458. [CrossRef] [PubMed]

6. Szosland, D. Shift work and metabolic syndrome, diabetes mellitus and ischaemic heart disease. *Int. J. Occup. Med. Environ. Health* **2010**, *23*, 287–291. [CrossRef] [PubMed]

7. Garaulet, M.; Madrid, J.A. Chronobiological aspects of nutrition, metabolic syndrome and obesity. *Adv. Drug Deliv. Rev.* **2010**, *62*, 967–978. [CrossRef] [PubMed]

8. Scheer, F.A.J.L.; Morris, C.J.; Shea, S.A. The internal circadian clock increases hunger and appetite in the evening independent of food intake and other behaviors. *Obesity* **2013**, *21*, 421–423. [CrossRef] [PubMed]

9. Kroke, A.; Manz, F.; Kersting, M.; Remer, T.; Sichert-Hellert, W.; Alexy, U.; Lentze, M.J. The DONALD Study. History, current status and future perspectives. *Eur. J. Nutr.* **2004**, *43*, 45–54. [CrossRef] [PubMed]

10. Sichert-Hellert, W.; Kersting, M.; Chahda, C.; Schäfer, R.; Kroke, A. German food composition database for dietary evaluations in children and adolescents. *J. Food Compos. Anal.* **2007**, *20*, 63–70. [CrossRef]

11. Deurenberg, P.; Pieters, J.J.; Hautvast, J.G. The assessment of the body fat percentage by skinfold thickness measurements in childhood and young adolescence. *Br. J. Nutr.* **1990**, *63*, 293–303. [CrossRef] [PubMed]

12. Slaughter, M.H.; Lohman, T.G.; Boileau, R.A.; Horswill, C.A.; Stillman, R.J.; Van Loan, M.D.; Bemben, D.A. Skinfold equations for estimation of body fatness in children and youth. *Hum. Biol.* **1988**, *60*, 709–723. [PubMed]

13. Sichert-Hellert, W.; Kersting, M.; Schoch, G. Underreporting of energy intake in 1 to 18 years old German children and adolescents. *Zeitschrift fur Ernahrungswissenschaft* **1998**, *37*, 242–251. [CrossRef] [PubMed]

14. Cole, T.J. Modeling postnatal exposures and their interactions with birth size. *J. Nutr.* **2004**, *134*, 201–204. [PubMed]

15. Willett, W.C.; Howe, G.R.; Kushi, L.H. Adjustment for total energy intake in epidemiologic studies. *Am. J. Clin. Nutr.* **1997**, *65*, 1220–1231.

16. Maldonado, G.; Greenland, S. Simulation study of confounder-selection strategies. *Am. J. Epidemiol.* **1993**, *138*, 923–936. [PubMed]

17. Kirkwood, B.R.; Sterne, J.A.C. *Essential Medical Statistics*, 2nd ed.; Blackwell Science: Malden, MA, USA, 2003; pp. 315–342.

18. Victora, C.G.; Huttly, S.R.; Fuchs, S.C.; Olinto, M.T. The role of conceptual frameworks in epidemiological analysis: A hierarchical approach. *Int. J. Epidemiol.* **1997**, *26*, 224–227. [CrossRef] [PubMed]

19. Cole, T.J.; Bellizzi, M.C.; Flegal, K.M.; Dietz, W.H. Establishing a standard definition for child overweight and obesity worldwide: International survey. *BMJ* **2000**, *320*, 1240–1243. [CrossRef] [PubMed]

20. McCarthy, H.D.; Cole, T.J.; Fry, T.; Jebb, S.A.; Prentice, A.M. Body fat reference curves for children. *Int. J. Obes.* **2006**, *30*, 598–602. [CrossRef] [PubMed]

21. De Stavola, B.L.; Nitsch, D.; dos Santos Silva, I.; McCormack, V.; Hardy, R.; Mann, V.; Cole, T.J.; Morton, S.; Leon, D.A. Statistical issues in life course epidemiology. *Am. J. Epidemiol.* **2006**, *163*, 84–96. [CrossRef] [PubMed]

22. Chandler-Laney, P.C.; Morrison, S.A.; Goree, L.L.T.; Ellis, A.C.; Casazza, K.; Desmond, R.; Gower, B.A. Return of hunger following a relatively high carbohydrate breakfast is associated with earlier recorded glucose peak and nadir. *Appetite* **2014**, *80*, 236–241. [CrossRef] [PubMed]

23. Ludwig, D.S.; Majzoub, J.A.; Al-Zahrani, A.; Dallal, G.E.; Blanco, I.; Roberts, S.B. High glycemic index foods, overeating, and obesity. *Pediatrics* **1999**, *103*, E26. [CrossRef] [PubMed]

24. Warren, J.M.; Henry, C.; Jeya, K.; Simonite, V. Low glycemic index breakfasts and reduced food intake in preadolescent children. *Pediatrics* **2003**, *112*, e414. [CrossRef] [PubMed]

25. Morgan, L.M.; Aspostolakou, F.; Wright, J.; Gama, R. Diurnal variations in peripheral insulin resistance and plasma non-esterified fatty acid concentrations: A possible link? *Ann. Clin. Biochem.* **1999**, *36*, 447–450. [CrossRef] [PubMed]

26. Morris, C.J.; Yang, J.N.; Garcia, J.I.; Myers, S.; Bozzi, I.; Wang, W.; Buxton, O.M.; Shea, S.A.; Scheer, F.A.J.L. Endogenous circadian system and circadian misalignment impact glucose tolerance via separate mechanisms in humans. *Proc. Natl. Acad. Sci. USA* **2015**, *112*, E2225–E2234. [CrossRef] [PubMed]

27. Goran, M.I.; Gower, B.A. Longitudinal study on pubertal insulin resistance. *Diabetes* **2001**, *50*, 2444–2450. [CrossRef] [PubMed]

28. Jeffery, A.N.; Metcalf, B.S.; Hosking, J.; Streeter, A.J.; Voss, L.D.; Wilkin, T.J. Age before stage: Insulin resistance rises before the onset of puberty: A 9-year longitudinal study (EarlyBird 26). *Diabetes Care* **2012**, *35*, 536–541. [CrossRef] [PubMed]

29. Bolli, G.B.; Gerich, J.E. The "dawn phenomenon"—A common occurrence in both non-insulin-dependent and insulin-dependent diabetes mellitus. *N. Engl. J. Med.* **1984**, *310*, 746–750. [CrossRef] [PubMed]

30. Schmidt, M.I.; Lin, Q.X.; Gwynne, J.T.; Jacobs, S. Fasting early morning rise in peripheral insulin: Evidence of the dawn phenomenon in nondiabetes. *Diabetes Care* **1984**, *7*, 32–35. [CrossRef] [PubMed]

31. Marin, G.; Rose, S.R.; Kibarian, M.; Barnes, K.; Cassorla, F. Absence of dawn phenomenon in normal children and adolescents. *Diabetes Care* **1988**, *11*, 393–396. [CrossRef] [PubMed]

32. Arslanian, S.; Ohki, Y.; Becker, D.J.; Drash, A.L. Demonstration of a dawn phenomenon in normal adolescents. *Hormone Res.* **1990**, *34*, 27–32. [CrossRef] [PubMed]

33. Moran, A.; Jacobs, D.R.; Steinberger, J.; Cohen, P.; Hong, C.-P.; Prineas, R.; Sinaiko, A.R. Association between the insulin resistance of puberty and the insulin-like growth factor-I/growth hormone axis. *J. Clin. Endocrinol. Metab.* **2002**, *87*, 4817–4820. [CrossRef] [PubMed]

34. Roenneberg, T.; Allebrandt, K.V.; Merrow, M.; Vetter, C. Social jetlag and obesity. *Curr. Biol.* **2012**, *22*, 939–943. [CrossRef] [PubMed]

35. Roenneberg, T.; Kuehnle, T.; Pramstaller, P.P.; Ricken, J.; Havel, M.; Guth, A.; Merrow, M. A marker for the end of adolescence. *Curr. Biol.* **2004**, *14*, R1038–R1039. [CrossRef] [PubMed]

36. Cairns, A.; Harsh, J. Changes in sleep duration, timing, and quality as children transition to kindergarten. *Behav. Sleep Med.* **2014**, *12*, 507–516. [CrossRef] [PubMed]

37. Werner, H.; LeBourgeois, M.K.; Geiger, A.; Jenni, O.G. Assessment of chronotype in four- to eleven-year-old children: Reliability and validity of the Children's Chronotype Questionnaire (CCTQ). *Chronobiol. Int.* **2009**, *26*, 992–1014. [CrossRef] [PubMed]

38. He, F.; Bixler, E.O.; Liao, J.; Berg, A.; Imamura Kawasawa, Y.; Fernandez-Mendoza, J.; Vgontzas, A.N.; Liao, D. Habitual sleep variability, mediated by nutrition intake, is associated with abdominal obesity in adolescents. *Sleep Med.* **2015**, *16*, 1489–1494. [CrossRef] [PubMed]

39. Kjeldsen, J.S.; Hjorth, M.F.; Andersen, R.; Michaelsen, K.F.; Tetens, I.; Astrup, A.; Chaput, J.-P.; Sjödin, A. Short sleep duration and large variability in sleep duration are independently associated with dietary risk factors for obesity in Danish school children. *Int. J. Obes.* **2014**, *38*, 32–39. [CrossRef] [PubMed]

40. Morris, C.J.; Garcia, J.I.; Myers, S.; Yang, J.N.; Trienekens, N.; Scheer, F.A.J.L. The human circadian system has a dominating role in causing the morning/evening difference in diet-induced thermogenesis. *Obesity* **2015**, *23*, 2053–2058. [CrossRef] [PubMed]

41. De Castro, J.M. The time of day of food intake influences overall intake in humans. *J. Nutr.* **2004**, *134*, 104–111. [PubMed]

42. Cecil, J.E.; Palmer, C.N.A.; Wrieden, W.; Murrie, I.; Bolton-Smith, C.; Watt, P.; Wallis, D.J.; Hetherington, M.M. Energy intakes of children after preloads: Adjustment, not compensation. *Am. J. Clin. Nutr.* **2005**, *82*, 302–308. [PubMed]

43. Birch, L.L.; Deysher, M. Caloric compensation and sensory specific satiety: Evidence for self regulation of food intake by young children. *Appetite* **1986**, *7*, 323–331. [PubMed]
44. Moreno, L.A.; Joyanes, M.; Mesana, M.I.; González-Gross, M.; Gil, C.M.; Sarría, A.; Gutierrez, A.; Garaulet, M.; Perez-Prieto, R.; Bueno, M.; et al. Harmonization of anthropometric measurements for a multicenter nutrition survey in Spanish adolescents. *Nutrition* **2003**, *19*, 481–486. [CrossRef]
45. Vicente-Rodríguez, G.; Rey-López, J.P.; Mesana, M.I.; Poortvliet, E.; Ortega, F.B.; Polito, A.; Nagy, E.; Widhalm, K.; Sjöström, M.; Moreno, L.A. Reliability and intermethod agreement for body fat assessment among two field and two laboratory methods in adolescents. *Obesity* **2012**, *20*, 221–228. [CrossRef] [PubMed]

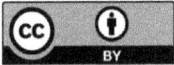

nutrients

MDPI

Review

Matching Meals to Body Clocks—Impact on Weight and Glucose Metabolism

Amy T. Hutchison [1,2], **Gary A. Wittert** [1,2] and **Leonie K. Heilbronn** [1,2,3,*]

[1] Adelaide Medical School, The University of Adelaide, Adelaide SA 5000, Australia; amy.hutchison@adelaide.edu.au (A.T.H.); gary.wittert@adelaide.edu.au (G.A.W.)
[2] South Australian Health and Medical Research Institute (SAHMRI), North Terrace, Adelaide SA 5005, Australia
[3] Robinson Research Institute, The University of Adelaide, North Adelaide SA 5006, Australia
[*] Correspondence: leonie.heilbronn@adelaide.edu.au

Received: 10 January 2017; Accepted: 24 February 2017; Published: 2 March 2017

Abstract: The prevalence of type 2 diabetes continues to rise worldwide and is reaching pandemic proportions. The notion that this is due to obesity, resulting from excessive energy consumption and reduced physical activity, is overly simplistic. Circadian de-synchrony, which occurs when physiological processes are at odds with timing imposed by internal clocks, also promotes obesity and impairs glucose tolerance in mouse models, and is a feature of modern human lifestyles. The purpose of this review is to highlight what is known about glucose metabolism in animal and human models of circadian de-synchrony and examine the evidence as to whether shifts in meal timing contribute to impairments in glucose metabolism, gut hormone secretion and the risk of type 2 diabetes. Lastly, we examine whether restricting food intake to discrete time periods, will prevent or reverse abnormalities in glucose metabolism with the view to improving metabolic health in shift workers and in those more generally at risk of chronic diseases such as type 2 diabetes and cardiovascular disease.

Keywords: circadian rhythm; glucose metabolism; time-restricted feeding; type 2 diabetes; chronic disease risk

1. Overview

The rate of type 2 diabetes is rapidly increasing worldwide, and is predicted to be the main contributor to disease burden in Australia by 2023 [1]. Obesity, particularly abdominal obesity and fatty liver are major contributors to the development of type 2 diabetes. In addition to the effects of energy imbalance and suboptimal nutrient consumption, accumulating evidence suggests that circadian de-synchrony, defined as when physiological processes are out of alignment with internal clocks, may be a contributing, and modifiable, factor in the development of type 2 diabetes [2].

Almost all living organisms display circadian rhythms that cycle within a 24-h period. Disruption of circadian rhythms, either as a result of shifting the light/dark cycle, or from genetic manipulations (e.g., knockout of essential clock genes encoding circadian rhythmicity), result in metabolic disturbances that include weight gain, impaired glucose tolerance and reduced lifespan in mouse models [3,4]. In humans, shift workers are at increased risk of developing metabolic disorders, including obesity and type 2 diabetes [5–8]. However, associations do not show causation, and shift workers are also more likely to have a lower socio-economic status, smoke, consume more alcohol, and have a higher dietary fat intake [9]. In this review, we discuss the role of circadian de-synchrony, and interactions between this and the pattern of meal consumption, in weight gain, and glucose metabolism in mouse models and humans. We examine the evidence for whether small shifts in meal timing (such as skipping breakfast, or eating erratically, without consistent daily meal times) negatively impact glycaemic control and lipid metabolism. The current evidence for a benefit of time restricted feeding, a dietary pattern whereby food intake is confined to short windows of time, is also interrogated and implications for translation to practice presented.

2. Circadian Rhythms and Impacts on Metabolism

Circadian rhythms oscillate with near 24-h rhythmicity under constant conditions, and are entrainable by external cues. Central to the maintenance of the circadian clock is the suprachiasmatic nucleus (SCN) in the brain which is entrained by the light/dark cycle, via retinal photoreceptors in the retino-hypothalamic tract. The SCN is also entrained by the sleep/wake cycle, physical activity, and fasting and feeding periods [10–12]. Circadian clocks have now been identified in almost all tissues and cell types, where they regulate local metabolic processes, including glucose and lipid homeostasis, hormone release, immune response, gastrointestinal motility and digestive processes [13]. Whilst these "peripheral clocks" receive input from the SCN, their phase is sensitive to other external factors including nutrient availability [14].

The molecular basis of circadian timing is provided by transcriptional/translational feedback loops centred on the transcriptional activators; circadian locomotor output cycles kaput (CLOCK) and brain and muscle ARNT-like 1 (BMAL1), which act as positive elements in the feedback loop. CLOCK and BMAL1 drive transcription of six repressor encoding genes, three period genes (*per1, per2, per3*), two crypto-chrome genes (*cry1 and cry2*), the transcription factor *Rev-Erbα* and one promoter gene *RORα* [15]. This core molecular clock cycles with a near 24-h periodicity and more than 25% of the transcriptome, proteasome, and more recently the phospho-proteasome [16], has been shown to cycle in temporally orchestrated waves. Over the past decade, many studies have shown that whole-body, or tissue-specific, knockout of circadian clock genes will induce profound changes in metabolism. These findings include increased adiposity, impaired glucose tolerance and reduced lifespan [3,4]. Many of these gene knockouts also display aberrations in feeding patterns, and eat more during the day, which may independently contribute to changes in metabolism [3,4].

3. Metabolic Consequences of Circadian De-Synchrony (Humans)

Epidemiological studies show that shift workers are at increased risk of developing obesity and type 2 diabetes [17]. One prospective study in women showed that the increased risk of type 2 diabetes was only partly mediated by greater weight gain in shift workers [18]. Interestingly, the prevalence of metabolic syndrome was also higher in men who had previously engaged in shift work versus those who had never performed shift work [19]. This could indicate that these disturbances in metabolism are not entirely reversible.

In humans, metabolic studies of simulated shift work show that shift work induces major disturbances in metabolism, independently of sleep restriction. Circadian misalignment that is induced by a 28 h "day", increased blood glucose levels in healthy adults, even in the presence of increased insulin secretion. This protocol was sufficient to temporarily induce pre-diabetes in 3 out of 8 individuals [20]. Whilst this study shows that circadian misalignment impairs glucose control, a 28 h "day" cycle is not representative of typical shift-work. In another study, individuals were randomly assigned to a "circadian alignment" protocol, where they slept from 11 p.m. to 7 a.m. from day 1–7, or a "circadian misalignment" protocol, where they slept from 11pm to 7am from day 1–3, but were then shifted 12 h to sleep from 11 a.m. to 7 p.m. for days 4–8. In the circadian alignment condition, glucose tolerance declined over the day from breakfast (8 a.m.) to dinner (8 p.m.), congruent with typical circadian changes in insulin secretion and resistance, discussed later in this review. However, under the circadian misalignment protocol, glucose tolerance was lower, presumably as a result of lowered insulin sensitivity. Critically, prolonged exposure to circadian misalignment resulted in poorer glucose tolerance [21]. Both meals and sleep times were shifted, with a meal consumed at around midnight in the circadian misalignment condition. Despite attempts to match sleep between conditions, sleep duration and quality were reduced in the misalignment condition.

The separate contributions of eating late at night, vs. exposure to light and not sleeping at night, have not yet been reported in humans.

Metabolic Consequences of Circadian De-Synchrony (Pre-Clinical Models)

Feeding and fasting periods are important external synchronisers for peripheral oscillators. Studies in mice have shown that fasting for 24-h flattens more than 80% of rhythmically expressed transcripts in the liver [22]. One mechanism through which this occurs is by activation of $5'$ AMP-activated protein kinase (AMPK), which phosphorylates *cry*, targeting it for degradation. Fasting also inhibits mechanistic target of rapamycin (mTOR) activity, which impacts *per* stability [23], and induces circardian de-synchrony.

Studies have shown that feeding rodents solely during the day (when this nocturnal animal would normally sleep), increases body weight as compared to animals fed ad libitum [24]. Similar responses have been observed in mice that are fed a high fat diet, with significantly more weight gain and poorer glucose tolerance in mice that are fed during the day versus mice that are fed at night [25]. Interestingly, feeding mice three discrete "meals" in a configuration that mimics typical human meal times (the mouse equivalent of 7 a.m., 12 p.m. and 8 p.m., with slightly more calories provided at lunch and dinner than breakfast) led to a phase advancement of the peripheral clock [26]. The metabolic impacts of this were not assessed, but there was no effect on body weight. However, the short duration and the necessity of implementing a 20% caloric restriction overall to ensure timely meal completion, could have influenced this response.

Mice that are fed a high-fat diet (HFD), ad libitum, display dampened diurnal rhythms in food intake, and eat more during the resting phase [24]. This abnormal pattern of eating, and the lack of a defined fasting period disrupts the cyclic pattern of expression of peripheral clocks and downstream targets, and may explain at least some of the metabolic consequences that are observed as a result of a high fat diet [27,28]. Whilst discussion of the effects of nutrients on circadian rhythms is beyond the scope of this review, and this has been extensively reviewed by others [29], it is important to acknowledge that nutrients have the potential to act as zeitgebers. As such, the composition of the diet may impact the degree of de-synchrony that occurs. However, evidence in humans is scant, and requires further investigation.

4. Glucose Metabolism, Gut Hormones and Circadian Rhythms

Like many other systems, postprandial glycaemia is under circadian regulation [30]. In humans, meal tests that are performed in the evening result in a hyperglycaemic response vs. identical meals that are given in the morning, even when there are identical fasting lengths between meals [31–33]. This impairment in glucose tolerance in the evening is the result of reduced insulin secretion, as well as peripheral and hepatic insulin resistance [32,34–36], which occurs independent of the sleep/wake and feeding/fasting cycles [36,37].

Anorexigenic hormones including glucagon-like peptide-1 (GLP-1), glucose-inhibitory peptide (GIP), peptide YY (PYY) and amylin, glucagon and insulin, and the orexigenic hormone ghrelin, also oscillate around anticipated meals. These gut hormones play a critical role in modulating gastric emptying, and the glycaemic response to meals. At night, gastric emptying slows [21]. Whether there are circadian rhythms in the release of gut hormones is still poorly described, although GLP-1 has received considerable interest. In a series of in vitro and in vivo experiments, a clear circadian pattern in the release of GLP-1 from rat and human intestinal L cells has been reported [38–40]. This pattern is altered by circadian disruptors, including constant light exposure, a Western diet and altered meal patterning (i.e., feeding during the day in rats). In rodents, clear diurnal GLP-1 rhythmicity is observed, in phase with insulin, with peak responses occurring when feeding is limited [39]. This response is entrained, since animals that are fed during the day (simulating a night-shift) showed a shift in GLP-1 peak, and a disturbed relationship between GLP-1, insulin and glucose concentrations [39]. In addition, exposure to constant light and feeding a high-fat, high-sucrose 'Western' diet, abrogated the normal rhythmic patterns of GLP-1 and insulin release and impaired glucose tolerance [38,39].

In humans, circadian-like patterns of GLP-1 levels, as well as a reduction in the amplitude of GLP-1 release in individuals with obesity and type 2 diabetes have been observed. However, these initial studies did not account for inter-meal intervals, or the caloric loads of the meals administered [41–43]. Subsequent studies that controlled these conditions, and fed participants identical mixed-nutrient test meals, 12 h apart, also showed rhythmic patterns in basal and post-prandial GLP-1 and insulin concentrations [40]. In contrast with rodents, GLP-1 and insulin responses did not change in parallel, with highest GLP-1 secretion observed at 2300 h whereas the highest insulin response was noted at 1100 h [40]. This study showed that exposure to 22 h of constant light dampened the patterns of GLP-1 and insulin release, in association with insulin resistance. Interestingly, these changes were not observed in participants maintained under the same sleep-deprivation protocol but within the normal light–dark period, which suggests a direct effect of light. Collectively, the data in both rodents and humans demonstrate a functional role of GLP-1 in the peripheral metabolic clock, and suggest that altered release of GLP-1, may be one mechanism that contributes to the metabolic perturbations that result from circadian de-synchrony. Further research is required to extend these observations in humans, and to establish the roles of irregular light-dark cycles on these pathways.

5. Can Smaller Misalignments in Meal Timing Impair Metabolic Processes?

As discussed, shift work, and eating significant amounts of food at night impairs glucose tolerance. However, many individuals do not entirely switch eating patterns from day to night. It is unclear whether smaller misalignments in meal timing, such as skipping breakfast, or consuming late night snacks, will induce similar impairments. It is also important to identify whether social jetlag, or eating and sleeping later on "weekends" is sufficient to impact metabolic health. Gill et al. [44] recently performed an observational study in 156 non-shift workers to examine typical human eating patterns. In this study, participants downloaded a smartphone application (app) and were asked to take a photo of each meal/beverage, just prior to consuming it, for 3 weeks. This time stamped when each food was eaten, and this information was uploaded to the investigators. There was a large variation in the number of meal events (4–15/day), and the average inter-meal interval was 3 h. More than half of the cohort reported eating over a 15 h time period each day (e.g., 0700–2200 h), with 75% of energy intake occurring in the afternoon and evening. This evidence is concerning given our knowledge that food intake entrains peripheral clocks, and that the eating during the day increases the risk of type 2 diabetes in mouse [27]. A recent study in humans examined the metabolic impacts of an identical 40% overfeeding diet as 3 meals per day or 3 meals and 3 snacks per day. Although, no differences in weight gain were observed, this study showed that increased meal frequency, in the presence of caloric excess, increased abdominal adipose tissue deposition, increased hepatic triglyceride content, reduced insulin-induced suppression of non-esterified fatty acid (NEFA) and reduced hepatic insulin sensitivity [45]. Of note, the snacks were consumed after each meal, and thus individuals in the snacking arm ate for longer each day, and later at night, which may have influenced this response.

Given the known circadian oscillations in GLP1, insulin release and glycaemia, eating more food earlier in the day has been hypothesised to be optimal for overall glycaemic control in individuals with type 2 diabetes. A study in which a hypo-energetic diet was prescribed as a high energy breakfast (08:00 h, 3000 kJ), standard lunch (13:00 h, 2500 kJ) and low energy dinner (21:00 h, 900 kJ), or the reverse protocol, was prescribed to individuals with type 2 diabetes for one week each [46]. Postprandial lunchtime glycaemia was lowest and insulin and GLP-1 concentrations were highest, when participants had followed the high energy breakfast protocol. This suggests that eating more breakfast could produce optimal glucose control. However, this difference could also be the result of consuming more kilojoules at breakfast (i.e., a greater preload effect). In individuals with type 2 diabetes, skipping breakfast increases the peak glycaemic response to a subsequent lunch meal [47]. This is expected, given the well described literature of the second meal effect, i.e., the effect that the prior meal has on reducing the glycaemic response to the next meal [48]. However, skipping breakfast also increased the postprandial glycaemic response to a subsequent dinner meal, which was unexpected [47]. Skipping breakfast also reduced postprandial insulin and GLP-1 secretion and increased NEFA and glucagon concentrations at the subsequent dinner meal. This study was conducted over the course of a single day in individuals who regularly ate breakfast. There is some evidence to suggest that there is entrainment in the response to specific meal patterns over time [49].

6. Matching Food Intake with Body Clocks

Time restricted feeding (TRF) describes a dieting approach whereby food is available ad libitum for a short window of time each day. Mice that are fed a high-fat diet, under ad libitum conditions display dampened diurnal rhythms in food intake and resting metabolic rate. Conversely, providing mice with a high fat diet under time-restricted conditions (i.e., for 9–12 h), solely during the night, resets peripheral clocks, and abrogates many of the metabolic consequences of a HFD. This includes restoring diurnal oscillations in resting energy expenditure and hepatic glucose metabolism [27]. A similar response has been observed in diet-induced obese mice, with TRF reducing hyperinsulinemia, hepatic steatosis, and inflammation [50]. Interestingly, when lean animals were switched to a TRF-HFD but allowed ad libitum access to a high fat diet for 2 consecutive days per week, (simulating a "weekend"), lean body weights and metabolic profiles were maintained [50]. A number of TRF studies have shown positive effects in various rodent models of metabolic disease, with the most commonly selected time being 8 h of food access, during the active phase [28,51]. These studies suggest that TRF will negate the metabolic consequences of poor dietary habits, at least in mouse.

The impacts of TRF in humans are less clear, and prospective randomised controlled trials testing this concept are limited. From the epidemiological data, individuals who report consuming more than one third of daily energy intake at the evening meal have double the risk of obesity as compared to individuals who report consuming more than a third of energy intake by 1200 h [52]. Eating lunch after 1500 h was also predictive of poorer weight loss and changes in markers of insulin sensitivity during a 20-week dietary intervention, independently of self-reported 24-h caloric intake [53]. In a randomised trial, participants assigned to consume more of their allotted kilojoules at breakfast lost more weight compared with those who consumed the majority of kilojoules at dinner [54]. Similarly, a hypoenergetic diet consumed as breakfast and lunch produced greater reductions in weight, hepatic lipid content, and greater improvements in glucose tolerance versus 6 meals/day in individuals with type 2 diabetes after 12 weeks [55]. Of note, those in the 2 meal per day condition would have fasted for longer prior to metabolic testing, which may have compounded the observed differences. Together, with the evidence presented above, it appears that consuming more energy in the morning, as opposed to later in the day, is beneficial for glycaemic control. However, it is unclear whether this is causal in the development of type 2 diabetes, and longer term randomised controlled trials comparing the metabolic impacts of this are necessary to definitively answer this question.

There are many observational studies of individuals who undertake the Islamic ritual of fasting during the month of Ramadan [56–62]. Ramadan is essentially a time restricted feeding protocol that requires individuals to abstain from eating and drinking during daylight hours. Given the animal data presented, the switch to a predominately night time pattern of food consumption that characterises Ramadan, could be predicted to adversely impact metabolic health. Conversely, most studies report favourable improvements in blood lipids, including reductions in total and low density lipoprotein (LDL)-cholesterol, triglycerides, and increases in high density lipoprotein (HDL)-cholesterol [56,57,60–62]. Some of these health benefits may be due a mild energy restriction, and modest weight loss that is typically observed in response to Ramadan fasting [56,57,61,62]. However, postprandial hyperglycaemia [63], increased fasting blood glucose and deterioration in glycaemic control [57,64] have also been reported. We speculate that implementing a TRF protocol at night will be beneficial for regulation of body weight, and cardiovascular outcomes, but not for glycaemic control.

One controlled study has examined the effects of implementing an evening TRF protocol on metabolic health outcomes. In this study, lean individuals were asked to limit all food intakes to a 4-h window early in the evening (1700–2100 h), vs. eating the same diet as breakfast, lunch and dinner for 8-weeks each [65,66]. All food intakes were monitored within a metabolic kitchen. Despite eating identical foods, the TRF condition resulted in small but significant reductions in body weight and fat mass, and improved cardiovascular profiles, including increased HDL and reduced triacylglycerol [65]. These changes were independent of diet composition, since dietary cholesterol and fatty acids were carefully matched in each dietary condition. In spite of modest weight loss in the TRF condition, fasting blood glucose levels were increased, and impaired glucose tolerance [66]. There were no differences in insulin response. This study demonstrates that limiting energy intake to late in the day is detrimental for glucose control in humans. This outcome may have been influenced by the greater number of kilojoules that were consumed closer to the time of testing in one condition (i.e., 100% calories between 1700 and 2100, vs. 30%–40% in the 3 meals/day condition). Alternatively, the glucose test was performed at a time that participants were no longer accustomed to eating, which could have impacted results [49]. In a similarly styled study, healthy, lean men underwent an alternate day fasting protocol, fasting from 2200 h until 1800 h the following day. This 20 h/day fast meant that re-feeding occurred later in the day. Despite this pattern of meal intake, insulin sensitivity was increased, although no changes in body weight, fasting blood glucose or insulin were noted [67]. The reason for the disparate results are unclear, but may be related to participant characteristics or the amount of energy consumed in the evening.

Two other TRF protocols have also been piloted to date. In one, 8 individuals who were obese and reported eating for at least 14 h/day were recruited [44]. Individuals were instructed to limit food intakes to 10–11 h/day, with no other dietary instruction. TRF resulted in 3.3 kg weight loss after 16 weeks, which was maintained for 12 months. Of note, the precise TRF schedule was self-selected, and participants shortened both ends of their day (avg. 1000–2030 h), and there was no control group. In another study, lean healthy men ate ad libitum vs. 13 h/day TRF (0600–1900) for 2 weeks each. The TRF study condition resulted in less food consumption, and a −0.4 kg weight loss, compared with a gain of +0.6 kg under ad libitum conditions [68]. Metabolic health outcomes were not reported in either publication, which makes it difficult to establish whether beneficial health effects, beyond weight loss, exist. The limited number of studies, with small sample sizes, lack of adequate controls, as well as the lack of data reporting the effects of TRF in individuals who are obese highlights the necessity of further research in this area.

A final aspect that remains is whether eating erratically will alter glucose control. To our knowledge two studies in humans have partially investigated this concept. Participants were asked to eat between 3–9 meals per day, or eat 6 meals/day at the same time each day for 2 weeks each. The irregular meal pattern caused insulin resistance in response to a high-carbohydrate breakfast meal in women who are lean [69] and obese [70], although fasting blood glucose was not different between meal conditions. These studies suggest that erratic eating patterns may also induce insulin resistance, but longer term studies are required.

7. Conclusions

There is a general belief that consumption of more energy throughout the day is preferable to evening consumption. Few studies have examined this prospectively in humans, or for any length of time. Nonetheless, time restricted feeding has shown promise as a tool to mitigate the metabolic sequelae of diet induced obesity in mouse models. Good quality evidence for TRF as a dietary approach to improve glucose control in humans is lacking. Controlled trials are necessary, and must determine if there is adaptation in the approach, whilst keeping in mind the practicality of translating this approach into the community.

Acknowledgments: Leonie K. Heilbronn is funded by a Future Fellowship, Australian Research Council (FT120100027).

Conflicts of Interest: The authors declare no conflict of interest.

References

1. AIoHaW. Australia's health. In *Australia's Health Series 2012*; Australian Institute of Health: Canberra, Australian, 2012.
2. Peschke, E.; Bähr, I.; Mühlbauer, E. Experimental and clinical aspects of melatonin and clock genes in diabetes. *J. Pineal Res.* **2015**, *59*, 1–23. [CrossRef] [PubMed]
3. Turek, F.W.; Joshu, C.; Kohsaka, A.; Lin, E.; Ivanova, G.; McDearmon, E.; Laposky, A.; Losee-Olson, S.; Easton, A.; Jensen, D.R.; et al. Obesity and metabolic syndrome in circadian Clock mutant mice. *Science* **2005**, *308*, 1043–1045. [CrossRef] [PubMed]
4. Rudic, R.D.; McNamara, P.; Curtis, A.M.; Boston, R.C.; Panda, S.; Hogenesch, J.B.; Fitzgerald, G.A. BMAL1 and CLOCK, two essential components of the circadian clock, are involved in glucose homeostasis. *PLoS Biol.* **2004**, *2*, e377. [CrossRef] [PubMed]
5. Knutsson, A. Health disorders of shift workers. *Occup. Med. (Lond.)* **2003**, *53*, 103–108. [CrossRef] [PubMed]
6. Lowden, A.; Moreno, C.; Holmback, U.; Lennernas, M.; Tucker, P. Eating and shift work-effects on habits, metabolism and performance. *Scand. J. Work Environ. Health* **2010**, *36*, 150–162. [CrossRef] [PubMed]
7. Zimberg, I.Z.; Fernandes Junior, S.A.; Crispim, C.A.; Tufik, S.; de Mello, M.T. Metabolic impact of shift work. *Work* **2012**, *41* (Suppl. 1), 4376–4383. [PubMed]
8. Banks, S.; Dorrian, J.; Grant, C.; Coates, A. Circadian Misalignment and Metabolic Consequences: Shiftwork and Altered Meal Times. In *Modulation of Sleep by Obesity, Diabetes, Age, and Diet*; Watson, R.R., Ed.; Academic Press: London, UK, 2014; pp. 155–162.
9. Howell, M.J.; Schenck, C.H.; Crow, S.J. A review of nighttime eating disorders. *Sleep Med. Rev.* **2009**, *13*, 23–34. [CrossRef] [PubMed]
10. Hastings, M.H.; Reddy, A.B.; Maywood, E.S. A clockwork web: Circadian timing in brain and periphery, in health and disease. *Nat. Rev. Neurosci.* **2003**, *4*, 649–661. [CrossRef] [PubMed]
11. Schibler, U.; Ripperger, J.; Brown, S.A. Peripheral circadian oscillators in mammals: Time and food. *J. Biol. Rhythms* **2003**, *18*, 250–260. [CrossRef] [PubMed]
12. Brown, S.A.; Zumbrunn, G.; Fleury-Olela, F.; Preitner, N.; Schibler, U. Rhythms of mammalian body temperature can sustain peripheral circadian clocks. *Curr. Biol.* **2002**, *12*, 1574–1583. [CrossRef]
13. Garaulet, M.; Madrid, J.A. Chronobiological aspects of nutrition, metabolic syndrome and obesity. *Adv. Drug Deliv. Rev.* **2010**, *62*, 967–978. [CrossRef] [PubMed]
14. Marcheva, B.; Ramsey, K.M.; Peek, C.B.; Affinati, A.; Maury, E.; Bass, J. Circadian clocks and metabolism. *Handb. Exp. Pharmacol.* **2013**, 127–155.
15. Garaulet, M.; Ordovas, J.M.; Madrid, J.A. The chronobiology, etiology and pathophysiology of obesity. *Int. J. Obes.* **2010**, *34*, 1667–1683. [CrossRef] [PubMed]
16. Robles, M.S.; Humphrey, S.J.; Mann, M. Phosphorylation Is a Central Mechanism for Circadian Control of Metabolism and Physiology. *Cell Metab.* **2016**. [CrossRef] [PubMed]
17. Karlsson, B.; Alfredsson, L.; Knutsson, A.; Andersson, E.; Toren, K. Total mortality and cause-specific mortality of Swedish shift- and dayworkers in the pulp and paper industry in 1952–2001. *Scand. J. Work Environ. Health* **2005**, *31*, 30–35. [CrossRef] [PubMed]
18. Pan, A.; Schernhammer, E.S.; Sun, Q.; Hu, F.B. Rotating night shift work and risk of type 2 diabetes: Two prospective cohort studies in women. *PLoS Med.* **2011**, *8*, e1001141. [CrossRef] [PubMed]
19. Puttonen, S.; Viitasalo, K.; Harma, M. The relationship between current and former shift work and the metabolic syndrome. *Scand. J. Work Environ. Health* **2012**, *38*, 343–348. [CrossRef] [PubMed]
20. Scheer, F.A.; Hilton, M.F.; Mantzoros, C.S.; Shea, S.A. Adverse metabolic and cardiovascular consequences of circadian misalignment. *Proc. Natl. Acad. Sci. USA* **2009**, *106*, 4453–4458. [CrossRef] [PubMed]
21. Morris, C.J.; Yang, J.N.; Garcia, J.I.; Myers, S.; Bozzi, I.; Wang, W.; Buxton, O.M.; Shea, S.A.; Scheer, F.A. Endogenous circadian system and circadian misalignment impact glucose tolerance via separate mechanisms in humans. *Proc. Natl. Acad. Sci. USA* **2015**, *112*, E2225–E2534. [CrossRef] [PubMed]
22. Vollmers, C.; Gill, S.; DiTacchio, L.; Pulivarthy, S.R.; Le, H.D.; Panda, S. Time of feeding and the intrinsic circadian clock drive rhythms in hepatic gene expression. *Proc. Natl. Acad. Sci. USA* **2009**, *106*, 21453–21458. [CrossRef] [PubMed]

23. Vendelbo, M.H.; Moller, A.B.; Christensen, B.; Nellemann, B.; Clasen, B.F.; Nair, K.S.; Jørgensen, J.O.; Jessen, N.; Møller, N. Fasting increases human skeletal muscle net phenylalanine release and this is associated with decreased mTOR signaling. *PLoS ONE* **2014**, *9*, e102031. [CrossRef] [PubMed]

24. Kohsaka, A.; Laposky, A.D.; Ramsey, K.M.; Estrada, C.; Joshu, C.; Kobayashi, Y.; Turek, F.W.; Bass, J. High-fat diet disrupts behavioral and molecular circadian rhythms in mice. *Cell Metab.* **2007**, *6*, 414–421. [CrossRef] [PubMed]

25. Arble, D.M.; Bass, J.; Laposky, A.D.; Vitaterna, M.H.; Turek, F.W. Circadian timing of food intake contributes to weight gain. *Obesity (Silver Spring)* **2009**, *17*, 2100–2102. [CrossRef] [PubMed]

26. Kuroda, H.; Tahara, Y.; Saito, K.; Ohnishi, N.; Kubo, Y.; Seo, Y.; Fuse, Y.; Ohura, Y.; Hirao, A.; Shibata, S. Meal frequency patterns determine the phase of mouse peripheral circadian clocks. *Sci. Rep.* **2012**, *2*, 711. [CrossRef] [PubMed]

27. Hatori, M.; Vollmers, C.; Zarrinpar, A.; DiTacchio, L.; Bushong, E.A.; Gill, S.; Leblanc, M.; Chaix, A.; Joens, M.; Fitzpatrick, J.A.; et al. Time-restricted feeding without reducing caloric intake prevents metabolic diseases in mice fed a high-fat diet. *Cell Metab.* **2012**, *15*, 848–860. [CrossRef] [PubMed]

28. Sherman, H.; Genzer, Y.; Cohen, R.; Chapnik, N.; Madar, Z.; Froy, O. Timed high-fat diet resets circadian metabolism and prevents obesity. *FASEB J.* **2012**, *26*, 3493–3502. [CrossRef] [PubMed]

29. Ribas-Latre, A.; Eckel-Mahan, K. Interdependence of nutrient metabolism and the circadian clock system: Importance for metabolic health. *Mol. Metab.* **2016**, *5*, 133–152. [CrossRef] [PubMed]

30. Kalsbeek, A.; la Fleur, S.; Fliers, E. Circadian control of glucose metabolism. *Mol. Metab.* **2014**, *3*, 372–383. [CrossRef] [PubMed]

31. Sonnier, T.; Rood, J.; Gimble, J.M.; Peterson, C.M. Glycemic control is impaired in the evening in prediabetes through multiple diurnal rhythms. *J. Diabetes Complicat.* **2014**, *28*, 836–843. [CrossRef] [PubMed]

32. Morris, C.J.; Purvis, T.E.; Mistretta, J.; Scheer, F.A. Effects of the internal circadian system and circadian misalignment on glucose tolerance in chronic shift workers. *J. Clin. Endocrinol. Metab.* **2016**, *101*, 101–1074. [CrossRef] [PubMed]

33. Bo, S.; Musso, G.; Beccuti, G.; Fadda, M.; Fedele, D.; Gambino, R.; Gentile, L.; Durazzo, M.; Ghigo, E.; Cassader, M. Consuming more of daily caloric intake at dinner predisposes to obesity. A 6-year population-based prospective cohort study. *PLoS ONE* **2014**, *9*, e108467. [CrossRef] [PubMed]

34. Morgan, L.M.; Aspostolakou, F.; Wright, J.; Gama, R. Diurnal variations in peripheral insulin resistance and plasma non-esterified fatty acid concentrations: a possible link? *Ann. Clin. Biochem.* **1999**, *36 Pt 4*, 447–450. [CrossRef] [PubMed]

35. Saad, A.; Dalla Man, C.; Nandy, D.K.; Levine, J.A.; Bharucha, A.E.; Rizza, R.A.; Basu, R.; Carter, R.E.; Cobelli, C.; Kudva, Y.C.; et al. Diurnal pattern to insulin secretion and insulin action in healthy individuals. *Diabetes* **2012**, *61*, 2691–2700. [CrossRef] [PubMed]

36. Van Cauter, E.; Blackman, J.D.; Roland, D.; Spire, J.P.; Refetoff, S.; Polonsky, K.S. Modulation of glucose regulation and insulin secretion by circadian rhythmicity and sleep. *J. Clin. Investig.* **1991**, *88*, 934–942. [CrossRef] [PubMed]

37. Van Cauter, E.; Polonsky, K.S.; Scheen, A.J. Roles of circadian rhythmicity and sleep in human glucose regulation. *Endocr Rev.* **1997**, *18*, 716–738. [CrossRef] [PubMed]

38. Gil-Lozano, M.; Wu, W.K.; Martchenko, A.; Brubaker, P.L. High-Fat Diet and Palmitate Alter the Rhythmic Secretion of Glucagon-Like Peptide-1 by the Rodent L-cell. *Endocrinology* **2016**, *157*, 586–599. [CrossRef] [PubMed]

39. Gil-Lozano, M.; Mingomataj, E.L.; Wu, W.K.; Ridout, S.A.; Brubaker, P.L. Circadian secretion of the intestinal hormone GLP-1 by the rodent L cell. *Diabetes* **2014**, *63*, 3674–3685. [CrossRef] [PubMed]

40. Gil-Lozano, M.; Hunter, P.M.; Behan, L.A.; Gladanac, B.; Casper, R.F.; Brubaker, P.L. Short-term sleep deprivation with nocturnal light exposure alters time-dependent glucagon-like peptide-1 and insulin secretion in male volunteers. *Am. J. Physiol. Endocrinol. Metab.* **2016**, *310*, E41–E50. [CrossRef] [PubMed]

41. Elliott, R.M.; Morgan, L.M.; Tredger, J.A.; Deacon, S.; Wright, J.; Marks, V. Glucagon-like peptide-1 (7-36)amide and glucose-dependent insulinotropic polypeptide secretion in response to nutrient ingestion in man: acute post-prandial and 24-h secretion patterns. *J. Endocrinol.* **1993**, *138*, 159–166. [CrossRef] [PubMed]

42. Mingrone, G.; Nolfe, G.; Gissey, G.C.; Iaconelli, A.; Leccesi, L.; Guidone, C.; Nanni, G.; Holst, J.J. Circadian rhythms of GIP and GLP1 in glucose-tolerant and in type 2 diabetic patients after biliopancreatic diversion. *Diabetologia* **2009**, *52*, 873–881. [CrossRef] [PubMed]

43. Galindo Munoz, J.S.; Jimenez Rodriguez, D.; Hernandez Morante, J.J. Diurnal rhythms of plasma GLP-1 levels in normal and overweight/obese subjects: lack of effect of weight loss. *J. Physiol. Biochem.* **2015**, *71*, 17–28. [CrossRef] [PubMed]
44. Gill, S.; Panda, S. A Smartphone App Reveals Erratic Diurnal Eating Patterns in Humans that Can Be Modulated for Health Benefits. *Cell Metabolism.* **2015**, *22*, 789–798. [CrossRef] [PubMed]
45. Koopman, K.E.; Caan, M.W.; Nederveen, A.J.; Pels, A.; Ackermans, M.T.; Fliers, E.; la Fleur, S.E.; Serlie, M.J. Hypercaloric diets with increased meal frequency, but not meal size, increase intrahepatic triglycerides: A randomized controlled trial. *Hepatology* **2014**, *60*, 545–553. [CrossRef] [PubMed]
46. Jakubowicz, D.; Wainstein, J.; Ahrén, B.; Bar-Dayan, Y.; Landau, Z.; Rabinovitz, H.R.; Froy, O. High-energy breakfast with low-energy dinner decreases overall daily hyperglycaemia in type 2 diabetic patients: A randomised clinical trial. *Diabetologia* **2015**, *58*, 912–919. [CrossRef] [PubMed]
47. Jakubowicz, D.; Wainstein, J.; Ahren, B.; Landau, Z.; Bar-Dayan, Y.; Froy, O. Fasting Until Noon Triggers Increased Postprandial Hyperglycemia and Impaired Insulin Response After Lunch and Dinner in Individuals With Type 2 Diabetes: A Randomized Clinical Trial. *Diabetes Care* **2015**, *38*, 1820–1826. [CrossRef] [PubMed]
48. Clark, C.A.; Gardiner, J.; McBurney, M.I.; Anderson, S.; Weatherspoon, L.J.; Henry, D.N.; Hord, N.G. Effects of breakfast meal composition on second meal metabolic responses in adults with Type 2 diabetes mellitus. *Eur. J. Clin. Nutr.* **2006**, *60*, 1122–1129. [CrossRef] [PubMed]
49. Thomas, E.A.; Higgins, J.; Bessesen, D.H.; McNair, B.; Cornier, M.A. Usual breakfast eating habits affect response to breakfast skipping in overweight women. *Obesity (Silver Spring)* **2015**, *23*, 750–759. [CrossRef] [PubMed]
50. Chaix, A.; Zarrinpar, A.; Miu, P.; Panda, S. Time-restricted feeding is a preventative and therapeutic intervention against diverse nutritional challenges. *Cell Metab.* **2014**, *20*, 991–1005. [CrossRef] [PubMed]
51. Chung, T.T.; Gunganah, K.; Monson, J.P.; Drake, W.M. Circadian variation in serum cortisol during hydrocortisone replacement is not attributable to changes in cortisol-binding globulin concentrations. *Clin. Endocrinol. (Oxf.)* **2016**, *84*, 496–500. [CrossRef] [PubMed]
52. Wang, J.B.; Patterson, R.E.; Ang, A.; Emond, J.A.; Shetty, N.; Arab, L. Timing of energy intake during the day is associated with the risk of obesity in adults. *J. Hum. Nutr. Diet.* **2014**, *27* (Suppl. 2), 255–262. [CrossRef] [PubMed]
53. Garaulet, M.; Gomez-Abellan, P.; Alburquerque-Bejar, J.J.; Lee, Y.C.; Ordovas, J.M.; Scheer, F.A.J.L. Timing of food intake predicts weight loss effectiveness. *Int. J. Obes.* **2013**, *37*, 604–611. [CrossRef] [PubMed]
54. Jakubowicz, D.; Barnea, M.; Wainstein, J.; Froy, O. High caloric intake at breakfast vs. dinner differentially influences weight loss of overweight and obese women. *Obesity (Silver Spring)* **2013**, *21*, 2504–2512. [CrossRef] [PubMed]
55. Kahleova, H.; Belinova, L.; Malinska, H.; Oliyarnyk, O.; Trnovska, J.; Skop, V.; Kazdova, L.; Dezortova, M.; Hajek, M.; Tura, A.; et al. Eating two larger meals a day (breakfast and lunch) is more effective than six smaller meals in a reduced-energy regimen for patients with type 2 diabetes: a randomised crossover study. *Diabetologia* **2014**, *57*, 1552–1560. [CrossRef] [PubMed]
56. Nematy, M.; Alinezhad-Namaghi, M.; Rashed, M.M.; Mozdehifard, M.; Sajjadi, S.S.; Akhlaghi, S.; Sabery, M.; Mohajeri, S.A.; Shalaey, N.; Moohebati, M.; et al. Effects of Ramadan fasting on cardiovascular risk factors: A prospective observational study. *Nutr. J.* **2012**, *11*, 69. [CrossRef] [PubMed]
57. Temizhan, A.; Tandogan, I.; Donderici, O.; Demirbas, B. The effects of Ramadan fasting on blood lipid levels. *Am. J. Med.* **2000**, *109*, 341–342. [CrossRef]
58. Aksungar, F.B.; Eren, A.; Ure, S.; Teskin, O.; Ates, G. Effects of intermittent fasting on serum lipid levels, coagulation status and plasma homocysteine levels. *Ann. Nutr. Metab.* **2005**, *49*, 77–82. [CrossRef] [PubMed]
59. Ziaee, V.; Razaei, M.; Ahmadinejad, Z.; Shaikh, H.; Yousefi, R.; Yarmohammadi, L.; Bozorgi, F.; Behjati, M.J. The changes of metabolic profile and weight during Ramadan fasting. *Singap. Med. J.* **2006**, *47*, 409–414.
60. Zare, A.; Hajhashemi, M.; Hassan, Z.M.; Zarrin, S.; Pourpak, Z.; Moin, M.; Salarilak, S.; Masudi, S.; Shahabi, S. Effect of Ramadan fasting on serum heat shock protein 70 and serum lipid profile. *Singap. Med. J.* **2011**, *52*, 491–495.
61. Adlouni, A.; Ghalim, N.; Benslimane, A.; Lecerf, J.M.; Saile, R. Fasting during Ramadan induces a marked increase in high-density lipoprotein cholesterol and decrease in low-density lipoprotein cholesterol. *Ann. Nutr. Metab.* **1997**, *41*, 242–249. [CrossRef] [PubMed]

62. Fakhrzadeh, H.; Larijani, B.; Sanjari, M.; Baradar-Jalili, R.; Amini, M.R. Effect of Ramadan fasting on clinical and biochemical parameters in healthy adults. *Ann. Saudi Med.* **2003**, *23*, 223–226. [PubMed]

63. Monnier, L.; El Azrak, A.; Lessan, N.; Rochd, D.; Colette, C.; Bonnet, F. Ramadan and diabetes: What we see, learn and understand from continuous glucose monitoring. *Diabetes Metab.* **2015**, *41*, 456–462. [CrossRef] [PubMed]

64. Norouzy, A.; Mohajeri, S.M.; Shakeri, S.; Yari, F.; Sabery, M.; Philippou, E.; Varasteh, A.R.; Nematy, M. Effect of Ramadan fasting on glycemic control in patients with Type 2 diabetes. *J. Endocrinol. Investig.* **2012**, *35*, 766–771.

65. Stote, K.S.; Baer, D.J.; Spears, K.; Paul, D.R.; Harris, G.K.; Rumpler, W.V.; Strycula, P.; Najjar, S.S.; Ferrucci, L.; Ingram, D.K. A controlled trial of reduced meal frequency without caloric restriction in healthy, normal-weight, middle-aged adults. *Am. J. Clin. Nutr.* **2007**, *85*, 981–988. [PubMed]

66. Carlson, O.; Martin, B.; Stote, K.S.; Golden, E.; Maudsley, S.; Najjar, S.S.; Ferrucci, L.; Ingram, D.K.; Longo, D.L.; Rumpler, W.V. Impact of reduced meal frequency without caloric restriction on glucose regulation in healthy, normal-weight middle-aged men and women. *Metabolism* **2007**, *56*, 1729–1734. [CrossRef] [PubMed]

67. Halberg, N.; Henriksen, M.; Soderhamn, N.; Stallknecht, B.; Ploug, T.; Schjerling, P.; Dela, F. Effect of intermittent fasting and refeeding on insulin action in healthy men. *J. Appl. Physiol.* **2005**, *99*, 2128–2136. [CrossRef] [PubMed]

68. LeCheminant, J.D.; Christenson, E.; Bailey, B.W.; Tucker, L.A. Restricting night-time eating reduces daily energy intake in healthy young men: a short-term cross-over study. *Br. J. Nutr.* **2013**, *110*, 2108–2113. [CrossRef] [PubMed]

69. Farshchi, H.R.; Taylor, M.A.; Macdonald, I.A. Regular meal frequency creates more appropriate insulin sensitivity and lipid profiles compared with irregular meal frequency in healthy lean women. *Eur. J. Clin. Nutr.* **2004**, *58*, 1071–1077. [CrossRef] [PubMed]

70. Farshchi, H.R.; Taylor, M.A.; Macdonald, I.A. Beneficial metabolic effects of regular meal frequency on dietary thermogenesis, insulin sensitivity, and fasting lipid profiles in healthy obese women. *Am. J. Clin. Nutr.* **2005**, *81*, 16–24. [PubMed]

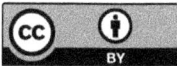

nutrients

MDPI

Review

The Impact of Shiftwork on Skeletal Muscle Health

Brad Aisbett [1,2,*]**, Dominique Condo** [1,2]**, Evelyn Zacharewicz** [1] **and Séverine Lamon** [1,2]

[1] School of Exercise and Nutrition Sciences, Deakin University, Geelong 3220, Australia;
    dominique.condo@deakin.edu.au (D.C.); e.zacharewicz@deakin.edu.au (E.Z.);
    severine.lamon@deakin.edu.au (S.L.)
[2] Institute for Physical Activity and Nutrition (I-PAN), Deakin University, Geelong 3220, Australia
*   Correspondence: brad.aisbett@deakin.edu.au; Tel.: +61-3-9244-6474

Received: 30 November 2016; Accepted: 3 March 2017; Published: 8 March 2017

Abstract: (1) Background: About one in four workers undertake shift rosters that fall outside the traditional 7 a.m.–6 p.m. scheduling. Shiftwork alters workers' exposure to natural and artificial light, sleep patterns, and feeding patterns. When compared to the rest of the working population, shiftworkers are at a greater risk of developing metabolic impairments over time. One fundamental component of metabolic health is skeletal muscle, the largest organ in the body. However, cause-and-effect relationships between shiftwork and skeletal muscle health have not been established; (2) Methods: A critical review of the literature was completed using online databases and reference lists; (3) Results: We propose a conceptual model drawing relationships between typical shiftwork consequences; altered light exposure, sleep patterns, and food and beverage consumption, and drivers of skeletal muscle health—protein intake, resistance training, and hormone release. At present, there is no study investigating the direct effect of shiftwork on skeletal muscle health. Instead, research findings showing that acute consequences of shiftwork negatively influence skeletal muscle homeostasis support the validity of our model; (4) Conclusion: Further research is required to test the potential relationships identified in our review, particularly in shiftwork populations. Part of this testing could include skeletal muscle specific interventions such as targeted protein intake and/or resistance-training.

Keywords: protein intake; resistance training; sleep; hormones

1. Introduction

In North America, continental Europe, and Australia, more than 15% of the workforce undertake shifts that include work hours outside 7 a.m. to 6 p.m. [1]. These workers deliver essential 24-h services for communities, including healthcare, construction, and emergency response [2–5]. To maintain these 24-h services, shiftworkers endure continual acute and chronic risks to their health and safety [6]. In the short-term, sleep deprivation and disturbances lead to impaired decision making and vigilance on the job, which can increase the risk of workplace accidents [7]. Disruptions to sleep and waking habits can also adversely influence social and family relationships [8], which can diminish job retention [9] and quality of life. Shiftworkers frequently exposed to irregular working hours also face significantly greater risks of developing diabetes [10], obesity [11], and cancer [12].

Together with the short- and long-term health and safety risks they face, the essential role that shiftworking populations serve in their communities makes them a high priority research area. To this end, considerable research has already focused on shiftworkers' sleep impairments [6], and associated risk of short-term injuries [7] and longer-term metabolic diseases [10,11,13,14]. One area that has received relatively little attention, but is pertinent to both short-term work capacity and long-term metabolic health is the impact of shiftwork on skeletal muscle health. Skeletal muscle is a major metabolic tissue that is not only essential for all human movement, but also constitutes a critical storage organ for essential substrates and plays a major role in energy production and metabolism [15,16]. Maintaining skeletal muscle health over a lifespan underpins physical work capacity [17] and is particularly relevant for many shiftworking populations who must perform physically demanding tasks and/or maintain standing or upright postures across shifts lasting eight or more hours [18]. Disruption in muscle homeostasis is associated with metabolic and chronic diseases that are overrepresented in shiftworking populations [10,11,13,14]; however, no cause-and-effect relationship has been established between shiftwork and poor skeletal muscle health.

The review will begin by defining shiftwork schedules and typical shiftwork industries. Thereafter, we will provide an overview of skeletal muscle physiology, and briefly describe the major drivers of skeletal muscle health. We will then propose a conceptual framework for the direct and indirect pathways through which shiftwork could impair skeletal muscle health (Figure 1). The bulk of the review will draw on available evidence supporting our hypothesis that shiftwork and its acute consequences impair skeletal muscle health. These sections will focus on the direct impacts of circadian disruption on skeletal muscle regulation as well as the impact of shiftwork and sleep disruption on food and beverage choices, and hormonal changes. The review will conclude with nutrition- and exercise-based targeted intervention areas that interested research groups may trial as part of a new research agenda for shiftworkers' health.

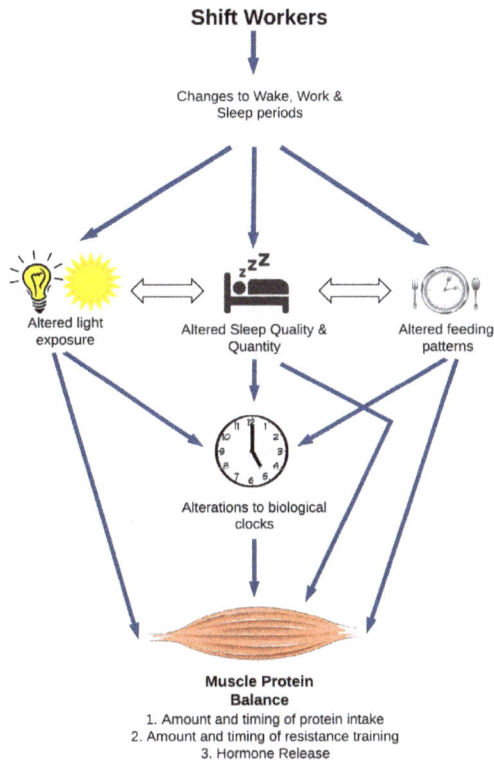

Figure 1. A model for the potential impact of shiftwork on skeletal muscle health.

1.1. Shiftwork

For the purposes of this review, shiftwork will comprise working hours that exist outside of the traditional 7 a.m. to 6 p.m. scheduling [1]. The various types of shiftwork patterns have been recently described in seminal reviews by Wright et al. [1] and Kecklund and Axelsson [6]. Briefly, night-shift hours typically range from 9 p.m. to 8 a.m.; evening shifts from 2 p.m. to 12 a.m.; and early morning shifts include any work starting between 4 and 7 a.m. [1]. Early morning and night shifts acutely lead to shorter sleep periods, whilst evening shiftwork is associated with the longest sleep durations [6]. Such rosters are typical of nursing, medicine and paramedicine, maintenance and factory work, aviation, and emergency services [1,5,6,18]. Many sectors use a rotating shift system where workers will rotate through a period of day to evening (where applicable) to night shift. The number of consecutive shifts of each type impacts sleep, with longer rotations (i.e., four to seven consecutive shifts of the same type) leading to ~25 min more sleep than faster rotations [6]. Changing from a day to night shift can lead to a period of total sleep deprivation, particularly on the first night shift [19]. The exposure to total sleep deprivation is also typical for emergency service workers who may be called to an incident (e.g., road crash, storm, or wildfire) in the afternoon or early evening after working all day [2–4]. In some emergency service jurisdictions, workers are able to rest or sleep at the station or in their homes until an emergency response is required [5]. In these environments, workers face disrupted sleep and partial sleep restriction that can evoke different physiological responses when compared to total sleep deprivation [5]. In this review, we will strive to draw on studies using actual or simulated shiftwork schedules to understand their potential impacts on skeletal muscle health. As disrupted sleep is a typical consequence of many schedules, we will also draw on experimental evidence using complete sleep deprivation and partial sleep restriction models. Special care will be taken to alert the reader of the potential impact that different types of shiftwork could have on skeletal muscle health in both acute and chronic settings.

1.2. Skeletal Muscle Health

A fundamental component of human metabolic health, physical work capacity, and quality of life is skeletal muscle health [17]. Skeletal muscle is a very plastic tissue able to rapidly modify its structure, function, and metabolism in response to internal and external stress signals. Comprising 40% of the total body mass [17], skeletal muscle is the largest human organ. It primarily functions as a structural support unit, enabling the body to maintain posture and perform gross and fine motor movements [20]. Skeletal muscle is composed of a heterogeneous collection of muscle fibres. Each fibre is a multinucleated muscle cell constituted of myofibrils, the proteinic structure made of actin and myosin that allows for muscle contraction. The different types of muscle fibres allow for the wide variety of capabilities of this organ; with fast-twitch fibres (type II) producing a contractile response that is faster but subjected to higher fatigability than slow twitch fibres (type I). Skeletal muscle is also a critical storage organ for essential substrates and plays a major role in energy production and metabolism [15,16]. Numerous substrates including muscle glycogen, blood glucose, and free fatty acids derived from muscle or adipose tissue can be used to generate ATP, the main source of energy that sustains muscle contraction [21]. Disruption in muscle energy metabolism is associated to metabolic disorders, including obesity and diabetes, and neurodegenerative conditions such as motor neuron disease. Of particular interest for this review, skeletal muscle houses 50%–75% of the body's total protein pool [17]. Skeletal muscle proteins are constantly built up (protein synthesis) and broken down (protein degradation) [17]. In normal physiological conditions, the amount of proteins synthetized in the muscle balances the amount of proteins degraded in the muscle, resulting in steady muscle mass [22]. Protein degradation can exceed protein synthesis during periods of serious disease, immobilization, and aging [23], leading to a net loss of muscle mass. In addition, muscle protein metabolism is disrupted during periods of malnutrition and starvation, where the muscle becomes a vital substitute fuel supply for the brain and immune system [17]. Compromising muscle protein metabolism results in a net loss of muscle mass [24–26] and prevents optimal muscle function. Low muscle mass is a hallmark of numerous metabolic challenges. These include chronic and metabolic disorders, such as cancer, AIDS, and neuromuscular conditions [23]. Maintaining the balance between protein synthesis and protein degradation over a lifespan is therefore critical for physical performance, metabolic health, and general wellbeing [17]. The muscle protein metabolism balance is tightly regulated by a combination of anabolic (pro-protein synthesis) and catabolic (pro-protein degradation) stimuli including (1) the ingestion of dietary protein (anabolic); (2) resistance exercise (anabolic) and (3) circulating signaling molecules, including metabolic hormones and myokines (anabolic or catabolic) [17].

2. A Model for Shiftwork and Skeletal Muscle Health

The overarching hypothesis of this review is that shiftwork may significantly impair skeletal muscle health through multiple physiological pathways, resulting in a reduction of protein synthesis and an augmentation of protein degradation in the muscle (Figure 1). At the top of Figure 1, shiftwork alters the sleep-wake cycle of the worker. In this review, we will focus on three typical consequences of the altered sleep-wake cycle, namely altered light exposure, sleep, and feeding patterns. Altered light exposure refers to the reduction in natural night and increase in artificial light, particularly at night. Shiftworkers' sleep patterns are characterized by a reduced quality and quantity of sleep and, depending on their schedule, a shift in their main sleep including (for some) sleeping primarily during day time hours. Similarly, shiftworkers' eating patterns move with their altered sleep-wake cycle, but shiftworkers also make different food and beverage choices than daytime workers. There are also several interactions between these sub-categories. Individually and collectively, changes in light, sleep, and feeding patterns can all influence the body's circadian clocks depicted in the middle of Figure 1. This image refers to the suprachiasmatic nucleus (SCN), the central clock of the body that governs tissue homeostasis. In addition, skeletal muscle possesses its own intrinsic biological clock, which is also sensitive to the changes in light exposure, wake, sleep, and dietary patterns experienced by shiftworkers [27]. The regulation of muscle homeostasis is multi-factorial, with protein intake, resistance training, and hormonal patterns independently influencing muscle protein balance. Beyond impacts on the central and peripheral circadian clocks, alterations to light, sleep, and feeding patterns may also directly impact muscle protein balance. Here we will primarily focus on the studies reporting muscle data. Human experimental data will be prioritized and supplemented, where appropriate, with evidence from animal studies. While this approach limits the number of studies discussed in our review, our intent is to stay focused on new contributions to the already large body of research addressing shiftworkers' health.

2.1. Direct Effects of Circadian Disruption on Skeletal Muscle Tissue

Skeletal muscle fibres possess their own intrinsic biological clock, which relies on a multi-level transcriptional and translational feedback loop system involving the core clock genes *Clock*, *Bmal1*, *Cry1/2*, and *Per 1/2* (reviewed in [28,29]). The muscle biological clock is primarily studied in rodent models. While the obvious limitations to this approach should be kept in mind, novel data are often only available from mouse and rat models. In mice, seventeen percent of all genes display circadian-like regulation patterns in skeletal muscle [30], including *Myod1*, a muscle-specific transcription factor playing a key role in muscle development [31]. These genes are involved in all aspects of muscle biology, including growth, function, and metabolism [28,29,32], where nearly 30% of all genes directly regulated by *Clock* are involved in energy metabolism [30]. It follows that disruptions in the circadian clock are strongly associated to skeletal muscle health. For example, a functional biological clock is essential to the normal secretion of basal myokines in vitro [33] and to the maintenance of muscle structure and function in rodents [27,31]. A series of recent animal studies have linked the specific loss-of-function of one of the core clock genes to a range of muscle phenotypes, including muscle atrophy, structural impairments, altered metabolism, altered regeneration, and reduction in force and endurance (reviewed in [32]).

Few human studies have investigated the direct relationships between the acute impacts of shiftwork (e.g., altered light exposure, sleep, and feeding patterns; Figure 1) and skeletal muscle health. One night of complete sleep deprivation decreased the mRNA levels of the clock genes *Bmal1* and

Cry1 in 15 healthy men [34]; however, whether light exposure during the trial or sleep deprivation itself drove these changes is unknown. The possible interplay between sleep restriction, diet, and skeletal muscle health has been evidenced in less controlled field studies. Nindl et al. [35] showed that soldiers who were only permitted 1–3 h sleep per night during a physically intense four-day training period lost 3% fat free mass. These soldiers were also subjected to severe caloric restriction each day. Unpacking the relative contribution of the sleep and calorie restriction was not possible. However, a more recent study showed that sleep loss could moderate the relative impact of calorie restriction on skeletal muscle health [36]. Nedeltcheva et al. [36] showed that participants following a 14-day calorie restricted diet lost 60% more muscle mass when sleep restricted (5.5 h sleep per night) than those who slept normally (8.5 h sleep per night).

In the relative absence of human data, the proposed association between the acute impacts of shiftwork and skeletal muscle health can be supported by rodent studies. In rats submitted to 96 h of rapid eye movement (REM) sleep deprivation, there was a significant decrease in tiblias anterior muscle mass [37], gastrocnemius mass/tibia length ratio [38], average fibre cross-sectional area (CSA, a direct measure of muscle size) [37], and type II (fast-twitch) fibre CSA [38]. The phosphorylation levels of the molecular markers of muscle protein synthesis were reduced, indicating a reduction in muscle protein synthesis with sleep deprivation. Conversely, the activity of the ubiquitin proteasome system increased, indicating greater protein degradation [38]. Sleep-deprivation induced muscle atrophy could be partially restored by a 96-h recovery period [37]. Work from the same group confirmed that a decrease in average muscle fibre CSA induced by sleep-deprivation was specific to glycolytic and mixed muscles and that 96 h of paradoxical sleep deprivation significantly reduced fat deposition in all types of muscle, possibly as a direct consequence of a negative energy balance [39]. Rats subjected to sleep deprivation for 18 h per day demonstrated an increase in the *Mhc1* gene and protein expression (a protein that is characteristic of slow-twitch fibres) and a decrease in the *Mhc2* gene and protein expression (a protein that is characteristic of fast-twitch fibres) in the masseter muscle after 7 and 14 days; values that returned to baseline levels after 21 days of sleep deprivation [40]. In contrast, rats subjected to 3–14 days of sleep deprivation did not display an increase in oxidative stress in skeletal muscle [41]. More recently, a mouse study using continuous light exposure confirmed that a functional circadian system is required to maintain skeletal muscle health. A six-month period of light exposure induced a number of muscle dysfunctions, including reduced grip strength and grip hanging duration; impairments that were mostly reversed when the animals were returned to a normal day/night cycle. It was proposed that these changes were mediated by changes in SCN neural activity [42]. More work is required to reconcile the acute and sustained impacts that sleep deprivation and/or changes in light exposure has on skeletal muscle, particularly in humans.

2.2. Shiftwork, Sleep Disruption, and Food and Beverage Choices

As presented in Figure 1, shiftwork alters workers' sleep-wake patterns, which in turns leads to changes in their food and beverage consumption. Figure 2 focuses on the potential pathways through which changes in food and beverage intake could impair skeletal muscle health.

Protein ingestion is one of the three primary drivers of protein synthesis in skeletal muscle [17]. As muscle tissue houses 50%–75% of the body's total protein pool [17], dietary protein supplies the materials needed to replenish and remodel muscle cells by increasing systemic amino acid availability and improving insulin sensitivity [43]. The type, amount, and timing of protein ingestion can be modulated to increase protein synthesis rates and improve net protein balance within skeletal muscle [44]. Twenty to 30 g of high quality protein containing approximately 10 g of essential amino acids is required to maximally stimulate maximal protein synthesis [45,46]. Protein intakes of 0–10 g produced significantly lower protein synthesis, with no additional benefit observed when >30 g was ingested [45,46]. Moderate amounts of protein spread evenly throughout the day causes a 25% increase in muscle protein synthesis compared to a skewed intake towards the end of the day. Therefore, low or irregular protein intake can result in a negative protein balance, with protein degradation surpassing protein synthesis and promoting net muscle loss. The amino acid profile and rate of digestibility can also influence protein synthesis. Protein sources consisting of essential amino acids doubled protein synthesis rates compared to equal amounts of non-essential amino acids [47]. Leucine, a branched chain amino acid, is particularly efficient as it stimulates muscle protein synthesis both directly and indirectly through the secretion of insulin from the pancreatic β cells [48]. Finally, rapidly digestible proteins such as whey result in a greater stimulation of post prandial muscle protein synthesis when compared to slowly digestible proteins such as casein [49].

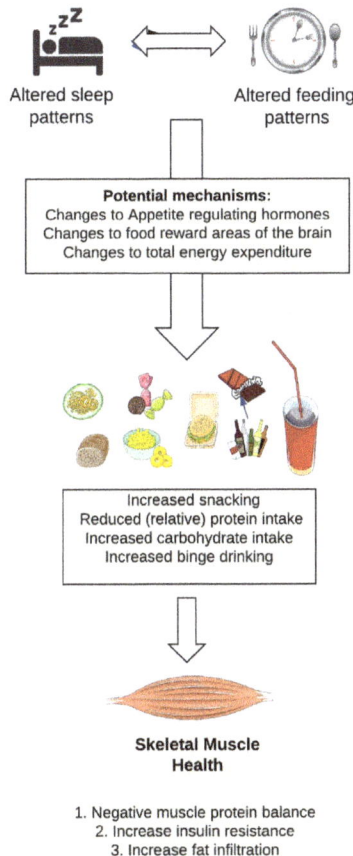

Figure 2. A model of how the altered sleep and feeding patterns of shiftworkers could impair skeletal muscle health.

The diets of shiftworkers have been reviewed by Lowden et al. [50]. These authors did not specifically focus on protein intake in shiftworkers, though some evidence suggested high ingestion of animal protein and fats by nightshift workers. A more consistent pattern is that despite little difference in energy intake between different work groups, fat and refined carbohydrates comprise a greater portion of shiftworkers' diets compared to daytime workers. Such dietary patterns can increase the risk of insulin resistance, promoting muscle protein degradation, favoring fat infiltration in the muscle and negatively impacting skeletal muscle health (Figure 2).

As shiftwork disrupts workers' sleep patterns, studies documenting food choices following sleep deprivation and sleep restriction may provide further insight into the links between shiftwork, diet, and skeletal muscle health. Sleep loss generally increases the preference for foods with a high carbohydrate content including sweets, salty, and starchy foods compared to vegetables, fruit, and high protein foods [51–54]. Across two weeks of sleep restriction (i.e., 5 h sleep per night) [55] or following one night of total sleep deprivation [56], participants increased their ad-libitum food and energy intake, particularly through increased snacking. Sleep restriction also impacts food-purchasing behaviours, influencing longer-term food intake. After one night of total sleep deprivation and following a calorie controlled breakfast, one study reported an increase in the purchase of higher calorie foods, including sweet and fatty food items, and total grams of food within the same budget compared to a night of sleep [57]. Neurological factors may contribute to explain these results, with imaging studies showing a greater response in the food reward areas of the brain to unhealthy food items compared to healthy food items following sleep restriction [58,59].

The mechanisms by which shiftwork may alter dietary choices could also include alterations in appetite regulating hormones, leptin (appetite-inhibiting hormone), and ghrelin (appetite-stimulating hormone [60]); however, direct evidence is lacking. Men working dayshifts recorded lower concentrations of leptin compared to other shifts [61]. However, early morning shiftworkers had lower ghrelin concentrations over the day, consumed less total energy, and reported lower appetite ratings when compared to day and night shiftworkers [61]. These potentially conflicting findings are further confounded by the direct impact of sleep restriction (common to many shiftworkers) on the same hormones. For instance, a randomised crossover study found reduced leptin and increased ghrelin following two consecutive nights of sleep restriction (4 h in bed) when compared to sleep extension (10 h in bed), under strict calorie control in the form of intravenous glucose [52]. It follows that hunger and appetite were increased following sleep restriction and were proportional to the increased ghrelin to leptin ratio [52]. Other studies have reported inconsistent results, with either increases in leptin following a sleep restriction period [55,62], no change in satiety [62], or no difference in leptin or ghrelin levels following sleep restriction, despite an increased calorie intake [51]. Teasing out the relationships between the different types of shiftwork, changes to appetite hormones, and food reward centers in the brain should be a focus of future research. Only then can the precise mechanisms for the changes in dietary patterns observed in shiftworkers be understood and targeted interventions be designed.

Shiftworking also influences alcohol consumption [63,64]. Dorrian and colleagues [63,64] reported that whilst shiftworkers do not drink more than those on standard work rosters, they are at increased risk of 'binge' drinking; that is, periods of heavy drinking followed by abstinence. Workers on 12-h rotating shifts consumed more drinks in a single 24-h period compared to those on 8-h rotating shifts [63]. These findings also align with a recent systematic review demonstrating a positive relationship between long working hours and alcohol consumption [65]. For the current review, an increased risk of binge drinking, perhaps during 'down periods' between shift 'blocks', could pose significant risks to skeletal muscle health. Recently, Parr and colleagues [66] have shown that heavy alcohol consumption reduces muscle protein synthesis rates and increases protein degradation [67] following a bout of combined resistance and endurance exercise. These participants were however well-rested, night-time sleepers so it is unclear whether the observed impairments of alcohol on skeletal muscle growth could be further exaggerated by the changes in sleep patterns (incl. sleep restriction) encountered by shiftworkers.

2.3. Shiftwork, Sleep Disruption, and Hormonal Changes

Hormones are circulating molecules that transmit physiological signals to organs, including to skeletal muscle. By binding to specific receptors expressed at the surface of the muscle fibre, hormones trigger the activation of molecular transduction pathways that regulate cell metabolism, structure, and function. In this section, we will draw on the small group of studies describing the hormonal profile exhibited by shiftworking populations. This pool of research will be supplemented by experimental evidence demonstrating the direct impact of sleep deprivation or restriction on the major anabolic and catabolic hormones, including testosterone, insulin and insulin like growth factor 1 (IGF-1), and cortisol.

2.3.1. Testosterone

Testosterone is a key regulator of skeletal muscle mass that directly promotes muscle protein synthesis [68] while also repressing the negative effect of genes activating protein breakdown [69]. Plasma testosterone levels rise with the onset of sleep and peak after the first REM sleep opportunity. At least 3 h of normal sleep are required to induce this rise [70]. Concentrations remain high until waking and then decrease gradually during the day. Early, underpowered field studies investigating the secretory pattern of testosterone in shiftworkers during and following their night shift reported decreased nocturnal [71] and diurnal [72] testosterone concentrations in serum. More recently, Jensen et al. [73] reported that police officers completing 2, 4, and 7 consecutive nights of night shift (coupled with equivalent recovery days) did not experience any change to their testosterone profiles. However, the authors did not report whether total testosterone (e.g., area under the curve) was affected. A study comparing sex hormone profiles in a heterogeneous population of night-versus day workers revealed that night workers had higher levels of androgen hormones, including testosterone, than day workers. However, this trend was not apparent when looking at males only. The testosterone peak was significantly delayed in night workers, independently of sex [74].

The direct relationship between sleep and testosterone in experimental settings has received more attention. Total sleep deprivation, sleep restriction, and fragmented sleep over a 24-h period, which could relate to the work of emergency response or on-call workers [2–5], respectively lower testosterone levels [71,72] and delay the normal nocturnal blood testosterone rise [75]. The nocturnal rise in testosterone appears dependent on REM sleep with the amplitude of this rise being significantly lower in participants who did not have any REM sleep opportunity [75]. Sustained sleep restriction, which is also representative of some shiftworking conditions, impairs testosterone release as well. After five nights of sleep restriction (4 h sleep per night), there was a trend ($p = 0.09$) for a reduction in total daytime testosterone [76]. Failure to reach statistical significance may reflect that the study was slightly underpowered, the period of sleep restriction was not long enough, or that the total testosterone measure was not sufficiently sensitive to pick up diurnal patterns. Indeed, eight nights of sleep restriction (5 h sleep per night) led to significantly decreased testosterone levels during waking hours, with differences being especially apparent between 2 p.m. and 10 p.m. [77]. Finally, a study compared the effects of shifting sleep (day sleep) and control conditions (night sleep) on circulating testosterone levels. Testosterone concentrations generally raised during sleep and dropped during waking, with small circadian effects being reported [78]. On balance, it appears that shiftwork, and total and sustained sleep restriction can all impair testosterone release, which may fail to promote muscle protein synthesis and preserve skeletal muscle health in affected populations.

2.3.2. Insulin and Insulin-Like Growth Factor 1 (IGF-1)

Insulin is a central regulator of skeletal muscle health and metabolism. This peptidic hormone concurrently increases the postprandial transport and delivery of amino acids to skeletal muscle, activates muscle protein synthesis, and inhibits muscle protein degradation [79]. Maintaining optimal insulin function is essential for metabolic health. Insulin resistance, a metabolic disorder that is characteristic of diabetes and obesity, blunts muscle protein synthesis and promotes muscle protein degradation. By favouring fatty acid uptake in the muscle, insulin resistance also augments fat infiltration into the muscle, leading to a negative muscle protein balance and decreased muscle mass [80,81].

The adverse impact of shiftwork and sleep restriction on insulin resistance is suggested through the consistent associations existing between shiftwork, sleep restriction, diabetes, and obesity [6]. Drawing on evidence from 38 meta-analyses and 24 systematic reviews, Kecklund and Axelsson [6] reported that diabetes (relative risk (RR) ratio: 1.09 (95% CI: 1.05 to 1.12)) was more prevalent in shiftworking than in control populations. While no data focused on shiftwork per se, sleep restriction studies returned a RR of 1.25 (95% CI: 1.14 to 1.3) for obesity/weight gain. In experimental settings, Buxton et al. [82] demonstrated reduced insulin sensitivity following as little as one week of sleep restriction (5 h per night) in 20 healthy men. Supporting this finding, five nights of sleep restriction (4 h per night) led to reduced whole body and peripheral insulin sensitivity that was associated with an increase in fasting non-esterified fatty acid in 14 healthy participants [83].

IGF-1 is another positive regulator of muscle protein synthesis that is the main activator of the Akt/mTOR pathway in muscle, while also carrying out signaling in other anabolic pathways [84]. Controlled human studies investigating the direct effects of sleep deprivation or restriction on IGF-1 levels are lacking; however, 25 h of sleep deprivation induced significant decreases in free IGF-1 concentrations, while one night of recovery efficiently restored basal circulating IGF-1 levels [85]. Whether chronic changes in IGF-1 concentrations are associated with shiftwork schedules still needs to be investigated.

2.3.3. Cortisol

Cortisol is the major hormone released through activation of the hypothalamic-pituitary-adrenal axis in response to psychological or physiological stressors [86] in humans. Elevated cortisol levels upset skeletal muscle protein balance by suppressing protein synthesis and promoting protein breakdown [84]. Cortisol inhibits IGF-1 production in skeletal muscle, while up regulating key inhibitors of protein synthesis [84]. Furthermore, cortisol stimulates the major protein degradation pathways, including the ubiquitin–proteasome system [84]. Under normal conditions, cortisol release follows a diurnal pattern characterized by a peak upon morning wakening, followed by a decline across the day, reaching its lowest level ~3–5 h after night-time sleep onset [86]. Across a variety of occupations and work rosters, shiftwork disrupts this diurnal pattern. Studies in police, nursing, and other emergency services demonstrated cortisol dysregulation after short- and longer-term exposure to shift- and, in particular, night-work rosters [87–89]. The impairment is typically characterized as suppressed cortisol awakening response, followed by a slower rate of decline, which can lead to an elevated night-time cortisol levels [89,90]. Depending on the number of samples collected, this flatter diurnal patterning can lead to a higher overall cortisol release across the day [30,91].

The abnormal cortisol pattern is related to the circadian misalignment caused by the irregular waking hours required of shiftworkers. Furthermore, workers suffering shortened sleep, through working longer shifts or rotating between roster-types also demonstrate cortisol release impairments [90]. Animal models also provide evidence that increased exposure to artificial light, an acute consequence of shiftwork (Figure 1), is associated with disrupted cortisol secretion patterns [92]. Relevant to our model, the dysregulation of cortisol release in shiftworkers could impair their skeletal muscle health by favoring a negative protein balance. These relationships between sleep disruptions, increased cortisol release and progressive muscle wasting have been very recently implicated in the development of sarcopenia [93]. We propose that the circadian misalignment and sleep disruption incurred by shiftworkers could also impair skeletal muscle health, independent of age.

3. Potential Countermeasures to Preserve Skeletal Muscle Health in Shiftworkers

The current review hypothesizes that shiftwork, through altered light exposure, disruptions to sleep, and changes in food intake patterns may impair skeletal muscle health. These populations may therefore need evidence-based strategies to help promote and preserve this fundamental human tissue, essential for short-term physical capacity and long-term metabolic health. Identifying and implementing successful countermeasures will not only benefit the individual shiftworker, but also improve the health of this essential workforce, underpinning the essential services they provide communities.

There have been several reviews dedicated to improving shiftworker health (e.g., Wright Jr. et al. [1] and Kecklund and Axelsson [6]). Many of these reviews target the factors identified in Figure 1 and therefore, strategies targeting circadian adjustment through manipulating light exposure, improving sleep quantity and quality, and overall diet, could also benefit skeletal muscle health. Rather than revisit these strategies, this final section will focus on countermeasures that target two of the main drivers of skeletal muscle synthesis—protein intake and resistance training. To do so, we will draw on experimental studies in humans and rodents completed in conditions that approximate one or more aspects of shiftwork (e.g., altered sleep timing).

Dietary protein is an established, potent stimulator of muscle protein synthesis [17]. Res et al. [94] reported that in humans, a 40-g mixed protein beverage drank 30 min prior to sleep significantly increased overnight muscle protein synthesis as well as the circulation of essential amino acids when compared to a control group. Although these findings were observed in participants permitted a full night's sleep, they do highlight the potential protective impact of protein ingestion for the skeletal muscle health of shiftworkers. This possibility is further supported by recent findings using rodent models. In rats, 96 h of sleep deprivation significantly decreased testosterone levels and elevated corticosterone (the predominant glucocorticoid in rats) levels [38]. Supplementation by the essential amino acid Leucine did not protect against these hormonal changes; however, it was able to counteract the sleep deprivation-induced reduction in muscle fibre CSA in type IIb, but not in type IIa muscle fibres. Leucine supplementation also rescued the sleep deprivation-induced decrease in markers of muscle protein synthesis, but not the sleep deprivation-induced increase in markers of protein degradation [38]. Although no study has replicated these findings in humans, additional protein ingestion does represent a plausible and practical countermeasure to help shiftworkers to preserve their skeletal muscle. Research into the timing and dose of the protein required to optimise skeletal muscle health across a range of shiftworking conditions is a worthwhile focus for future investigations.

Resistance training is another primary stimulator of muscle protein synthesis [95]. Therefore, it may represent an effective countermeasure to the decrease in muscle protein synthesis and increase in muscle protein breakdown we have proposed for shiftworking populations (Figure 1). We are unaware of any studies that have explored the direct impact of resistance training on skeletal muscle health in shiftworkers or in human participants following a period of sleep deprivation or restriction. There are, however, some allied findings in rodents to prompt further investigation into this countermeasure. Monico-Netto et al. [39] tested rats' responses to 96 h of sleep deprivation, eight-week resistance training, and 96 h sleep deprivation following the eight-week resistance training protocol. Resistance training alone increased muscle mass and CSA, while sleep deprivation alone significantly reduced muscle mass and CSA. When combined, resistance training attenuated the changes in muscle morphology and attenuated the reduction in circulating levels of anabolic hormones that were induced by sleep deprivation. In addition, resistance training was able to blunt, but not fully suppress, the sleep deprivation induced increase in corticosterone levels and protected against the increase of some, but not all, muscle protein degradation markers. These findings have yet to be replicated in human participants. The concurrent impact of chronic sleep restriction (and other sleep disruptions common to shiftwork) and resistance training is also yet to be explored, but the findings of Monico-Netto et al. [39] are promising and should prompt further research in humans and, in particular, shiftworking populations.

For researchers and practitioners implementing resistance training programs in shiftworking populations, research using acute periods of total sleep deprivation and partial sleep restriction provide some insights that could be used to optimize training prescription. Reilly and Piercy [96] showed that participants found their sub-maximal bench press exercise at 3 a.m. was significantly more demanding (i.e., associated with a higher rating of perceived exertion) than when the same load was lifted at 3 p.m. The experimental design was not continued to examine a training effect, nor could the impact of the time of day be separated from the sleep deprivation incurred by keeping participants up until 3 a.m. However, given that perceived exertion is a key driver of self-selected work intensity, then shiftworkers training following impaired sleep may not be able to (a) lift as much load in their training and/or (b) progressively overload their training load sufficiently to optimize protein synthesis.

Nutrients **2017**, *9*, 248

Secondly, the increased exertion of training, especially if coupled with a lack of progression, could de-motivate shiftworkers to undertake resistance training. To counter these potential impairments, workplaces should consider the positive influence that exercising in pairs or teams may have on motivation and exertion [97,98], two drivers of physical activity and training that are impaired by sleep restriction [96,99]. Indeed, in a highly competitive team weight-lifting environment, Blumert et al. [100] found that maximal strength is not impaired by 24 h of complete sleep deprivation. We have also shown that firefighters working in teams will maintain their physical performance on important tasks without a decrease in motivation or perceived exertion [101]. Neither of these acute sleep restriction or deprivation environments are a true proxy for the chronic sleep disruptions commonplace for shiftworkers. However, researchers seeking to trial resistance training programs with shiftworking clients should strongly consider the value of exercising in groups or with partners to buffer the normal drop in motivation or perceived exertion associated with sleep deprivation and restriction.

4. Conclusions

The current review hypothesized that shiftwork may significantly impair skeletal muscle health through multiple physiological pathways resulting in a reduction of protein synthesis and an augmentation of protein degradation in the muscle. Our conceptual model explored relationships between typical shiftwork consequences; altered light exposure, sleep patterns, and food and beverage consumption, and drivers of skeletal muscle health—protein intake, resistance training, and hormone release. To date, no study has directly investigated the skeletal muscle health of shiftworkers. In the absence of direct evidence, we drew from some experimental findings that altered light, sleep, and eating patterns can directly influence skeletal muscle homeostasis. Emerging data from human and rodent laboratory experiments suggests that targeted protein ingestion and/or resistance training may be viable strategies to preserve skeletal muscle health for shiftworkers. Further research is required to test the potential relationships identified in our review, including the efficacy of the proposed interventions.

Acknowledgments: The authors wish to acknowledge Olivia Knowles for excellent technical assistance. Séverine Lamon is supported by a Discovery Early Career Research Award (DECRA) from the Australian Research Council (ARC) (DE150100538).

Author Contributions: All authors (B.A., D.C., E.Z. and S.L.) contributed to the following areas: conception and design of the work, interpretation of literature for the work, drafting the work and revising it critically and the final approval for the version to be published The authors agree to be accountable for all aspects of the work, ensuring that questions related to the accuracy or integrity of any part of the work are appropriately investigated and resolved.

Conflicts of Interest: The authors declare no conflict of interest.

References

1. Wright, K.P., Jr.; Bogan, R.K.; Wyatt, J.K. Shift work and the assessment and management of shift work disorder (swd). *Sleep Med. Rev.* **2013**, *17*, 41–54. [CrossRef] [PubMed]
2. Alterman, T.; Luckhaupt, S.E.; Calvert, G.M.; Dahlhamer, J.M.; Ward, B.W. Prevalence rates of work organization characteristics among workers in the U.S.: Data from the 2010 national health interview survey. *Am. J. Ind. Med.* **2013**, *56*, 647–659. [CrossRef] [PubMed]
3. Eurofound. Sixth European Working Conditions Survey. 2015. Available online: http://www.eurofound.europa.eu/surveys/data-visualisation/sixth-europeanworking-conditions-survey-2015 (accessed on 2 November 2016).
4. Australian Bureau of Statistics. Australian Labour Market Statistics, October 2010. Available online: www.abs.gov.au (accessed on 2 November 2016).
5. Ferguson, S.A.; Paterson, J.L.; Jay, S.M.; Hall, S.J.; Aisbett, B. On-call work: To sleep or not to sleep? It depends. *Chronobiol. Int.* **2016**, *33*, 678–684. [CrossRef] [PubMed]
6. Kecklund, G.; Axelsson, J. Health consequences of shift work and insufficient sleep. *BMJ (Clin. Res. Ed.)* **2016**, *355*, i5210. [CrossRef] [PubMed]

7. Wagstaff, A.S.; Sigstad Lie, J.-A. Shift and night work and long working hours—A systematic review of safety implications. *Scand. J. Work Environ. Health* **2011**, *37*, 173–185. [CrossRef] [PubMed]

8. Bambra, C.; Whitehead, M.; Sowden, A.; Akers, J.; Petticrew, M. "A hard day's night?" The effects of compressed working week interventions on the health and work-life balance of shift workers: A systematic review. *J. Epidemiol. Community Health* **2008**, *62*, 764–777. [CrossRef] [PubMed]

9. Harma, M. Workhours in relation to work stress, recovery and health. *Scand. J. Work Environ. Health* **2006**, *32*, 502–514. [CrossRef] [PubMed]

10. Gan, Y.; Yang, C.; Tong, X.Y.; Sun, H.L.; Cong, Y.J.; Yin, X.X.; Li, L.Q.; Cao, S.Y.; Dong, X.X.; Gong, Y.H.; et al. Shift work and diabetes mellitus: A meta-analysis of observational studies. *Occup. Environ. Med.* **2015**, *72*, U91. [CrossRef] [PubMed]

11. Van Drongelen, A.; Boot, C.R.L.; Merkus, S.L.; Smid, T.; van der Beek, A.J. The effects of shift work on body weight change—A systematic review of longitudinal studies. *Scand. J. Work Environ. Health* **2011**, *37*, 263–275. [CrossRef] [PubMed]

12. Lin, X.; Chen, W.; Wei, F.; Ying, M.; Wei, W.; Xie, X. Night-shift work increases morbidity of breast cancer and all-cause mortality: A meta-analysis of 16 prospective cohort studies. *Sleep Med.* **2015**, *16*, 1381–1387. [CrossRef] [PubMed]

13. Anothaisintawee, T.; Reutrakul, S.; van Cauter, E.; Thakkinstian, A. Sleep disturbances compared to traditional risk factors for diabetes development: Systematic review and meta-analysis. *Sleep Med. Rev.* **2015**, *30*, 11–24. [CrossRef] [PubMed]

14. Proper, K.I.; van de Langenberg, D.; Rodenburg, W.; Vermeulen, R.C.H.; van der Beek, A.J.; van Steeg, H.; van Kerkhof, L.W.M. The relationship between shift work and metabolic risk factors: A systematic review of longitudinal studies. *Am. J. Prev. Med.* **2016**, *50*, e147–e157. [CrossRef] [PubMed]

15. Fielding, R.A.; Ralston, S.H.; Rizzoli, R. Emerging impact of skeletal muscle in health and disease. *Calcif. Tissue Int.* **2015**, *96*, 181–182. [CrossRef] [PubMed]

16. Jensen, J.; Rustad, P.I.; Kolnes, A.J.; Lai, Y.C. The role of skeletal muscle glycogen breakdown for regulation of insulin sensitivity by exercise. *Front. Physiol.* **2011**, *2*, 112. [CrossRef] [PubMed]

17. Rasmussen, B.B.; Phillips, S.M. Contractile and nutritional regulation of human muscle growth. *Exerc. Sport Sci. Rev.* **2003**, *31*, 127–131. [CrossRef] [PubMed]

18. Wolkow, A.; Ferguson, S.; Aisbett, B.; Main, L. Effects of work-related sleep restriction on acute physiological and psychological stress responses and their interactions: A review among emergency service personnel. *Int. J. Occup. Med. Environ. Health* **2015**, *28*, 183–208. [CrossRef] [PubMed]

19. Vedaa, Ø.; Harris, A.; Bjorvatn, B.; Waage, S.; Sivertsen, B.; Tucker, P.; Pallesen, S. Systematic review of the relationship between quick returns in rotating shift work and health-related outcomes. *Ergonomics* **2016**, *59*, 1–14. [CrossRef] [PubMed]

20. Bassel-Duby, R.; Olson, E.N. Signaling pathways in skeletal muscle remodeling. *Annu. Rev. Biochem.* **2006**, *75*, 19–37. [CrossRef] [PubMed]

21. Hargreaves, M. Skeletal muscle metabolism during exercise in humans. *Clin. Exp. Pharmacol. Physiol.* **2000**, *27*, 225–228. [CrossRef] [PubMed]

22. Russell, A.P. Molecular regulation of skeletal muscle mass. *Clin. Exp. Pharmacol. Physiol.* **2010**, *37*, 378–384. [CrossRef] [PubMed]

23. Short, K.R.; Nair, K.S. Muscle protein metabolism and the sarcopenia of aging. *Int. J. Sport Nutr. Exerc. Metab.* **2001**, *11*, 119–127. [CrossRef]

24. Bodine, S.C.; Stitt, T.N.; Gonzalez, M.; Kline, W.O.; Stover, G.L.; Bauerlein, R.; Zlotchenko, E.; Scrimgeour, A.; Lawrence, J.C.; Glass, D.J.; et al. Akt/mtor pathway is a crucial regulator of skeletal muscle hypertrophy and can prevent muscle atrophy in vivo. *Nat. Cell Biol.* **2001**, *3*, 1014–1019. [CrossRef] [PubMed]

25. Ferrando, A.A.; Tipton, K.D.; Bamman, M.M.; Wolfe, R.R. Resistance exercise maintains skeletal muscle protein synthesis during bed rest. *J. Appl. Physiol.* **1997**, *82*, 807–810. [PubMed]

26. Rommel, C.; Bodine, S.C.; Clarke, B.A.; Rossman, R.; Nunez, L.; Stitt, T.N.; Yancopoulos, G.D.; Glass, D.J. Mediation of igf-1-induced skeletal myotube hypertrophy by pi(3)k/akt/mtor and pi(3)k/akt/gsk3 pathways. *Nat. Cell Biol.* **2001**, *3*, 1009–1013. [CrossRef] [PubMed]

27. Schroder, E.A.; Harfmann, B.D.; Zhang, X.; Srikuea, R.; England, J.H.; Hodge, B.A.; Wen, Y.; Riley, L.A.; Yu, Q.; Christie, A.; et al. Intrinsic muscle clock is necessary for musculoskeletal health. *J. Physiol.* **2015**, *593*, 5387–5404. [CrossRef] [PubMed]

28. Harfmann, B.D.; Schroder, E.A.; Esser, K.A. Circadian rhythms, the molecular clock, and skeletal muscle. *J. Biol. Rhythm.* **2015**, *30*, 84–94. [CrossRef] [PubMed]

29. Lefta, M.; Wolff, G.; Esser, K.A. Circadian rhythms, the molecular clock, and skeletal muscle. *Curr. Top. Dev. Biol.* **2011**, *96*, 231–271. [PubMed]

30. Miller, B.H.; McDearmon, E.L.; Panda, S.; Hayes, K.R.; Zhang, J.; Andrews, J.L.; Antoch, M.P.; Walker, J.R.; Esser, K.A.; Hogenesch, J.B.; et al. Circadian and clock-controlled regulation of the mouse transcriptome and cell proliferation. *Proc. Natl. Acad. Sci. USA* **2007**, *104*, 3342–3347. [CrossRef] [PubMed]

31. Andrews, J.L.; Zhang, X.; McCarthy, J.J.; McDearmon, E.L.; Hornberger, T.A.; Russell, B.; Campbell, K.S.; Arbogast, S.; Reid, M.B.; Walker, J.R.; et al. Clock and bmal1 regulate myod and are necessary for maintenance of skeletal muscle phenotype and function. *Proc. Natl. Acad. Sci. USA* **2010**, *107*, 19090–19095. [CrossRef] [PubMed]

32. Chatterjee, S.; Ma, K. Circadian clock regulation of skeletal muscle growth and repair. *F1000Research* **2016**, *5*, 1549. [CrossRef] [PubMed]

33. Perrin, L.; Loizides-Mangold, U.; Skarupelova, S.; Pulimeno, P.; Chanon, S.; Robert, M.; Bouzakri, K.; Modoux, C.; Roux-Lombard, P.; Vidal, H.; et al. Human skeletal myotubes display a cell-autonomous circadian clock implicated in basal myokine secretion. *Mol. Metab.* **2015**, *4*, 834–845. [CrossRef] [PubMed]

34. Cedernaes, J.; Osler, M.E.; Voisin, S.; Broman, J.E.; Vogel, H.; Dickson, S.L.; Zierath, J.R.; Schioth, H.B.; Benedict, C. Acute sleep loss induces tissue-specific epigenetic and transcriptional alterations to circadian clock genes in men. *J. Clin. Endocrinol. Metab.* **2015**, *100*, E1255–E1261. [CrossRef] [PubMed]

35. Nindl, B.C.; Leone, C.D.; Tharion, W.J.; Johnson, R.F.; Castellani, J.W.; Patton, J.F.; Montain, S.J. Physical performance responses during 72 h of military operational stress./performances physiques lors de 72 h d'operation militaire. *Med. Sci. Sports Exerc.* **2002**, *34*, 1814–1822. [CrossRef] [PubMed]

36. Nedeltcheva, A.V.; Kilkus, J.M.; Imperial, J.; Schoeller, D.A.; Penev, P.D. Insufficient sleep undermines dietary efforts to reduce adiposity. *Ann. Intern. Med.* **2010**, *153*, 435–441. [CrossRef] [PubMed]

37. Dattilo, M.; Antunes, H.K.; Medeiros, A.; Monico-Neto, M.; Souza Hde, S.; Lee, K.S.; Tufik, S.; de Mello, M.T. Paradoxical sleep deprivation induces muscle atrophy. *Muscle Nerve* **2012**, *45*, 431–433. [CrossRef] [PubMed]

38. De Sa Souza, H.; Antunes, H.K.; Dattilo, M.; Lee, K.S.; Monico-Neto, M.; de Campos Giampa, S.Q.; Phillips, S.M.; Tufik, S.; de Mello, M.T. Leucine supplementation is anti-atrophic during paradoxical sleep deprivation in rats. *Amino Acids* **2016**, *48*, 949–957. [CrossRef] [PubMed]

39. Monico-Neto, M.; Antunes, H.K.; Lee, K.S.; Phillips, S.M.; Giampa, S.Q.; Souza Hde, S.; Dattilo, M.; Medeiros, A.; de Moraes, W.M.; Tufik, S.; et al. Resistance training minimizes catabolic effects induced by sleep deprivation in rats. *Appl. Physiol. Nutr. Metab.* **2015**, *40*, 1143–1150. [CrossRef] [PubMed]

40. Cao, R.; Huang, F.; Wang, P.; Chen, C.; Zhu, G.; Chen, L.; Wu, G. Chronic sleep deprivation alters the myosin heavy chain isoforms in the masseter muscle in rats. *Br. J. Oral Maxillofac. Surg.* **2015**, *53*, 430–435. [CrossRef] [PubMed]

41. Gopalakrishnan, A.; Ji, L.L.; Cirelli, C. Sleep deprivation and cellular responses to oxidative stress. *Sleep* **2004**, *27*, 27–35. [PubMed]

42. Lucassen, E.A.; Coomans, C.P.; van Putten, M.; de Kreij, S.R.; van Genugten, J.H.; Sutorius, R.P.; de Rooij, K.E.; van der Velde, M.; Verhoeve, S.L.; Smit, J.W.; et al. Environmental 24-hr cycles are essential for health. *Curr. Biol.* **2016**, *26*, 1843–1853. [CrossRef] [PubMed]

43. Motil, K.J.; Matthews, D.E.; Bier, D.M.; Burke, J.F.; Munro, H.N.; Young, V.R. Whole-body leucine and lysine metabolism: Response to dietary protein intake in young men. *Am. J. Physiol. Endocrinol. Metab.* **1981**, *240*, E712–E721.

44. Paddon-Jones, D.; Rasmussen, B.B. Dietary protein recommendations and the prevention of sarcopenia. *Curr. Opin. Clin. Nutr. Metab. Care* **2009**, *12*, 86–90. [CrossRef] [PubMed]

45. Symons, T.B.; Sheffield-Moore, M.; Wolfe, R.R.; Paddon-Jones, D. Moderating the portion size of a protein-rich meal improves anabolic efficiency in young and elderly. *J. Am. Diet. Assoc.* **2009**, *109*, 1582–1586. [CrossRef] [PubMed]

46. Moore, D.R.; Robinson, M.J.; Fry, J.L.; Tang, J.E.; Glover, E.I.; Wilkinson, S.B.; Prior, T.; Tarnopolsky, M.A.; Phillips, S.M. Ingested protein dose response of muscle and albumin protein synthesis after resistance exercise in young men. *Am. J. Clin. Nutr.* **2008**, *89*, 161–168. [CrossRef] [PubMed]

47. Børsheim, E.; Tipton, K.D.; Wolf, S.E.; Wolfe, R.R. Essential amino acids and muscle protein recovery from resistance exercise. *Am. J. Physiol. Endocrinol. Metab.* **2002**, *283*, E648–E657. [CrossRef] [PubMed]

48. Duan, Y.; Li, F.; Liu, H.; Li, Y.; Liu, Y.; Kong, X.; Zhang, Y.; Deng, D.; Tang, Y.; Feng, Z.; et al. Nutritional and regulatory roles of leucine in muscle growth and fat reduction. *Front. Biosci. (Landmark Ed.)* **2015**, *20*, 796–813. [PubMed]

49. Tipton, K.; Elliott, T.; Cree, M.; Wolf, S.E.; Sanford, A.; Wolfe, R.R. Ingestion of casein and whey proteins result in muscle anabolism after resistance exercise. *Med. Sci. Sports Exerc.* **2004**, *36*, 2073–2081. [CrossRef] [PubMed]

50. Arne, L.; Moreno, C.; Holmbäck, U.; Lennernäs, M.; Tucker, P. Eating and shift work—Effects on habits, metabolism and performance. *Scand. J. Work Environ. Health* **2010**, *36*, 150–162.

51. Nedeltcheva, A.V.; Kessler, L.; Imperial, J.; Penev, P.D. Exposure to recurrent sleep restriction in the setting of high caloric intake and physical inactivity results in increased insulin resistance and reduced glucose tolerance. *J. Clin. Endocrinol. Metab.* **2009**, *94*, 3242–3250. [CrossRef] [PubMed]

52. Spiegel, K.; Tasali, E.; Penev, P.; Van Cauter, E. Brief communication: Sleep curtailment in healthy young men is associated with decreased leptin levels, elevated ghrelin levels, and increased hunger and appetite. *Ann. Intern. Med.* **2004**, *141*, 846–850. [CrossRef] [PubMed]

53. Beebe, D.W.; Simon, S.; Summer, S.; Hemmer, S.; Strotman, D.; Dolan, L.M. Dietary intake following experimentally restricted sleep in adolescents. *Sleep* **2013**, *36*, 827–834. [CrossRef] [PubMed]

54. Spaeth, A.M.; Dinges, D.F.; Goel, N. Sex and race differences in caloric intake during sleep restriction in healthy adults. *Am. J. Clin. Nutr.* **2014**, *100*, 559–566. [CrossRef] [PubMed]

55. Markwald, R.R.; Melanson, E.L.; Smith, M.R.; Higgins, J.; Perreault, L.; Eckel, R.H.; Wright, K.P. Impact of insufficient sleep on total daily energy expenditure, food intake, and weight gain. *Proc. Natl. Acad. Sci. USA* **2013**, *110*, 5695–5700. [CrossRef] [PubMed]

56. Hogenkamp, P.S.; Nilsson, E.; Nilsson, V.C.; Chapman, C.D.; Vogel, H.; Lundberg, L.S.; Zarei, S.; Cedernaes, J.; Rångtell, F.H.; Broman, J.-E.; et al. Acute sleep deprivation increases portion size and affects food choice in young men. *Psychoneuroendocrinology* **2013**, *38*, 1668–1674. [CrossRef] [PubMed]

57. Chapman, C.; Nilsson, E.; Nilsson, V.; Cedernaes, J.; Rångtell, F.; Vogel, H.; Dickson, S.; Broman, J.; Hogenkamp, P.; Schiöth, H.; et al. Acute sleep deprivation increases food purchasing in men. *Obesity (Silver Spring, Md.)* **2013**, *21*, E555–E560. [CrossRef] [PubMed]

58. St-Onge, M.P.; Wolfe, S.; Sy, M.; Shechter, A.; Hirsch, J. Sleep restriction increases the neuronal response to unhealthy food in normal-weight individuals. *Int. J. Obes. (2005)* **2014**, *38*, 411–416. [CrossRef] [PubMed]

59. St-Onge, M.-P.; McReynolds, A.; Trivedi, Z.B.; Roberts, A.L.; Sy, M.; Hirsch, J. Sleep restriction leads to increased activation of brain regions sensitive to food stimuli. *Am. J. Clin. Nutr.* **2012**, *95*, 818–824. [CrossRef] [PubMed]

60. Gangwisch, J.E. Epidemiological evidence for the links between sleep, circadian rhythms and metabolism. *Obes. Rev. Off. J. Int. Assoc. Study Obes.* **2009**, *10*, 37–45. [CrossRef] [PubMed]

61. Crispim, C.A.; Waterhouse, J.; Dâmaso, A.R.; Zimberg, I.Z.; Padilha, H.G.; Oyama, L.M.; Tufik, S.; de Mello, M.T. Hormonal appetite control is altered by shift work: A preliminary study. *Metabolism* **2011**, *60*, 1726–1735. [CrossRef] [PubMed]

62. Van Leeuwen, W.M.A.; Hublin, C.; Sallinen, M.; Härmä, M.; Hirvonen, A.; Porkka-Heiskanen, T. Prolonged sleep restriction affects glucose metabolism in healthy young men. *Int. J. Endocrinol.* **2010**, *2010*, 7. [CrossRef] [PubMed]

63. Dorrian, J.; Heath, G.; Sargent, C.; Banks, S.; Coates, A. Alcohol use in shiftworkers. *Accid. Anal. Prev.* **2017**, *99*, 395–400. [CrossRef] [PubMed]

64. Dorrian, J.; Skinner, N. Alcohol consumption patterns of shiftworkers compared with dayworkers. *Chronobiol. Int.* **2012**, *29*, 610–618. [CrossRef] [PubMed]

65. Virtanen, M.; Jokela, M.; Nyberg, S.T.; Madsen, I.E.H.; Lallukka, T.; Ahola, K.; Alfredsson, L.; Batty, G.D.; Bjorner, J.B.; Borritz, M.; et al. Long working hours and alcohol use: Systematic review and meta-analysis of published studies and unpublished individual participant data. *BMJ (Clin. Res. Ed.)* **2015**, *350*, g7772. [CrossRef] [PubMed]

66. Parr, E.B.; Camera, D.M.; Areta, J.L.; Burke, L.M.; Phillips, S.M.; Hawley, J.A.; Coffey, V.G. Alcohol ingestion impairs maximal post-exercise rates of myofibrillar protein synthesis following a single bout of concurrent training. *PLoS ONE* **2014**, *9*, e88384. [CrossRef] [PubMed]

67. Smiles, W.J.; Parr, E.B.; Coffey, V.G.; Lacham-Kaplan, O.; Hawley, J.A.; Camera, D.M. Protein coingestion with alcohol following strenuous exercise attenuates alcohol-induced intramyocellular apoptosis and inhibition of autophagy. *Am. J. Physiol. Endocrinol. Metab.* **2016**, *311*, E836–E849. [CrossRef] [PubMed]

68. Urban, R.J.; Bodenburg, Y.H.; Gilkison, C.; Foxworth, J.; Coggan, A.R.; Wolfe, R.R.; Ferrando, A. Testosterone administration to elderly men increases skeletal muscle strength and protein synthesis. *Am. J. Physiol. Endocrinol. Metab.* **1995**, *269*, E820–E826.

69. Zhao, W.; Pan, J.; Wang, X.; Wu, Y.; Bauman, W.A.; Cardozo, C.P. Expression of the muscle atrophy factor muscle atrophy f-box is suppressed by testosterone. *Endocrinology* **2008**, *149*, 5449–5460. [CrossRef] [PubMed]

70. Wittert, G. The relationship between sleep disorders and testosterone in men. *Asian J. Androl.* **2014**, *16*, 262–265. [CrossRef] [PubMed]

71. Touitou, Y.; Motohashi, Y.; Reinberg, A.; Touitou, C.; Bourdeleau, P.; Bogdan, A.; Auzéby, A. Effect of shift work on the night-time secretory patterns of melatonin, prolactin, cortisol and testosterone. *Eur. J. Appl. Physiol. Occup. Physiol.* **1990**, *60*, 288–292. [CrossRef] [PubMed]

72. Chatterton, R.J.; Dooley, S. Reversal of diurnal cortisol rhythm and suppression of plasma testosterone in obstetric residents on cal. *J. Soc. Gynecol. Investig.* **1999**, *61*, 50–54. [CrossRef]

73. Jensen, M.A.; Hansen, A.M.; Kristiansen, J.; Nabe-Nielsen, K.; Garde, A.H. Changes in the diurnal rhythms of cortisol, melatonin, and testosterone after 2, 4, and 7 consecutive night shifts in male police officers. *Chronobiol. Int.* **2016**, 1–13. [CrossRef] [PubMed]

74. Papantoniou, K.; Pozo, O.J.; Espinosa, A.; Marcos, J.; Castano-Vinyals, G.; Basagana, X.; Juanola Pages, E.; Mirabent, J.; Martin, J.; Such Faro, P.; et al. Increased and mistimed sex hormone production in night shift workers. *Cancer Epidemiol. Biomark. Prev.* **2015**, *24*, 854–863. [CrossRef] [PubMed]

75. Luboshitzky, R.; Zabari, Z.; Shen-Orr, Z.; Herer, P.; Lavie, P. Disruption of the nocturnal testosterone rhythm by sleep fragmentation in normal men. *J. Clin. Endocrinol. Metab.* **2001**, *86*, 1134–1139. [CrossRef] [PubMed]

76. Reynolds, A.C.; Dorrian, J.; Liu, P.Y.; Van Dongen, H.P.A.; Wittert, G.A.; Harmer, L.J.; Banks, S. Impact of five nights of sleep restriction on glucose metabolism, leptin and testosterone in young adult men. *PLoS ONE* **2012**, *7*, e41218. [CrossRef] [PubMed]

77. Leproult, R.; van Cauter, E. Effect of 1 week of sleep restriction on testosterone levels in young healthy menfree. *JAMA* **2011**, *305*, 2173–2174. [CrossRef] [PubMed]

78. Axelsson, J.; Ingre, M.; Akerstedt, T.; Holmbäck, U. Effects of acutely displaced sleep on testosterone. *J. Clin. Endocrinol. Metab.* **2005**, *90*, 4530–4535. [CrossRef] [PubMed]

79. Dimitriadis, G.; Mitrou, P.; Lambadiari, V.; Maratou, E.; Raptis, S.A. Insulin effects in muscle and adipose tissue. *Diabetes Res. Clin. Pract.* **2011**, *93*, S52–S59. [CrossRef]

80. Abdul-Ghani, M.A.; de Fronzo, R.A. Pathogenesis of insulin resistance in skeletal muscle. *J. Biomed. Biotechnol.* **2010**. [CrossRef] [PubMed]

81. Nilsson, M.I.; Greene, N.P.; Dobson, J.P.; Wiggs, M.P.; Gasier, H.G.; Macias, B.R.; Shimkus, K.L.; Fluckey, J.D. Insulin resistance syndrome blunts the mitochondrial anabolic response following resistance exercise. *Am. J. Physiol. Endocrinol. Metab.* **2010**, *299*, E466–E474. [CrossRef] [PubMed]

82. Buxton, O.M.; Pavlova, M.; Reid, E.W.; Wang, W.; Simonson, D.C.; Adler, G.K. Sleep restriction for 1 week reduces insulin sensitivity in healthy men. *Diabetes* **2010**, *59*, 2126–2133. [CrossRef] [PubMed]

83. Rao, M.N.; Neylan, T.C.; Grunfeld, C.; Mulligan, K.; Schambelan, M.; Schwarz, J.-M. Subchronic sleep restriction causes tissue-specific insulin resistance. *J. Clin. Endocrinol. Metab.* **2015**, *100*, 1664–1671. [CrossRef] [PubMed]

84. Dattilo, M.; Antunes, H.K.M.; Medeiros, A.; Mônico Neto, M.; Souza, H.S.; Tufik, S.; de Mello, M.T. Sleep and muscle recovery: Endocrinological and molecular basis for a new and promising hypothesis. *Med. Hypotheses* **2011**, *77*, 220–222. [CrossRef] [PubMed]

85. Chennaoui, M.; Drogou, C.; Sauvet, F.; Gomez-Merino, D.; Scofield, D.E.; Nindl, B.C. Effect of acute sleep deprivation and recovery on insulin-like growth factor-i responses and inflammatory gene expression in healthy men. *Eur. Cytokine Netw.* **2014**, *25*, 52–57. [PubMed]

86. Hayes, L.D.; Bickerstaff, G.F.; Baker, J.S. Interactions of cortisol, testosterone, and resistance training: Influence of circadian rhythms. *Chronobiol. Int.* **2010**, *27*, 675–705. [CrossRef] [PubMed]

87. Hennig, J.; Kieferdorf, P.; Moritz, C.; Huwe, S.; Netter, P. Changes in cortisol secretion during shiftwork: Implications for tolerance to shiftwork? *Ergonomics* **1998**, *41*, 610–621. [CrossRef] [PubMed]

88. Charles, L.E.; Fekedulegn, D.; Burchfiel, C.M.; Hartley, T.A.; Andrew, M.E.; Violanti, J.M.; Miller, D.B. Shiftwork and diurnal salivary cortisol patterns among police officers. *J. Occup. Environ. Med.* **2016**, *58*, 542–549. [CrossRef] [PubMed]
89. Lac, G.; Chamoux, A. Biological and psychological responses to two rapid shiftwork schedules. *Ergonomics* **2004**, *47*, 1339–1349. [CrossRef] [PubMed]
90. Wirth, M.; Burch, J.; Violanti, J.; Burchfiel, C.; Fekedulegn, D.; Andrew, M.; Zhang, H.; Miller, D.B.; Héébert, J.R.; Vena, J.E. Shiftwork duration and the awakening cortisol response among police officers. *Chronobiol. Int. J. Biol. Med. Rhythm Res.* **2011**, *28*, 446–457. [CrossRef] [PubMed]
91. Golden, S.H.; Wand, G.S.; Malhotra, S.; Kamel, I.; Horton, K. Reliability of hypothalamic-pituitary-adrenal axis assessment methods for use in population-based studies. *Eur. J. Epidemiol.* **2011**, *26*, 525. [CrossRef] [PubMed]
92. Bedrosian, T.A.; Galan, A.; Vaughn, C.A.; Weil, Z.M.; Nelson, R.J. Light at night alters daily patterns of cortisol and clock proteins in female siberian hamsters. *J. Neuroendocrinol.* **2013**, *25*, 590–596. [CrossRef] [PubMed]
93. Piovezan, R.D.; Abucham, J.; Dos Santos, R.V.T.; Mello, M.T.; Tufik, S.; Poyares, D. The impact of sleep on age-related sarcopenia: Possible connections and clinical implications. *Ageing Res. Rev.* **2015**, *23*, 210–220. [CrossRef] [PubMed]
94. Res, P.T.; Groen, B.; Pennings, B.; Beelen, M.; Wallis, G.A.; Gijsen, A.P.; Senden, J.M.; van Loon, L.J. Protein ingestion before sleep improves postexercise overnight recovery. *Med. Sci. Sports Exerc.* **2012**, *44*, 1560–1569. [CrossRef] [PubMed]
95. Kumar, V.; Atherton, P.J.; Selby, A.; Rankin, D.; Williams, J.; Smith, K.; Hiscock, N.; Rennie, M.J. Muscle protein synthetic responses to exercise: Effects of age, volume, and intensity. *J. Gerontol. Ser. A Biol. Sci. Med. Sci.* **2012**, *67*, 1170–1177. [CrossRef] [PubMed]
96. Reilly, T.; Piercy, M. The effect of partial sleep deprivation on weight-lifting performance. *Ergonomics* **1994**, *37*, 107–115. [CrossRef] [PubMed]
97. Snyder, A.L.; Anderson-Hanley, C.; Arciero, P.J. Virtual and live social facilitation while exergaming: Competiveness moderates exercise intensity. *J. Sport Exerc. Psychol.* **2012**, *34*, 252–259. [CrossRef] [PubMed]
98. Anderson-Hanley, C.; Snyder, A.L.; Nimon, J.P.; Arciero, P.J. Social facilitation in virtual reality-enhanced exercise: Competitiveness moderates exercise effort of older adults. *Clin. Interv. Aging* **2011**, *6*, 275–280. [CrossRef] [PubMed]
99. Aisbett, B.; Wolkow, A.; Sprajcer, M.; Ferguson, S.A. "Awake, smoky, and hot": Providing an evidence-base for managing the risks associated with occupational stressors encountered by wildland firefighters. *Appl. Ergon.* **2012**, *43*, 916–925. [CrossRef] [PubMed]
100. Blumert, P.A.; Crum, A.J.; Ernsting, M.; Volek, J.S.; Hollander, D.B.; Haff, E.E.; Haff, G.G. The acute effects of twenty-four hours of sleep loss on the performance of national-caliber male collegiate weightlifters. *J. Strength Cond. Res. (Allen Press Publ. Serv. Inc.)* **2007**, *21*, 1146–1154. [CrossRef] [PubMed]
101. Vincent, G.; Ferguson, S.A.; Tran, J.; Larsen, B.; Wolkow, A.; Aisbett, B. Sleep restriction during simulated wildfire suppression: Effect on physical task performance. *PLoS ONE* **2015**, *10*, e0115329. [CrossRef] [PubMed]

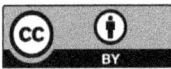

nutrients

MDPI

Article

Relationship between Self-Reported Dietary Nutrient Intake and Self-Reported Sleep Duration among Japanese Adults

Yoko Komada [1,2], Hajime Narisawa [1,2], Fumitaka Ueda [3], Hitomi Saito [3], Hiroyuki Sakaguchi [3], Makoto Mitarai [4], Rina Suzuki [4], Norihisa Tamura [1,2], Shigeru Inoue [5] and Yuichi Inoue [1,2,*]

[1] Department of Somnology, Tokyo Medical University, 6-1-1 Shinjuku, Shinjuku-ku, Tokyo 160-8402, Japan; ykoma@tokyo-med.ac.jp (Y.K.); haji.nari@gmail.com (H.N.); tamura65@tokyo-med.ac.jp (N.T.)

[2] Japan Somnology Center, Neuropsychiatric Research Institute, 1-24-10 Yoyogi, Shibuya-ku, Tokyo 151-0053, Japan

[3] Pharmaceutical and Healthcare Research Laboratories, FUJIFILM Corporation, 2-5-1 Suwa, Tama, Tokyo 206-0024, Japan; fumitaka.ueda@fujifilm.com (F.U.); hitomi.saito@fujifilm.com (H.S.); hiroyuki.sakaguchi@fujifilm.com (H.S.)

[4] Marketing Department, Maruha Nichiro Corporation, 3-2-20 Toyosu, Koto-ku, Tokyo 135-8608, Japan; m-mitarai@maruha-nichiro.co.jp (M.M.); ri-suzuki@maruha-nichiro.co.jp (R.S.)

[5] Department of Preventive Medicine and Public Health, Tokyo Medical University, 6-1-1 Shinjuku, Shinjuku-ku, Tokyo 160-8402, Japan; inoue@tokyo-med.ac.jp

[*] Correspondence: inoue@somnology.com; Tel.: +81-3-3351-6141; Fax +81-3-3351-6208

Received: 7 November 2016; Accepted: 8 February 2017; Published: 13 February 2017

Abstract: Several studies have reported that short sleep duration is a risk factor for obesity and metabolic disease. Moreover, both sleep duration and sleep timing might independently be associated with dietary nutrient intake. In this study, we investigated the associations between self-reported sleep duration and dietary nutrient intake, with and without adjustments for variations in sleep timing (i.e., the midpoint of sleep). We conducted a questionnaire survey, comprising a validated brief self-administered diet history questionnaire (BDHQ) and the Japanese version of the Pittsburgh Sleep Quality Index (PSQI) among 1902 healthy Japanese adults and found that the dietary intakes of several nutrients correlated with sleep duration among men regardless of adjustment for the midpoint of sleep. Particularly, (1) small but significant correlations were observed between sleep duration and the percentage of energy from protein, regardless of adjustment for the midpoint of sleep; (2) energy-adjusted intakes of sodium, vitamin D, and vitamin B12 also significantly correlated with sleep duration; and (3) intakes of bread, pulses, and fish and shellfish correlated with sleep duration. In contrast, no significant correlations were observed between sleep duration and dietary intakes among women. This study revealed that after controlling for the midpoint of sleep, sleep duration correlated significantly with the dietary intake of specific nutrients and foods in a population of Japanese men.

Keywords: sleep duration; midpoint of sleep; dietary nutrients; nutrition; food

1. Introduction

In recent years, laboratory and epidemiologic evidence has identified short sleep duration as a risk factor for the development of obesity and metabolic disease [1–4]. Indeed, in humans, sleep duration plays an important role in regulating the levels of leptin and ghrelin, which are among the key modulators of appetite and energy expenditure [1,5]. Several studies have shown associations of repetitive partial sleep deprivation and/or chronic short sleep duration with a significant decrease in leptin levels and an increase in ghrelin levels [4,6,7]. This might be related to an increase in subjective hunger experienced by self-restricted individuals [1].

Several studies have investigated the association between sleep duration and dietary intake. In a NHANES (National Health and Nutrition Examination Survey)-based study, Grandner et al. found that relative to normal sleepers (7–8 h), short sleepers (5–6 h) reported higher intakes of absolute protein, carbohydrate, and total fat but a lower intake of dietary fiber, whereas very short sleepers (<5 h) reported lower intakes of protein, carbohydrates, dietary fiber, and total fats [8]. In an analysis of Chinese adults, individuals with a self-reported short sleep duration (<7 h) had a lower carbohydrate intake and higher fat intake, compared to normal-duration sleepers (7–9 h) [9]. Kant et al. also observed that both short and long sleepers reported receiving lower percentages of energy from protein, compared to normal duration sleepers in the NHANES [10].

Several previous studies have therefore emphasized the relationship between short sleep duration and poor dietary intake. A recent report suggested that in addition to sleep duration, sleep timing exhibited an important correlation with obesity [11]. Individuals with later sleep timing were 1.5 times more likely to be obese than were individuals with an early sleep timing, despite reasonably similar sleep durations [11]. Regarding nutrient intake, two recent studies showed the influence of sleep timing on the dietary intakes of certain nutrients [12,13]. A cross-sectional study of a large representative sample of the Finnish population also revealed that individuals with later sleep timing exhibited less healthy dietary habits, such as lower vitamin and higher fat consumption, compared to individuals with earlier sleep timing [12]. Another study of young Japanese women found that later sleep timing (i.e., later midpoint of sleep) was significantly associated with a lower percentage of energy intake from protein and carbohydrates; a lower energy-adjusted intake of cholesterol, potassium, calcium, magnesium, iron, zinc, vitamin A, vitamin D, thiamin, riboflavin, vitamin B6, and folate; and a higher percentage of energy intake from alcohol and fat [13].

Considering the results of the above-mentioned studies, we hypothesized that both sleep duration and sleep timing are associated with dietary nutrient intake. To test this hypothesis, we conducted a survey of sleep and dietary nutrient intake in a Japanese adult population. Our primary aim was to identify the existence of an association between the self-reported sleep duration and the intakes of specific dietary nutrients, after adjusting for variations in sleep timing.

2. Methods

2.1. Ethical Approval

This study was approved by the ethics committee of Tokyo Medical University (No. 2586), and written informed consent was obtained from all study participants.

2.2. Patient Selection

A total of 2007 healthy individuals, aged between 30 and 69 years, participated in this cross-sectional survey. Participants were recruited via study advertisements run by a Clinical Research Organization. Individuals who met the following criteria were excluded from the present study: previous or current diagnosis of psychiatric disorders, history of neurologic illness, use of medication with known effects on sleep or daytime alertness, or shift worker. We also excluded those with self-reported extremely low or high energy intake (<725 or >3235 kcal/day) (n = 92), and those whose midpoint of sleep was outside the range of midnight to noon (n = 15). After these exclusions, the final sample included in the subsequent analyses comprised 1902 adults.

2.3. Demographic Variables

The participants filled out self-administered questionnaires containing questions related to demographics and lifestyle. The demographic items included age, sex, height, weight, current smoking habits (yes or no), current exercise routine ($\geq$2 times/week, $\geq$30 min/session; yes or no), family structure (living alone or living with other family members).

2.4. Assessment of Dietary Intake

Dietary intake during the preceding one month was assessed with a validated, self-administered, brief diet history questionnaire (BDHQ) [14]. The BDHQ is a four-page structured questionnaire that enquires about the consumption frequency of a total of 56 foods and beverages that are commonly consumed in the general Japanese population. Dietary intakes, in terms of energy and selected nutrients, were estimated by applying an ad hoc computer algorithm to the 56 foods and beverages of the BDHQ and the Standard Tables of Food Composition in Japan [15].

2.5. Assessment of Sleep Duration and Sleep Timing

Sleep duration was assessed using the Japanese version of the Pittsburgh Sleep Quality Index (PSQI) [16,17]. The PSQI is a self-rated questionnaire that measures sleep difficulty retrospectively for a one-month period, with a global score ranging from 0 to 21. Higher PSQI scores indicate a lower quality of sleep. In the PSQI, the subjects reported bedtimes, sleep onset latency, and rise times. Using these data, we calculated the sleep duration by subtracting the sleep onset time from the rise time and the midpoint of sleep as the halfway point between sleep onset time and rise time to determine sleep timing [13].

2.6. Statistical Analysis

The average values of dietary intake and anthropometric variables were calculated. For energy adjustment, we used the percentages of total energy intakes (% energy) from macronutrients and alcohol and the intakes per 1000 kcal (/1000 kcal) for other nutrients and food. In this study, we evaluated energy (kcal/day), alcohol (% energy), protein (% energy), total fat (% energy), carbohydrate (% energy), cholesterol (mg/1000 kcal), sodium (mg/1000 kcal), potassium (mg/1000 kcal), calcium (mg/1000 kcal), magnesium (mg/1000 kcal), iron (mg/1000 kcal), zinc (mg/1000 kcal), vitamin A (μg/1000 kcal), vitamin D (μg/1000 kcal), vitamin E (mg/1000 kcal), thiamin (mg/1000 kcal), riboflavin (mg/1000 kcal), vitamin B6 (mg/1000 kcal), vitamin B12 (μg/1000 kcal), folate (μg/1000 kcal), and vitamin C (mg/1000 kcal), as well as rice (g/1000 kcal), noodles (g/1000 kcal), bread (g/1000 kcal), confections (g/1000 kcal), potatoes (g/1000 kcal), fat and oil (g/1000 kcal), fruits (g/1000 kcal), vegetables (g/1000 kcal), pulses (g/1000 kcal), fish and shell fish (g/1000 kcal), meat (g/1000 kcal), eggs (g/1000 kcal), and milk and milk products (g/1000 kcal).

The Student's *t*-test was used to compare continuous variables, and the chi-square test was used to compare categorical variables between men and women. The multicolinearity effect was checked using VIF (Variance Inflation Factor) <10/tolerance tests >0.10. A Pearson's correlation analysis was performed to examine the relationships between sleep duration and dietary intakes. A partial correlation procedure was used to examine the linear relationships between these variables after controlling for the effects of other variables (age, sleep timing). All analyses were performed using the statistical software SPSS version 15.0 (SPSS Japan, Inc., Tokyo, Japan). *p*-values < 0.05 were considered statistically significant.

3. Results

The mean age of all the subjects was 48.0 (10.3) years (mean (standard deviation)), and 54.1% of the subjects were male. The mean body mass index (BMI) was 22.4 (3.3). The characteristics and dietary intakes, stratified by sex, are shown in Table 1. We observed significant differences in age (t(1900) = 15.2, p = 0.001), sleep latency (t(1900) = 6.3, p = 0.001), and rise time (t(1900) = 0.66, p = 0.036) between men and women. We further observed significant differences in the percentages of current smokers (χ^2(1) = 51.0, p = 0.001), subjects with a current exercise routine (χ^2(1) = 47.1, p = 0.001), subjects who lived alone (χ^2(1) = 43.0, p = 0.001), and occupational statuses (χ^2(3) = 432.4, p = 0.001). A residual analysis revealed that among men, the percentage of full-time workers was significantly higher and the percentages of part-time workers and homemakers were significantly lower than among women.

Table 1. Participant characteristics and dietary intakes, stratified by sex (*n* = 1902).

	All (*n* = 1902)		Male (*n* = 1029)		Female (*n* = 873)		*p*-Value
	Mean	SD	Mean	SD	Mean	SD	
Age, years	48.0	10.3	51.1	10.2	44.3	9.2	0.001
Body mass index, kg/m^2	22.4	3.3	23.3	3.1	21.4	3.4	0.063
Bedtime, h:min	23:58	1:26	0:03	1:28	23:52	1:23	0.544
Sleep latency, min	19.4	19.0	16.9	15.0	22.4	22.6	0.001
Rise time, h:min	6:46	1:28	6:47	1:32	6:45	1:22	0.036
Midpoint of sleep, h:min	3:32	1:21	3:34	1:24	3:29	1:16	0.059
Sleep duration, h:min	6:26	1:05	6:23	1:04	6:30	1:07	0.311
Current smoking, %	22.0		28.3		14.7		0.001
Current exercise routine, %	27.7		34.2		20.1		0.001
Living alone, %	16.6		21.8		10.5		0.001
Occupation							
Full-time worker	61.8		77.9		42.6		0.001
Part-time worker	8.5		3.0		15.1		
Homemaker	11.6		0.0		25.3		
Unemployed	18.2		19.1		17.0		
Energy, kcal/day	1772.0	527.0	1922.5	521.6	1596.7	478.8	0.001
Alcohol, % energy	5.5	9.0	7.8	10.1	2.8	6.5	0.001
Nutrients							
Protein, % energy	14.5	2.9	13.9	2.7	15.3	3.0	0.001
Total fat, % energy	25.4	5.8	24.1	5.8	27.0	5.6	0.001
Carbohydrate, % energy	53.2	8.8	52.8	9.5	53.8	8.1	0.012
Cholesterol, mg/1000 kcal	196.0	75.0	184.3	75.5	210.4	73.1	0.001
Sodium, mg/1000 kcal	2313.0	491.0	2293.2	483.7	2337.1	499.8	0.052
Potassium, mg/1000 kcal	1336.0	404.0	1245.8	351.9	1442.8	435.0	0.001
Calcium, mg/1000 kcal	275.0	108.0	255.0	99.7	300.6	112.6	0.001
Magnesium, mg/1000 kcal	134.0	32.0	129.3	28.3	141.7	35.0	0.001
Iron, mg/1000 kcal	4.1	1.1	3.9	1.0	4.4	1.2	0.001
Zinc, mg/1000 kcal	4.2	0.7	4.1	0.7	4.4	0.7	0.001
Vitamin A, μg/1000 kcal	374.0	230.0	357.2	218.1	395.6	243.6	0.001
Vitamin D, μg/1000 kcal	6.5	4.3	6.1	3.9	6.9	4.6	0.001
Vitamin E, mg/1000 kcal	3.8	1.1	3.5	1.0	4.1	1.1	0.001
Thiamin, mg/1000 kcal	0.37	0.1	0.37	0.1	0.43	0.1	0.001
Riboflavin, mg/1000 kcal	0.69	0.2	0.66	0.2	0.73	0.2	0.001
Vitamin B6, mg/1000 kcal	0.65	0.2	0.62	0.2	0.69	0.2	0.001
Vitamin B12, μg/1000 kcal	4.6	2.4	4.5	2.3	4.8	2.6	0.006
Folate, μg/1000 kcal	176.0	68.0	164.0	58.7	190.9	75.6	0.001
Vitamin C, mg/1000 kcal	58.0	29.0	53.5	26.5	64.8	31.0	0.001
Food Group (g/1000 kcal)							
Rice	147.0	76.0	152.1	76.6	142.0	75.6	0.004
Noodles	44.0	30.0	49.2	33.1	38.2	26.3	0.001
Bread	49.0	28.0	43.5	25.8	55.6	30.9	0.001
Confections	27.0	21.0	22.5	17.9	33.5	24.1	0.001
Potatoes	18.0	17.0	19.2	18.4	25.7	21.8	0.001
Fat and oil	5.9	2.6	5.8	2.6	6.0	2.8	0.092
Fruits	62.0	58.0	61.4	59.2	63.9	57.2	0.362
Vegetables	134.0	82.0	116.3	66.2	155.0	95.1	0.001
Pulses	34.0	26.0	30.2	23.1	39.5	29.0	0.001
Fish and Shell fish	36.0	22.0	35.2	20.5	38.3	24.3	0.002
Meat	37.0	20.0	35.8	18.3	40.4	21.8	0.001
Eggs	20.0	14.0	19.8	14.7	21.8	14.7	0.003
Milk and milk products	68.0	61.0	63.5	61.4	73.4	61.2	0.001

SD: standard deviation.

Table 2. Correlation between sleep duration and dietary intakes among men (n = 1029).

	Mean	SD	[1] r	[1] β	[2] r	[2] β	[3] r	[3] β
Energy, kcal/day	1922.5	521.6	0.052	−0.05	0.134	−0.06	0.139	−0.06
Alcohol, % energy	7.8	10.1	0.024	0.02	0.150	0.02	0.156	0.02
Nutrients								
Protein, % energy	13.9	2.7	**0.076b**	0.08	**0.126b**	0.07	**0.126b**	0.07
Total fat, % energy	24.1	5.8	0.031	0.03	0.032	0.03	0.052	0.03
Carbohydrate, % energy	52.8	9.5	**0.068b**	−0.07	0.182	−0.06	0.183	−0.06
Cholesterol, mg/1000 kcal	184.3	75.5	0.058	0.06	0.113	0.05	0.114	0.05
Sodium, mg/1000 kcal	2293.2	483.7	**0.087a**	0.09	**0.093a**	0.09	**0.115a**	0.08
Potassium, mg/1000 kcal	1245.8	351.9	0.004	0.00	0.220	−0.02	0.224	−0.01
Calcium, mg/1000 kcal	255.0	99.7	0.011	0.01	0.212	0.00	0.218	0.00
Magnesium, mg/1000 kcal	129.3	28.3	0.030	0.03	0.226	0.02	0.230	0.02
Iron, mg/1000 kcal	3.9	1.0	0.045	0.05	0.180	0.04	0.182	0.04
Zinc, mg/1000 kcal	4.1	0.7	0.048	0.05	0.048	0.05	0.056	0.05
Vitamin A, μg/1000 kcal	357.2	218.1	0.014	0.01	0.074	0.01	0.096	0.02
Vitamin D, μg/1000 kcal	6.1	3.9	**0.088a**	0.09	**0.218a**	0.08	**0.218a**	0.08
Vitamin E, mg/1000 kcal	3.5	1.0	0.022	0.02	0.132	0.01	0.133	0.01
Thiamin, mg/1000 kcal	0.4	0.1	0.036	0.04	0.130	0.03	0.131	0.03
Riboflavin, mg/1000 kcal	0.7	0.2	0.026	0.03	0.187	0.02	0.193	0.02
Vitamin B6, mg/1000 kcal	0.6	0.2	0.058	0.06	0.208	0.05	0.213	0.05
Vitamin B12, μg/1000 kcal	4.5	2.3	**0.093a**	0.09	**0.192a**	0.08	**0.192a**	0.08
Folate, μg/1000 kcal	164.0	58.7	0.020	0.02	0.209	0.01	0.222	0.01
Vitamin C, mg/1000 kcal	53.5	26.5	0.007	0.01	0.242	−0.01	0.243	−0.01
Food Group (g/1000 kcal)								
Rice	152.1	76.6	0.025	−0.03	0.193	−0.01	0.197	−0.01
Noodles	49.2	33.1	0.038	0.04	0.114	0.04	0.143	0.04
Bread	43.5	25.8	0.056	−0.06	0.074	−0.06	**0.092b**	−0.06
Confections	22.5	17.9	0.054	−0.05	0.062	−0.06	0.083	−0.06
Potatoes	19.2	18.4	0.005	−0.01	0.044	−0.01	0.045	−0.01
Fat and oil	5.8	2.6	0.008	0.01	0.132	0.02	0.136	0.01
Fruits	61.4	59.2	0.005	−0.01	0.166	−0.02	0.167	−0.02
Vegetables	116.3	66.2	0.005	0.01	0.170	−0.01	0.178	0.00
Pulses	30.2	23.1	**0.086a**	0.09	**0.134a**	0.08	**0.141a**	0.08
Fish and Shell fish	35.2	20.5	**0.096a**	0.10	**0.183a**	0.09	**0.183a**	0.09
Meat	35.8	18.3	0.016	0.02	0.133	0.02	0.134	0.02
Eggs	19.8	14.7	0.046	0.05	0.075	0.04	0.081	0.05
Milk and milk products	63.5	61.4	0.031	−0.03	0.093	−0.04	0.099	−0.03

SD: standard deviation; r: Pearson's correlation coefficient r; β: standardized coefficient β; [1]: Univariate regression analysis; [2]: Multivariate regression analysis (sleep duration, age); [3]: Multivariate regression analysis (sleep duration, age, midpoint of sleep); a: $p < 0.01$, b: $p < 0.05$, number in bold showed significant variables.

Table 3. Correlation between sleep duration and dietary intakes among women (*n* = 873).

	Mean	SD	[1] *r*	[1] β	[2] *r*	[2] β	[3] *r*	[3] β
Energy, kcal/day	1596.7	478.8	0.002	0.00	0.097	0.01	0.109	0.01
Alcohol, % energy	2.8	6.5	0.018	−0.02	0.031	−0.02	0.068	−0.02
Nutrients								
Protein, % energy	15.3	3.0	0.019	0.02	0.147	0.03	0.160	0.03
Total fat, % energy	27.0	5.6	0.051	−0.05	0.064	−0.05	0.068	−0.05
Carbohydrate, % energy	53.8	8.1	0.035	0.04	0.056	0.03	0.057	0.03
Cholesterol, mg/1000 kcal	210.4	73.1	0.026	0.03	0.043	0.03	0.081	0.03
Sodium, mg/1000 kcal	2337.1	499.8	0.049	0.05	0.097	0.06	0.099	0.06
Potassium, mg/1000 kcal	1442.8	435.0	0.039	−0.04	0.217	−0.02	0.222	−0.02
Calcium, mg/1000 kcal	300.6	112.6	0.047	−0.05	0.204	−0.03	0.208	−0.03
Magnesium, mg/1000 kcal	141.7	35.0	0.014	−0.01	0.231	0.01	0.234	0.00
Iron, mg/1000 kcal	4.4	1.2	0.008	−0.01	0.157	0.01	0.161	0.00
Zinc, mg/1000 kcal	4.4	0.7	0.048	0.05	0.119	0.06	0.137	0.06
Vitamin A, μg/1000 kcal	395.6	243.6	0.008	−0.01	0.037	−0.01	0.038	−0.01
Vitamin D, μg/1000 kcal	6.9	4.6	0.017	0.02	0.140	0.03	0.145	0.03
Vitamin E, mg/1000 kcal	4.1	1.1	0.018	−0.02	0.133	−0.01	0.146	−0.01
Thiamin, mg/1000 kcal	0.4	0.1	0.013	−0.01	0.160	0.00	0.166	0.00
Riboflavin, mg/1000 kcal	0.7	0.2	0.050	−0.05	0.177	−0.04	0.178	−0.04
Vitamin B6, mg/1000 kcal	0.7	0.2	0.021	−0.02	0.159	−0.01	0.166	−0.01
Vitamin B12, μg/1000 kcal	4.8	2.6	0.013	−0.01	0.131	0.00	0.131	0.00
Folate, μg/1000 kcal	190.9	75.6	0.015	−0.02	0.166	0.00	0.170	0.00
Vitamin C, mg/1000 kcal	64.8	31.0	0.013	−0.01	0.186	0.00	0.187	0.00
Food group (g/1000 kcal)								
Rice	142.0	75.6	0.045	0.05	0.090	0.04	0.106	0.04
Noodles	38.2	26.3	0.014	0.01	0.089	0.01	0.137	0.01
Bread	55.6	30.9	0.043	−0.04	0.043	−0.04	0.044	−0.04
Confections	33.5	24.1	0.029	−0.03	0.069	−0.03	0.093	−0.03
Potatoes	25.7	21.8	0.038	−0.04	0.051	−0.04	0.068	−0.04
Fat and oil	6.0	2.8	0.024	−0.02	0.060	−0.03	0.060	−0.03
Fruits	63.9	57.2	0.008	0.01	0.135	0.02	0.137	0.02
Vegetables	155.0	95.1	0.034	−0.03	0.138	−0.02	0.141	−0.02
Pulses	39.5	29.0	0.006	0.01	0.121	0.02	0.122	0.02
Fish and Shell fish	38.3	24.3	0.018	0.02	0.129	0.03	0.129	0.03
Meat	40.4	21.8	0.002	0.00	0.039	−0.01	0.046	−0.01
Eggs	21.8	14.7	0.002	0.00	0.020	0.00	0.094	0.00
Milk and milk products	73.4	61.2	**0.066b**	−0.07	0.132	−0.06	0.132	−0.06

SD: standard deviation, *r*: Pearson's correlation coefficient *r*; β: standardized coefficient β; [1]: Univariate regression analysis; [2]: Multivariate regression analysis (sleep duration, age); [3]: Multivariate regression analysis (sleep duration, age, midpoint of sleep); a: *p* < 0.01, b: *p* < 0.05, number in bold showed significant variables.

Total energy and alcohol (% energy) intakes were significantly higher in male versus female subjects. On the other hand, male subjects had significantly lower intakes of protein (% energy), fat (% energy), and carbohydrates (% energy), as well as energy-adjusted (per 1000 kcal) nutrients other than sodium. Regarding food-group intakes (g/1000 kcal), those of bread, confections, potatoes, vegetables, pulses, fish and shell fish, meat, eggs, milk, and milk products were significantly higher among women than among men, whereas the reverse was true for rice and noodles.

Data regarding total energy; % energy from alcohol, protein, fat, and carbohydrates; and energy-adjusted (per 1000 kcal) nutrient and food-group intakes by sex are presented in Tables 2 and 3, respectively. Regarding macronutrients, small but significant correlations were observed between sleep duration and the percentage of energy derived from protein, both with and without adjustments for the midpoint of sleep among men (*r* = 0.126, *p* < 0.05). The energy-adjusted intakes of sodium, vitamin D, and vitamin B12 correlated significantly with sleep duration in men after adjusting for the midpoint of sleep (sodium: *r* = 0.115, *p* < 0.01; vitamin D: *r* = 0.218, *p* < 0.01; vitamin B12: *r* = 0.192, *p* < 0.01).

Regarding food-group intakes, we observed significant correlations between sleep duration and the intakes of bread, pulses, and fish and shellfish among men, both with and without adjustment for the midpoint of sleep (bread: $r = 0.092$, $p < 0.05$; pulses: $r = 0.141$, $p < 0.01$; fish and shellfish: $r = 0.183$, $p < 0.01$).

In contrast, we observed no significant correlations between dietary intakes and sleep duration among women (Table 3).

4. Discussion

To the best of our knowledge, this is the first study to investigate the relationship between sleep duration and dietary intake of specific nutrients, while considering variations in sleep timing (i.e., the midpoint of sleep). In an earlier survey of a US population, energy intakes across sleep duration groups exhibited an inverse U-shaped distribution [8]. Another previous study also found an association of sleep deprivation with increased energy intake [7]. However, our results did not indicate a significant correlation between energy intakes and sleep duration. The reason for this discrepancy should be clarified in future studies.

We observed a significant sex-based difference in energy (kcal/day) intakes; specifically, male subjects had higher energy intakes. The observed sex-related differences in the intakes of several energy-adjusted nutrients, such as protein, calcium, and iron, are attributed to differences in total energy intake. After adjusting for the midpoint of sleep, we found that the intakes of specific dietary nutrients were correlated with sleep duration among men. The percentage of energy from protein and the energy-adjusted intakes of sodium, vitamin D, and vitamin B12 exhibited small but significant increases that correlated with sleep duration. In addition, the intakes of bread, pulses, and fish and shellfish were correlated with sleep duration, regardless of whether we adjusted for the midpoint of sleep. These results agree with those of a previous study that investigated the relationship between sleep duration and dietary intake in the NHANES; in that study, short sleepers reported lower intakes of protein, carbohydrates, dietary fiber, and total fats than did normal sleepers [8]. Another previous study of adolescents with short sleep durations observed decreased intakes of healthy foods such as vegetables, fruits, and fish, and increased intakes of unhealthy fast foods such as pizza, hamburgers, pasta dishes, and snack products [18]. Short sleep duration–induced changes in food preferences may be accompanied by changes in nutrient intakes, possibly consequent to changes in the secretion of appetite-related hormones such as leptin and ghrelin [5,6,19]. Previous studies also reported that total blood levels and circadian changes in cortisol, insulin, and thyroid-stimulating hormone levels were affected by a short sleep duration [20–22]. Additionally, a short sleep duration was found to enhance activity in brain reward and food-sensitive centers in response to unhealthy food stimuli [23]. A short sleep duration also led to extended hours of wakefulness, thus presenting additional opportunities for increased food intake [5]. Although these parameters were not evaluated objectively in the present study, they should be addressed in future studies. However, we observed no significant correlations between sleep duration and dietary intake among women in this study. We cannot clearly explain this sex-based difference. Previous studies either combined the data of men and women for analysis [8,12] or surveyed only women [13,24]. However, sex has been suggested as an important factor regarding food and nutrient intakes [25]. Our present study suggested a sex-based difference in the influence of sleep duration on dietary intake. Thus, the results of this study suggest a significant and independent association of sleep duration with dietary intakes of certain nutrients and foods in a Japanese adult male population after controlling for variations in the midpoint of sleep. Clock genes may influence the relationship between sleep timing and dietary intake. Circadian clocks, which are controlled by clock genes, regulate various biological rhythms, including sleep timing and the endocrine system [26]. In addition, mouse clock gene mutants exhibit increased alcohol intake [27]. Clock genes were also found to regulate metabolism [26]. In the meantime, periodic meal intake was found to be an important circadian clock entrainment signal in animals [28]. Furthermore, certain nutrients and food components, such as glucose, ethanol, caffeine, thiamine, and retinoic acid, can induce phase-shifts in circadian rhythms [29]. However, we could not identify if reverse causation occurred because this epidemiological study was cross-sectional. Further studies are required to understand the relationships between dietary intakes and circadian clocks in humans.

We should note several limitations of our study. First, information about both dietary nutrient intake and sleep duration was based on the participants' self-reports. However, the participants might have overestimated their vegetable intake and/or underestimated their intakes of sweets and high-fat foods [14] during the preceding month. Still, the BDHQ was validated and used in several previous studies. Therefore, we used self-reporting methods to obtain data from our large sample. Further studies involving biomarkers and digital dietary records of nutrient intake are warranted. We also did not obtain information about the participants' usage of caffeine, antidepressants, or other medications that could influence appetite and/or sleep. Furthermore, the sleep duration and midpoint of sleep were derived from the same questionnaire, despite the lack of a significant correlation between these two variables. The subjective sleep duration might also have been misclassified because of reporting errors, which warrants the use of an objective sleep measurement such as actigraphy. Second, the results of this study might have been affected by sampling bias, as health-conscious people may have been more likely to participate in this type of health survey. However, the mean nutrient and food intake values in this population were almost the same as those reported by similarly aged adults in the National Nutrition and Health Survey in Japan [30]. Therefore, the subjects of the present study may be representative of the general Japanese population, at least regarding the study variables.

5. Conclusions

This study found that sleep duration was significantly and independently associated with the dietary intakes of certain nutrients and foods in a Japanese adult male population after controlling for variations in the midpoint of sleep.

Acknowledgments: This study was supported by a grant from the Research Project on Development of Agricultural Products and Foods with Health-promoting benefits (NARO), Japan.

Author Contributions: Author Komada, Ueda, Saito, Sakaguchi, Mitarai, Suzuki and Inoue Y. designed the study and collected the data. Author Narisawa, Tamura, and Inoue S. provided summaries of previous research studies. Author Komada and Inoue Y. wrote the manuscript.

Conflicts of Interest: Department of Somnology, Tokyo Medical University, is supported by Philips Respironics GK, Alfresa Pharma Corporation, Otsuka Pharmaceutical Co., Ltd., and MSD K.K. Yoko Komada has received grant support from Alfresa Pharma Corporation, MSD K.K., Eisai Co., ltd. Yuichi Inoue has received clinically pertinent fees, and lecture fees and research funding from Nippon Boehringer Ingelheim, Takeda Pharmaceutical, Astellas Pharma, Philips Respironics, Alfresa Pharma, MSD, Pacific Medico, Otsuka Pharmaceutical, Eisai, Yoshitomiyakuhin, and Hisamitsu Pharmaceutical. This does not alter the authors' adherence to *Nutrients* policies on sharing data and materials.

References

1. Van Cauter, E.; Spiegel, K.; Tasali, E.; Leproult, R. Metabolic consequences of sleep and sleep loss. *Sleep Med.* **2008**, *9* (Suppl. 1), S23–S28. [CrossRef]
2. Magee, L.; Hale, L. Longitudinal associations between sleep duration and subsequent weight gain: A systematic review. *Sleep Med. Rev.* **2012**, *16*, 231–241. [CrossRef] [PubMed]
3. Owens, J. Insufficient sleep in adolescents and young adults: An update on causes and consequences. *Pediatrics* **2014**, *134*, e921–e932. [CrossRef] [PubMed]
4. Spiegel, K.; Tasali, E.; Penev, P.; Van Cauter, E. Brief communication: Sleep curtailment in healthy young men is associated with decreased leptin levels, elevated ghrelin levels, and increased hunger and appetite. *Ann. Intern. Med.* **2004**, *141*, 846–850. [CrossRef] [PubMed]
5. Dashti, H.S.; Scheer, F.A.; Jacques, P.F.; Lamon-Fava, S.; Ordovas, J.M. Short sleep duration and dietary intake: Epidemiologic evidence, mechanisms, and health implications. *Adv. Nutr.* **2015**, *6*, 648–659. [CrossRef] [PubMed]
6. Taheri, S.; Lin, L.; Austin, D.; Young, T.; Mignot, E. Short sleep duration is associated with reduced leptin, elevated ghrelin, and increased body mass index. *PLoS Med.* **2004**, *1*, e62. [CrossRef] [PubMed]

7. St-Onge, M.P. The role of sleep duration in the regulation of energy balance: Effects on energy intakes and expenditure. *J. Clin. Sleep Med.* **2013**, *9*, 73–80. [CrossRef] [PubMed]
8. Grandner, M.A.; Jackson, N.; Gerstner, J.R.; Knutson, K.L. Dietary nutrients associated with short and long sleep duration. Data from a nationally representative sample. *Appetite* **2013**, *64*, 71–80. [CrossRef] [PubMed]
9. Shi, Z.; McEvoy, M.; Luu, J.; Attia, J. Dietary fat and sleep duration in chinese men and women. *Int. J. Obes.* **2008**, *32*, 1835–1840. [CrossRef] [PubMed]
10. Kant, A.K.; Graubard, B.I. Association of self-reported sleep duration with eating behaviors of american adults: Nhanes 2005–2010. *Am. J. Clin. Nutr.* **2014**, *100*, 938–947. [CrossRef] [PubMed]
11. Olds, T.S.; Maher, C.A.; Matricciani, L. Sleep duration or bedtime? Exploring the relationship between sleep habits and weight status and activity patterns. *Sleep* **2011**, *34*, 1299–1307. [PubMed]
12. Kanerva, N.; Kronholm, E.; Partonen, T.; Ovaskainen, M.L.; Kaartinen, N.E.; Konttinen, H.; Broms, U.; Mannisto, S. Tendency toward eveningness is associated with unhealthy dietary habits. *Chronobiol. Int.* **2012**, *29*, 920–927. [CrossRef] [PubMed]
13. Sato-Mito, N.; Sasaki, S.; Murakami, K.; Okubo, H.; Takahashi, Y.; Shibata, S.; Yamada, K.; Sato, K. The midpoint of sleep is associated with dietary intake and dietary behavior among young Japanese women. *Sleep Med.* **2011**, *12*, 289–294. [CrossRef] [PubMed]
14. Kobayashi, S.; Murakami, K.; Sasaki, S.; Okubo, H.; Hirota, N.; Notsu, A.; Fukui, M.; Date, C. Comparison of relative validity of food group intakes estimated by comprehensive and brief-type self-administered diet history questionnaires against 16 day dietary records in Japanese adults. *Public Health Nutr.* **2011**, *14*, 1200–1211. [CrossRef] [PubMed]
15. Science and Technology Agency. *Standard Tables of Food Composition in Japan*; Printing Bureau of the Ministry of Finance: Tokyo, Japan, 2005. (In Japanese)
16. Buysse, D.J.; Reynolds, C.F., 3rd; Monk, T.H.; Berman, S.R.; Kupfer, D.J. The pittsburgh sleep quality index: A new instrument for psychiatric practice and research. *Psychiatry Res.* **1989**, *28*, 193–213. [CrossRef]
17. Doi, Y.; Minowa, M.; Uchiyama, M.; Okawa, M.; Kim, K.; Shibui, K.; Kamei, Y. Psychometric assessment of subjective sleep quality using the Japanese version of the Pittsburgh Sleep Quality Index (PSQI-J) in psychiatric disordered and control subjects. *Psychiatry Res.* **2000**, *97*, 165–172. [CrossRef]
18. Garaulet, M.; Ortega, F.B.; Ruiz, J.R.; Rey-Lopez, J.P.; Beghin, L.; Manios, Y.; Cuenca-Garcia, M.; Plada, M.; Diethelm, K.; Kafatos, A.; et al. Short sleep duration is associated with increased obesity markers in european adolescents: Effect of physical activity and dietary habits. The Helena study. *Int. J. Obes.* **2011**, *35*, 1308–1317. [CrossRef] [PubMed]
19. Markwald, R.R.; Melanson, E.L.; Smith, M.R.; Higgins, J.; Perreault, L.; Eckel, R.H.; Wright, K.P., Jr. Impact of insufficient sleep on total daily energy expenditure, food intake, and weight gain. *Proc. Natl. Acad. Sci. USA* **2013**, *110*, 5695–5700. [CrossRef] [PubMed]
20. Spiegel, K.; Knutson, K.; Leproult, R.; Tasali, E.; Van Cauter, E. Sleep loss: A novel risk factor for Insulin resistance and type 2 diabetes. *J. Appl. Physiol.* **2005**, *99*, 2008–2019. [CrossRef] [PubMed]
21. Spiegel, K.; Leproult, R.; L'Hermite-Baleriaux, M.; Copinschi, G.; Penev, P.D.; Van Cauter, E. Leptin levels are dependent on sleep duration: Relationships with sympathovagal balance, carbohydrate regulation, cortisol, and thyrotropin. *J. Clin. Endocrinol. Metab.* **2004**, *89*, 5762–5771. [CrossRef] [PubMed]
22. Chaput, J.P.; Despres, J.P.; Bouchard, C.; Tremblay, A. Short sleep duration is associated with reduced leptin levels and increased adiposity: Results from the quebec family study. *Obesity* **2007**, *15*, 253–261. [CrossRef] [PubMed]
23. St-Onge, M.P.; Wolfe, S.; Sy, M.; Shechter, A.; Hirsch, J. Sleep restriction increases the neuronal response to unhealthy food in normal-weight individuals. *Int. J. Obes.* **2014**, *38*, 411–416. [CrossRef] [PubMed]
24. Grandner, M.A.; Hale, L.; Moore, M.; Patel, N.P. Mortality associated with short sleep duration: The evidence, the possible mechanisms, and the future. *Sleep Med. Rev.* **2010**, *14*, 191–203. [CrossRef] [PubMed]
25. Zhang, J.; Temme, E.H.; Kesteloot, H. Sex ratio of total energy intake in adults: An analysis of dietary surveys. *Eur. J. Clin. Nutr.* **1999**, *53*, 542–551. [CrossRef] [PubMed]
26. Laposky, A.D.; Bass, J.; Kohsaka, A.; Turek, F.W. Sleep and circadian rhythms: Key components in the regulation of energy metabolism. *FEBS Lett.* **2008**, *582*, 142–151. [CrossRef] [PubMed]
27. Spanagel, R.; Rosenwasser, A.M.; Schumann, G.; Sarkar, D.K. Alcohol consumption and the body's biological clock. *Alcohol. Clin. Exp. Res.* **2005**, *29*, 1550–1557. [CrossRef] [PubMed]

28. Stephan, F.K. Broken circadian clocks: A clock gene mutation and entrainment by feeding. American journal of physiology. *Regul. Integr. Comp. Physiol.* **2003**, *285*, R32–R33. [CrossRef] [PubMed]

29. Froy, O. The relationship between nutrition and circadian rhythms in mammals. *Front. Neuroendocrinol.* **2007**, *28*, 61–71. [CrossRef] [PubMed]

30. The Ministry of Health, Labour and Welfare, Japan. National Health and Nutrition Survey Reports. Available online: http://www.mhlw.go.jp/bunya/kenkou/kenkou_eiyou_chousa.html (accessed on 1 November 2016).

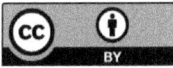

nutrients

MDPI

Article

Association between Serum Vitamin D Levels and Sleep Disturbance in Hemodialysis Patients

Bin Han *,†, **Fu-Xiang Zhu** †, **Chao Shi, Heng-Lan Wu and Xiao-Hong Gu**

Department of nephrology, First Affiliated Hospital of Jiaxing University, Jiaxing 314000, China;
zfxywh@163.com (F.-X.Z.); shichao@ymail.com (C.S.); wh1525487@sina.com (H.-L.W.);
zjl1499525408@sina.com (X.-H.G.)
* Correspondence: wmuhanbin@163.com; Tel.: +86-573-8208-3006
† These authors contributed equally to this work.

Received: 19 August 2016; Accepted: 7 February 2017; Published: 14 February 2017

Abstract: Sleep disturbance is a frequent and serious complication of hemodialysis (HD). Low serum vitamin D levels have been associated with sleep quality in non-HD subjects. Our aim was to examine the possible association between serum vitamin D levels and the presence of sleep disturbance in HD patients. We recruited 141 HD patients at the HD center of the First Affiliated Hospital of Jiaxing University during 2014–2015. Serum levels of 25-hydroxyvitamin D (25(OH)D) were determined by the competitive protein-binding assay. Sleep quality was measured using the Pittsburgh Sleep Quality Index (PSQI). Demographic, clinical and laboratory data were recorded. Meanwhile, 117 healthy control subjects were also recruited and underwent measurement of 25(OH)D. Eighty-eight patients (62.4%) had sleep disturbance (PSQI scores $\geq$ 5). Patients with sleep disturbance showed lower levels of 25(OH)D as compared to those without sleep disturbance (85.6 $\pm$ 37.4 vs. 39.1 $\pm$ 29.1 nmol/L, $p < 0.001$). In multivariate analyses, serum levels of 25(OH)D ($\leq$48.0 nmol/L) were independently associated with sleep disturbance in HD patients (OR 9.897, 95% CI 3.356–29.187, $p < 0.001$) after adjustment for possible variables. Our study demonstrates that low serum levels of vitamin D are independently associated with sleep disturbance in HD patients, but the finding needs to be confirmed in future experimental and clinical studies.

Keywords: vitamin; sleep disturbance; hemodialysis

1. Introduction

Sleep disturbance is extremely common in hemodialysis (HD) patients, with prevalence ranging from 41% to 83% [1–4]. The presence of sleep disturbance has been associated with reduced quality of life [3,5] and increased mortality [3,6] in HD patients. Moreover, it has been reported to be involved in the development of cardiovascular diseases in patients undergoing maintenance HD [7]. However, the pathogenesis of sleep disturbance in HD patients remains unclear.

As a fundamental micronutrient, vitamin D is extremely essential for human health [8]. A large body of preclinical studies has found the profusion of vitamin D receptors in specific areas of the brainstem that are thought to regulate sleep [9–11]. Furthermore, increasing clinical studies have shown that low serum levels of vitamin D are associated with poorer sleep, including low sleep efficiency and short sleep duration, in non-HD subjects, suggesting a potential role for vitamin D in maintaining healthy sleep [12,13]. Similarly, a significantly correlation between vitamin D levels and sleep quality has been found in patients with systemic lupus erythematosus (SLE) [14]. Recent uncontrolled clinical trials of vitamin D supplements in patients with sleep problems have reported improved sleep quality with higher levels of supplemental vitamin D [15,16].

At the global level, about one billion people have vitamin D insufficiency/deficiency [8]. In patients with chronic kidney disease (CKD) stage 5 on HD, the prevalence of vitamin D insufficiency/deficiency is up to 96.6% [17]. The presence of vitamin D anomalies has been associated with increased risk of cardiovascular outcomes and mortality in patients with end-stage renal disease (ESRD) on HD [18,19]. To date, however, no study has evaluated the potential relationship of vitamin D to sleep disturbance in HD patients. Given the involvement of vitamin D in sleep quality in non-HD subjects and the acknowledged high prevalence of vitamin D anomalies in HD patients, whether serum vitamin D levels are correlated with sleep disturbance in HD patients was examined.

2. Methods

2.1. Study Population

Patients undergoing maintenance HD with a frequency of three times per week were consecutively recruited at the HD center of the First Affiliated Hospital of Jiaxing University between 12 May 2014 and 20 June 2015. Eligibility criteria included: (i) Chinese ethnicity; (ii) aged over 18 years; (iii) receipt of maintenance HD therapy (single-pool Kt/V > 1.0) for at least 3 months; (iv) having the ability and willingness to give informed consent. Exclusion criteria were: (i) patients with severe visual or auditory impairment or cognitive dysfunction; (ii) patients with malignancy, autoimmune diseases or active infections; (iii) current treatment of immunosuppressants, immunomodulators or steroids; (iv) patients with a history of psychiatric disorders (clinical diagnosis or previous treatment); (v) concomitant chronic obstructive pulmonary disease and sleep apnea (clinical diagnosis or previous treatment); (vi) patients taking vitamin D supplementation or with osteoporosis. Meanwhile, 117 healthy volunteers without renal impairment, concomitant chronic obstructive pulmonary disease, sleep apnea, sleep complaints or a history of psychiatric disorders, were recruited from a health survey. Written informed consents were obtained from all participating subjects according to the principles of the Declaration of Helsinki (1989) and the study was approved by the Ethics Committee of the First Affiliated Hospital of Jiaxing University. The methods were carried out in accordance with the approved guidelines.

2.2. Clinical Variables

Demographic and clinical data including time on HD and dialysis shift were obtained through participant report and electronic medical records. Blood samples were collected according to a standard protocol between 8 a.m. and 10 a.m. each morning. Blood samples were obtained for all subjects and stored at $-80\,^{\circ}$C until measurement. All blood samples of the controls were collected at the end of August 2014. Serum 25-hydroxyvitamin D [25(OH)D] was chosen to measure vitamin D status for all subjects because of its widespread clinical application, standardized ranges and testing protocol. Serum 25(OH)D levels were test by using a competitive protein-binding assay at our hospital's laboratory. The intra-assay coefficient of variation was 7%–10%. Serum 25(OH)D in HD patients was recorded and divided into four quartiles ($\leq$26.0, 26.1–48.0, 48.1–84.0 and $\geq$84.1 nmol/L), as the raw 25(OH)D data were skewed. Blood pressure was measured at admission using an automated sphygmomanometer after at least 5 min of rest.

2.3. Measurement

Sleep quality was measured using the Pittsburgh Sleep Quality Index (PSQI) [20]. The self-administered questionnaire assesses individual's sleep quality during the past month and contains 19 items which yield seven components, including subjective sleep quality, sleep latency, sleep duration, sleep efficiency, sleep disturbance, use of sleep medications, and daytime dysfunction. Each component is scored from 0 to 3, which yields a total PSQI score from 0 to 21, with high PSQI score indicating poor sleep quality. According to Buysse et al., subjects with a PSQI score $\geq$5 are considered as "poor sleepers", while those with a score <5 are defined as "good sleepers". The Chinese Version of PSQI has been used in Taiwan [21].

2.4. Statistical Analysis

Data were analyzed using SPSS for windows (SPSS Inc., Chicago, IL, USA) version 17. All continuous variables are expressed as the mean $\pm$ standard deviation (SD). The categorical variables were compared using the Pearson χ^2 test. Student's t test or one-way analysis of variance (ANOVA) was used for normally distributed variables, while the Mann-Whitney U test was performed for parametric variables with non-normal distributions. Post hoc tests were conducted to determine the difference between groups, followed by Fisher's least significant difference (LSD) test. The association between serum 25(OH)D levels and sleep disturbance in HD patients was evaluated by logistic regression (Enter method) including all factors with $p < 0.05$ in the univariate analysis. The results were expressed as adjusted odds ratios (OR) with the corresponding 95% confidence intervals (CI). Level of statistical significance was defined as $p < 0.05$.

3. Results

3.1. Group Differences in Demographic and Clinical Information

A total of 141 HD patients (86 men, 55 women) with a mean age of 68 years were enrolled in the current study. The PSQI total score was 8.5 ± 4.3 and 88 patients (62.4%) were poor sleepers with PSQI global scores ≥ 5. The sub-scores were as follows: sleep quality, 1.2 ± 0.63; sleep onset latency, 1.4 ± 1.20; sleep duration, 1.54 ± 1.14; sleep efficacy, 0.29 ± 0.85; sleep disturbance 1.72 ± 0.79; daytime dysfunction, 2.23 ± 1.21. None of them received vitamin D supplementation and psychiatric drugs. There were no significant differences in mean age and gender (M/F) between HD patients and healthy volunteers. No between-season sampling differences were observed for the 25(OH)D levels in HD patients: spring ($n = 17$), 46.7 ± 30.7 nmol/L; summer ($n = 60$), 58.9 ± 37.5 nmol/L; fall ($n = 51$), 60.3 ± 41.8 nmol/L; and winter ($n = 13$), 44.2 ± 27.9 nmol/L ($p = 0.40$).

HD patients showed markedly lower serum 25(OH)D levels as compared to normal controls (56.6 ± 39.5 vs. 68.8 ± 19.9 nmol/L, $p = 0.002$). The serum 25(OH)D levels were significantly lower in poor sleepers than in good sleepers (39.1 ± 29.1 vs. 85.6 ± 37.4 nmol/L, $p < 0.001$). Furthermore, significant differences were observed between poor sleepers and good sleepers in 25(OH)D level quartiles of patients ($p < 0.001$). Indeed, the proportion of subjects in lower quartiles (≤ 26.0 and 26.1–48.0 nmol/L) was significantly higher in patients with sleep disturbance (both $p < 0.001$), while the proportion of subjects in higher quartiles (48.1–84.0 and ≥ 84.1 nmol/L) was significantly lower in patients with sleep disturbance (both $p < 0.001$) (Table 1).

When compared to good sleepers, the poor sleepers had spent a longer time on HD (2 (1–4) vs. 1 (1–2) years, $p < 0.001$), had a lower serum hemoglobin level (90.99 ± 18.30 vs. $109.96 + 11.05$ g/L, $p < 0.001$), a lower serum albumin level (32.54 ± 5.72 vs. 37.73 ± 3.63 g/L, $p < 0.001$), a lower serum calcium level (2.08 ± 0.21 vs. 2.24 ± 0.24 mmol/L, $p < 0.001$), a higher phosphate level (1.59 ± 0.57 vs. 1.56 ± 0.45 mmol/L, $p = 0.024$), and a lower HDL-C level ($0.87(0.72–1.11)$ vs. $1.03(0.84–1.21)$ mmol/L, $p = 0.004$) (Table 1).

3.2. Independent Characteristics of Patients with Sleep Disturbance

With all HD patients taken as a whole, the presence of sleep disturbance taken as a dependent variable, and quartile 3 and quartile 4 taken as the references used for levels of serum 25(OH)D in the logistic analysis, 25(OH)D levels (≤ 48.0 nmol/L) were independently associated with the presence of sleep disturbance in HD patients (OR 9.897, 95% CI 3.356–29.187, $p < 0.001$). Moreover, lower levels of hemoglobin, lower levels of albumin and higher levels of phosphorus were significantly associated with the presence of sleep disturbance in HD patients (OR 0.954, 95% CI 0.921–0.988, $p = 0.009$; OR 0.867, 95% CI 0.760–0.989, $p = 0.034$ and OR 3.423, 95% CI 1.061–11.044, $p = 0.039$, respectively) (Table 2).

Table 1. Demographic, clinical and laboratory characteristics of the sample.

Variables	Poor Sleepers (PSQI ≥ 5, *n* = 88)	Good Sleepers (PSQI < 5, *n* = 53)	Normal Controls (*n* = 117)
Gender (M/F)	52/36	34/19	68/49
Age (years)	59.7 ± 15.3	62.8 ± 12.5	60.1 ± 14.0
BMI (kg/m²)	22.6 ± 3.4	21.7 ± 2.7	22.8 ± 2.9
Education level 1/2 [a]	21 (23.9)	16 (30.2)	
Widowed	11 (11.7)	3 (5.7)	
Current smoking	18 (20.5)	9 (17.0)	
Current drinking	11 (12.5)	6 (11.3)	
Cause of renal failure			
Diabetes	28 (31.8)	15 (28.3)	
Hypertension	28 (31.8)	11 (20.8)	
Glomerulonephritis	16 (18.2)	14 (26.4)	
Other	16 (18.2)	13 (24.5)	
Time on HD (years)	2 (1–4) [b]	1 (1–2)	
Dialysis shift (morning/evening)	54/34	23/20	
SBP (mmHg)	148.6 ± 27.3	141.6 ± 32.7	
DBP (mmHg)	76.9 ± 15.0	76.7 ± 15.0	
Hemoglobin (g/L)	91.0 ± 18.3 [b]	111.0 ± 11.1	
Albumin (g/L)	32.5 ± 5.7 [b]	37.7 ± 3.6	
Fasting glucose (mmol/L)	4.7 (4.0–5.9)	4.5 (3.9–6.8)	
Creatinine (FV)	600.6 ± 262.1	649.7 ± 255.1	
Uric acid (μmol/L)	358.3 ± 166.8	332.4 ± 121.0	
Calcium (mmol/L)	2.08 ± 0.21 [b]	2.24 ± 0.24	
Phosphate (mmol/L)	1.59 ± 0.57 [c]	1.56 ± 0.45	
iPTH (pg/mL)	239.9 (124.9–431.0)	211.9 (90.0–314.4)	
Triglyceride (mmol/L)	1.55 (1.17–2.25)	1.60 (1.11–2.65)	
Total cholesterol (mmol/L)	4.29 (3.57–5.11)	4.36 (3.70–5.60)	
LDL-C (mmol/L)	2.58 (1.98–3.09)	2.42 (1.94–3.07)	
HDL-C (mmol/L)	0.87 (0.72–1.11) [c]	1.03 (0.84–1.21)	
25(OH)D [d]			
Quartile 1	36 (40.9) [b]	3 (5.7)	
Quartile 2	28 (31.8) [b]	4 (7.5)	
Quartile 3	12 (13.6) [b]	23 (43.4)	
Quartile 4	12 (13.6) [b]	23 (43.4)	
25(OH)D (nmol/L)	39.1 ± 29.1 [b,e]	85.6 ± 37.4 [e]	68.8 ± 19.9

Data are expressed as number (percentage) or means (±SD) or medians (IQR). Abbreviations: PSQI, Pittsburgh Sleep Quality Index; BMI, body mass index; HD, hemodialysis; SBP, systolic blood pressure; DBP, diastolic blood pressure; iPTH, intact parathyroid hormone; LDL-C, low-density lipoprotein cholesterol; HDL-C, high-density lipoprotein cholesterol; 25(OH)D, 25-hydroxyvitamin D. [a] 1 Bachelor or above, 2 elementary school, Junior high school, senior high school; [b] $p < 0.001$ compared with good sleepers; [c] $p < 0.05$ compared with good sleepers; [d] $p < 0.001$ between poor sleepers and good sleepers in 25(OH)D level quartiles of patients; [e] $p < 0.001$ compared with normal controls.

Table 2. Characteristics associated with sleep disturbance in HD patients [a].

Variables	OR (95% CI)	*p* Value
25(OH)D [b]	9.897 (3.356–29.187)	<0.001
Time on HD		0.687
Hemoglobin	0.954 (0.921–0.988)	0.009
Albumin	0.867 (0.760–0.989)	0.034
Calcium		0.306
Phosphate	3.423 (1.061–11.044)	0.039
HDL-C		0.715

25(OH)D, 25-hydroxyvitamin D; HD, hemodialysis; OR, odds ratio; CI, confidence interval; HDL-C, high-density lipoprotein cholesterol. [a] Contains only the variables which were significant ($p < 0.05$) in the multivariable model; [b] Quartile 1 and quartile 2.

4. Discussion

To the best of our knowledge, this is the first study to analyze the association between serum levels of vitamin D and sleep quality in HD patients. We found that low serum levels of vitamin D were significantly associated with sleep disturbance in HD patients, which is similar to the findings of previous studies in elderly adults and patients with SLE [12–14]. Our finding might have important implications in providing novel proposals for the prevention and treatment of sleep disturbance in HD patients.

In the present study, we found that 62.4% of HD patients had sleep disturbance, which is consistent with the findings of recent research [4,22]. Currently, despite many available documents, it remains difficult to determine the true prevalence of sleep disturbance in HD patients, possibly due to these differences in study designs, the time of sleep evaluation, the source of patient recruitment, and race/ethnicity [23]. Our results also demonstrated that lower levels of hemoglobin, lower levels of albumin and higher levels of phosphorus were risk factors for the development of sleep disturbance in HD patients, which broadly agrees with the results of earlier studies [4,24,25].

We found that serum levels of vitamin D were significantly lower in poor sleepers than in good sleepers. Sleep disturbance is associated with increased food intake and obesity which is an important risk factor for vitamin D deficiency [26,27]. Nevertheless, there was no intergroup difference in BMI in our HD cohort. Since serum levels of vitamin D are directly related to sunlight exposure in humans [8], low vitamin D levels of the poor sleepers could result from decreased exposure to sunlight.

Importantly, we found that serum vitamin D levels were independently associated with the presence of sleep disturbance in HD patients. As mentioned earlier, a growing body of studies has reported low vitamin D levels with sleep disturbance in non-HD subjects [12–14]. Moreover, several uncontrolled clinical trials have demonstrated the positive effects of vitamin D supplementation on sleep quality in non-HD subjects [15,16]. The exact mechanisms by which vitamin D could affect sleep are unclear. In animal studies, vitamin D receptors have been found in specific regions of the central nervous system, some of which regulate sleep, including the anterior and posterior hypothalamus, the raphe nuclei, the midbrain central gray, and the nucleus reticularis pontis caudalis and oralis [9–11,28], which suggests vitamin D may play a role in individuals' sleep. Another possible explanation is the effect of vitamin D on the immune system. Vitamin D plays a key role in modulating the secretion of inflammatory cytokines, such as tumor necrosis factor-α (TNF-α), interleukin-6 (IL-6), and interleukin-1β (IL-1β) [29–31]. A growing body of evidence suggests the involvement of IL-1β, TNF-α, and other inflammatory cytokines in sleep regulation [32,33]. Plasma levels of IL-1, IL-6 and TNF-α are increased in maintenance HD patients [34,35], which correlates with a poor outcome in these patients [36,37]. Vitamin D deficiency is extremely common in HD patients and is an independent predictor of disease progression and mortality in these patients [17–19]. Therefore, these results mentioned above suggest that vitamin D might play an important role in sleep disturbance in HD patients.

Some limitations of the present study should be noted. First, the association between vitamin D levels and sleep traits has been reported to vary by race/ethnicity [23]. Subjects in our sample were recruited from the Han Chinese population. Therefore, our results may not be readily generalized to other populations. Second, the effects of other variables on vitamin D levels, such as dietary intake and lifestyle changes, were not considered in the current study. Finally, we did not perform an objective sleep assessment such as a polysomnography to prove our findings. Further studies with a polysomnogram or other objective measures are needed. However, the correlation between the PSQI and polysomnography has been shown to be significant in certain domains [38].

5. Conclusions

In summary, despite of these limitations, our study demonstrates an important association between serum levels of vitamin D and sleep disturbance in patients undergoing maintenance HD. However, the finding would have to be confirmed in future experimental and clinical studies.

Acknowledgments: This work was funded by a grant from the Jiaxing Municipal Sci-Tech Bureau Program (2016BY28005). The authors express their gratitude to all subjects who participated in the current study.

Author Contributions: The study was conceived and designed by B.H. and F.X.Z. C.S., X.H.G. and H.L.W. prepared the samples and analyzed the data. B.H. and F.X.Z. participated in interpreting and analyzing the data. B.H. wrote the paper. All authors reviewed the manuscript.

Conflicts of Interest: The authors declare no conflict of interest.

References

1. Pai, M.F.; Hsu, S.P.; Yang, S.Y.; Ho, T.I.; Lai, C.F.; Peng, Y.S. Sleep disturbance in chronic hemodialysis patients: The impact of depression and anemia. *Ren. Fail.* **2007**, *29*, 673–677. [CrossRef] [PubMed]
2. Parker, K.P. Sleep disturbances in dialysis patients. *Sleep Med. Rev.* **2003**, *7*, 131–143. [CrossRef] [PubMed]
3. Elder, S.J.; Pisoni, R.L.; Akizawa, T.; Fissell, R.; Andreucci, V.E.; Fukuhara, S.; Kurokawa, K.; Rayner, H.C.; Furniss, A.L.; Port, F.K.; et al. Sleep quality predicts quality of life and mortality risk in haemodialysis patients: Results from the dialysis outcomes and practice patterns study (dopps). *Nephrol. Dial. Transplant.* **2008**, *23*, 998–1004. [CrossRef] [PubMed]
4. Einollahi, B.; Motalebi, M.; Rostami, Z.; Nemati, E.; Salesi, M. Sleep quality among iranian hemodialysis patients: A multicenter study. *Nephro-Urol. Mon.* **2015**, *7*, e23849.
5. Turkmen, K.; Erdur, F.M.; Guney, I.; Gaipov, A.; Turgut, F.; Altintepe, L.; Saglam, M.; Tonbul, H.Z.; Abdel-Rahman, E.M. Sleep quality, depression, and quality of life in elderly hemodialysis patients. *Int. J. Nephrol. Renov. Dis.* **2012**, *5*, 135–142. [CrossRef] [PubMed]
6. Brekke, F.B.; Waldum, B.; Amro, A.; Osthus, T.B.; Dammen, T.; Gudmundsdottir, H.; Os, I. Self-perceived quality of sleep and mortality in norwegian dialysis patients. *Hemodial. Int.* **2014**, *18*, 87–94. [CrossRef] [PubMed]
7. Unruh, M.; Kurella Tamura, M.; Larive, B.; Rastogi, A.; James, S.; Schiller, B.; Gassman, J.; Chan, C.; Lockridge, R.; Kliger, A. Impact of sleep quality on cardiovascular outcomes in hemodialysis patients: Results from the frequent hemodialysis network study. *Am. J. Nephrol.* **2011**, *33*, 398–406. [CrossRef] [PubMed]
8. Holick, M.F. Vitamin D deficiency. *N. Engl. J. Med.* **2007**, *357*, 266–281. [CrossRef] [PubMed]
9. Musiol, I.M.; Stumpf, W.E.; Bidmon, H.J.; Heiss, C.; Mayerhofer, A.; Bartke, A. Vitamin D nuclear binding to neurons of the septal, substriatal and amygdaloid area in the siberian hamster (phodopus sungorus) brain. *Neuroscience* **1992**, *48*, 841–848. [CrossRef]
10. Stumpf, W.E.; Bidmon, H.J.; Li, L.; Pilgrim, C.; Bartke, A.; Mayerhofer, A.; Heiss, C. Nuclear receptor sites for vitamin D-soltriol in midbrain and hindbrain of siberian hamster (phodopus sungorus) assessed by autoradiography. *Histochemistry* **1992**, *98*, 155–164. [CrossRef] [PubMed]
11. Stumpf, W.E.; O'Brien, L.P. 1,25 (OH)2 vitamin D3 sites of action in the brain. An autoradiographic study. *Histochemistry* **1987**, *87*, 393–406. [CrossRef] [PubMed]
12. Massa, J.; Stone, K.L.; Wei, E.K.; Harrison, S.L.; Barrett-Connor, E.; Lane, N.E.; Paudel, M.; Redline, S.; Ancoli-Israel, S.; Orwoll, E.; et al. Vitamin D and actigraphic sleep outcomes in older community-dwelling men: The mros sleep study. *Sleep* **2015**, *38*, 251–257. [CrossRef] [PubMed]
13. Kim, J.H.; Chang, J.H.; Kim, D.Y.; Kang, J.W. Association between self-reported sleep duration and serum vitamin D level in elderly korean adults. *J. Am. Geriatr. Soc.* **2014**, *62*, 2327–2332. [CrossRef] [PubMed]
14 Gholamrezaei, A.; Bonakdar, Z.S.; Mirbagher, L.; Hosseini, N. Sleep disorders in systemic lupus erythematosus. Does vitamin D play a role? *Lupus* **2014**, *23*, 1054–1058. [CrossRef] [PubMed]
15. Gominak, S.C.; Stumpf, W.E. The world epidemic of sleep disorders is linked to vitamin D deficiency. *Med. Hypotheses* **2012**, *79*, 132–135. [CrossRef] [PubMed]
16. Huang, W.; Shah, S.; Long, Q.; Crankshaw, A.K.; Tangpricha, V. Improvement of pain, sleep, and quality of life in chronic pain patients with vitamin D supplementation. *Clin. J. Pain* **2013**, *29*, 341–347. [CrossRef] [PubMed]
17. Krassilnikova, M.; Ostrow, K.; Bader, A.; Heeger, P.; Mehrotra, A. Low dietary intake of vitamin D and vitamin D deficiency in hemodialysis patients. *J. Nephrol. Ther.* **2014**, *4*, 166. [CrossRef] [PubMed]
18. Ravani, P.; Malberti, F.; Tripepi, G.; Pecchini, P.; Cutrupi, S.; Pizzini, P.; Mallamaci, F.; Zoccali, C. Vitamin D levels and patient outcome in chronic kidney disease. *Kidney Int.* **2009**, *75*, 88–95. [CrossRef] [PubMed]
19. Schiller, A.; Gadalean, F.; Schiller, O.; Timar, R.; Bob, F.; Munteanu, M.; Stoian, D.; Mihaescu, A.; Timar, B. Vitamin D deficiency—Prognostic marker or mortality risk factor in end stage renal disease patients with diabetes mellitus treated with hemodialysis—A prospective multicenter study. *PLoS ONE* **2015**, *10*, e0126586. [CrossRef] [PubMed]
20. Buysse, D.J.; Reynolds, C.F., III; Monk, T.H.; Berman, S.R.; Kupfer, D.J. The pittsburgh sleep quality index: A new instrument for psychiatric practice and research. *Psychiatry Res.* **1989**, *28*, 193–213. [CrossRef]

21. Tsai, P.S.; Wang, S.Y.; Wang, M.Y.; Su, C.T.; Yang, T.T.; Huang, C.J.; Fang, S.C. Psychometric evaluation of the chinese version of the pittsburgh sleep quality index (cpsqi) in primary insomnia and control subjects. *Qual. Life Res.* **2005**, *14*, 1943–1952. [CrossRef] [PubMed]

22. Joshwa, B.; Khakha, D.C.; Mahajan, S. Fatigue and depression and sleep problems among hemodialysis patients in a tertiary care center. *Saudi J. Kidney Dis. Transplant.* **2012**, *23*, 729–735.

23. Bertisch, S.M.; Sillau, S.; de Boer, I.H.; Szklo, M.; Redline, S. 25-hydroxyvitamin D concentration and sleep duration and continuity: Multi-ethnic study of atherosclerosis. *Sleep* **2015**, *38*, 1305–1311. [CrossRef] [PubMed]

24. Ezzat, H.; Mohab, A. Prevalence of sleep disorders among esrd patients. *Ren. Fail.* **2015**, *37*, 1013–1019. [CrossRef] [PubMed]

25. Unruh, M.L.; Hartunian, M.G.; Chapman, M.M.; Jaber, B.L. Sleep quality and clinical correlates in patients on maintenance dialysis. *Clin. Nephrol.* **2003**, *59*, 280–288. [CrossRef] [PubMed]

26. Chaput, J.P. Sleep patterns, diet quality and energy balance. *Physiol. Behav.* **2014**, *134*, 86–91. [CrossRef] [PubMed]

27. Earthman, C.P.; Beckman, L.M.; Masodkar, K.; Sibley, S.D. The link between obesity and low circulating 25-hydroxyvitamin D concentrations: Considerations and implications. *Int. J. Obes.* **2012**, *36*, 387–396. [CrossRef] [PubMed]

28. Mizoguchi, A.; Eguchi, N.; Kimura, K.; Kiyohara, Y.; Qu, W.M.; Huang, Z.L.; Mochizuki, T.; Lazarus, M.; Kobayashi, T.; Kaneko, T.; et al. Dominant localization of prostaglandin d receptors on arachnoid trabecular cells in mouse basal forebrain and their involvement in the regulation of non-rapid eye movement sleep. *Proc. Natl. Acad. Sci. USA* **2001**, *98*, 11674–11679. [CrossRef] [PubMed]

29. Al-Rasheed, N.M.; Al-Rasheed, N.M.; Bassiouni, Y.A.; Hasan, I.H.; Al-Amin, M.A.; Al-Ajmi, H.N.; Mohamad, R.A. Vitamin D attenuates pro-inflammatory TNF-alpha cytokine expression by inhibiting NF-small ka, CyrillicB/p65 signaling in hypertrophied rat hearts. *J. Physiol. Biochem.* **2015**, *71*, 289–299. [CrossRef] [PubMed]

30. Roy, P.; Nadeau, M.; Valle, M.; Bellmann, K.; Marette, A.; Tchernof, A.; Gagnon, C. Vitamin D reduces LPS-induced cytokine release in omental adipose tissue of women but not men. *Steroids* **2015**, *104*, 65–71. [CrossRef] [PubMed]

31. Sommer, A.; Fabri, M. Vitamin D regulates cytokine patterns secreted by dendritic cells to promote differentiation of il-22-producing t cells. *PLoS ONE* **2015**, *10*, e0130395. [CrossRef] [PubMed]

32. Obal, F., Jr.; Krueger, J.M. Biochemical regulation of non-rapid-eye-movement sleep. *Front. Biosci.* **2003**, *8*, d520–d550. [PubMed]

33. Krueger, J.M.; Majde, J.A.; Rector, D.M. Cytokines in immune function and sleep regulation. *Handb. Clin. Neurol.* **2011**, *98*, 229–240. [PubMed]

34. Herbelin, A.; Urena, P.; Nguyen, A.T.; Zingraff, J.; Descamps-Latscha, B. Elevated circulating levels of interleukin-6 in patients with chronic renal failure. *Kidney Int.* **1991**, *39*, 954–960. [CrossRef] [PubMed]

35. Pereira, B.J.; Shapiro, L.; King, A.J.; Falagas, M.E.; Strom, J.A.; Dinarello, C.A. Plasma levels of IL-1 beta, TNF alpha and their specific inhibitors in undialyzed chronic renal failure, CAPD and hemodialysis patients. *Kidney Int.* **1994**, *45*, 890–896. [CrossRef] [PubMed]

36. Barreto, D.V.; Barreto, F.C.; Liabeuf, S.; Temmar, M.; Lemke, H.D.; Tribouilloy, C.; Choukroun, G.; Vanholder, R.; Massy, Z.A.; European Uremic Toxin Work Group. Plasma interleukin-6 is independently associated with mortality in both hemodialysis and pre-dialysis patients with chronic kidney disease. *Kidney Int.* **2010**, *77*, 550–556. [CrossRef] [PubMed]

37. Kimmel, P.L.; Phillips, T.M.; Simmens, S.J.; Peterson, R.A.; Weihs, K.L.; Alleyne, S.; Cruz, I.; Yanovski, J.A.; Veis, J.H. Immunologic function and survival in hemodialysis patients. *Kidney Int.* **1998**, *54*, 236–244. [CrossRef] [PubMed]

38. Backhaus, J.; Junghanns, K.; Broocks, A.; Riemann, D.; Hohagen, F. Test-retest reliability and validity of the pittsburgh sleep quality index in primary insomnia. *J. Psychosom. Res.* **2002**, *53*, 737–740. [CrossRef]

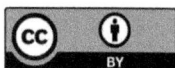

nutrients

MDPI

Article

Caffeine Consumption and Sleep Quality in Australian Adults

Emily J. Watson [1,*], Alison M. Coates [2], Mark Kohler [1] and Siobhan Banks [1]

[1] Centre for Sleep Research, University of South Australia, GPO Box 2471, Adelaide 5001, SA, Australia; Mark.Kohler@unisa.edu.au (M.K.); Siobhan.Banks@unisa.edu.au (S.B.)

[2] Alliance for Research in Exercise, Nutrition and Activity, University of South Australia, GPO Box 2471, Adelaide 5001, SA, Australia; alison.coates@unisa.edu.au

*   Correspondence: emily.watson@mymail.unisa.edu.au; Tel.: +61-8-8302-2453

Received: 24 May 2016; Accepted: 1 August 2016; Published: 4 August 2016

Abstract: Caffeine is commonly consumed to help offset fatigue, however, it can have several negative effects on sleep quality and quantity. The aim of this study was to determine the relationship between caffeine consumption and sleep quality in adults using a newly validated caffeine food frequency questionnaire (C-FFQ). In this cross sectional study, 80 adults (M $\pm$ SD: 38.9 $\pm$ 19.3 years) attended the University of South Australia to complete a C-FFQ and the Pittsburgh Sleep Quality Index (PSQI). Caffeine consumption remained stable across age groups while the source of caffeine varied. Higher total caffeine consumption was associated with decreased time in bed, as an estimate of sleep time ($r = -0.229$, $p = 0.041$), but other PSQI variables were not. Participants who reported poor sleep (PSQI global score $\geqslant$ 5) consumed 192.1 $\pm$ 122.5 mg (M $\pm$ SD) of caffeine which was significantly more than those who reported good sleep quality (PSQI global score < 5; 125.2 $\pm$ 62.6 mg; $p = 0.008$). The C-FFQ was found to be a quick but detailed way to collect population based caffeine consumption data. The data suggests that shorter sleep is associated with greater caffeine consumption, and that consumption is greater in adults with reduced sleep quality.

Keywords: sleep hygiene; caffeine intake; sleep quantity; sleep quality; caffeine food frequency questionnaire

1. Introduction

Caffeine is a widely consumed stimulant that is found in a variety of commonly consumed foods and beverages such as chocolate, soft drink (soda), tea, and coffee. Caffeine is commonly used as a fatigue countermeasure [1]. Due to its action on adenosine receptors [2,3] caffeine improves alertness [4]. The Australian Bureau of Statistics (ABS) showed that on average in 2011/2012 Australian adults aged 19–70 years had daily caffeine intakes ranging between 103 and 183 mg per day [5], with coffee being the most common source of caffeine [5]. Currently there are no consumption guidelines for caffeine in Australia. Therefore, it is important to examine the impact caffeine has on our sleep to make more informed recommendations on consumption and to better understand the impact in roles where caffeine consumption is higher.

While sleep need is individual and can differ from person to person, it is recommended that adults obtain 7–9 h per night [6]. Sleep has been shown to be important for many different cognitive and health reasons [7–10]. These benefits of sleep are not only dependent on total sleep time but also sleep quality, measured by variables such as sleep efficiency, and sleep onset latency. In adults there are a number of experimental studies investigating caffeine intake and its influence on sleep, with previous experimental studies finding that caffeine consumption can impact sleep quality [11,12]. Experimental laboratory studies have shown that when caffeine is ingested one to three hours before bedtime it decreases sleep efficiency [11–13], decreases total sleep time [11,12,14], and increases sleep onset latency [11–13]. It can also impact sleep architecture by reducing the amount of deep sleep [12,13]. However, the experimental nature of these studies does not take into account the impact of an individual's habitual caffeine intake or sleep patterns [15].

The effect of caffeine on sleep in university and general populations has been examined by several cross-sectional surveys and/or field studies [16–23]. In these studies increased caffeine consumption has been associated with decreased total sleep time [16,21], increased naps [16], decreased time in bed [17], increased sleep efficiency due to decreased time in bed [17], daytime sleepiness [20,22], and poor subjective sleep quality [22,23]. However, in other studies increased caffeine consumption does not impact total sleep time [17], daytime sleepiness [17] or Pittsburgh Sleep Quality Index (PSQI) global score [18,19,23]. Of these cross-sectional studies, only one looked at total caffeine consumption, i.e., all caffeinated beverages and caffeinated food consumed [18], while the others examined only caffeinated beverages [16,23] or a selection of caffeinated beverages [17,19–22]. Additionally, it was not always clear what question was asked to calculate caffeine consumption, or how the participants recorded their intake. Also many studies do not consider caffeine from chocolate or examine the separate sources of caffeine individually. This is important because different age groups may prefer particular sources of caffeine. Furthermore, all the previous questionnaire studies rely on an individual knowing what drinks/foods contain caffeine.

The mixed sleep patterns in caffeine users could be due to reporting inaccuracies. Few studies gather detailed information about caffeine consumption or sources of caffeine. To address this we have developed a caffeine food frequency questionnaire (C-FFQ) [24] that is short, does not rely on prior caffeine content knowledge, and gathers information about a wide variety of caffeine sources (coffee, tea, soft drink (soda) and chocolate beverages and foods). The overall aim of this study was to determine the relationship between caffeine consumption and sleep using this newly validated Caffeine Food Frequency Questionnaire (C-FFQ) [24] and self-reported sleep quality in adults. Specifically, this study aimed to: (1) identify what types of foods/beverages contribute to caffeine intake; (2) determine the impact of caffeine on different sleep quality variables (time in bed, sleep onset latency and sleep efficiency); and (3) determine the difference in caffeine intake between self-reported good and poor sleepers.

2. Materials and Methods

This cross-sectional study was designed to investigate the relationship between habitual caffeine consumption and sleep. It was conducted between March and August 2015 at the University of South Australia, Adelaide. The project was approved by the University of South Australia's Human Research Ethics Committee (HREC number: 30885).

2.1. Participants

Adults were recruited via University of South Australia web pages, social media, flyers, and word of mouth. Participants were ineligible for the study if they did not consume caffeine daily, were under the age of 18 years, not proficient in reading and writing in English, experiencing any sleep related conditions, have any conditions that affect caffeine intake, and not able to attend the University of South Australia. Participants were also excluded if they were taking any medications (prescription or over the counter, e.g., sleeping tablet, herbal supplement) to assist sleeping or alertness.

2.2. Procedure

All participants gave written informed consent before attending the University of South Australia. While at the University of South Australia participants were asked to complete questionnaires recalling caffeine consumption over the past week and sleep patterns over the past month.

2.3. Measures

Caffeine food frequency questionnaire (C-FFQ): The C-FFQ is a self-report, validated, and reliable questionnaire designed to assess the average daily caffeine consumption and the range of caffeinated products consumed [24]. The C-FFQ asks about beverages (e.g., energy drinks, soft drinks (soda), both hot and cold coffee and tea, and chocolate flavoured milk) and foods (e.g., chocolate) that were consumed in the previous week. The questionnaire requires participants to select the beverage or foods they consumed based on images of currently available products in Australia, indicating the specific brand, size, and the number of times over the last week each was consumed. Average daily total caffeine consumption and average daily caffeine amounts from beverage and food sources were expressed as mg/day.

Pittsburgh Sleep Quality Index (PSQI): The PSQI is a frequently used sleep quality questionnaire that has been shown to be reliable and valid in many populations [25–27]. The PSQI is a subjective measure of sleep which uses self-report to measure sleep quality and sleep disturbance over a one-month period. The PSQI contains 19 self-report questions and 5 questions rated by the bed partner or roommate. This study utilised only the self-rated questions which combine to form seven component scores [25]. The seven component scores include subjective sleep quality, sleep latency, sleep duration, habitual sleep efficiency, sleep disturbances, use of sleep medication, and daytime dysfunction. Each component has a range of 0–3 points. In all cases a score of 0 indicates the best outcome, while a score of 3 indicates the worst outcome. A global PSQI score is calculated from adding together all seven component scores to give an overall indication of sleep quality. The PSQI global score ranges from 0 to 21 points, with 0 indicating no difficulty and 21 severe difficulties. A global score of ≥ 5 indicates poor sleep quality [25]. This cut-off has been shown to have high specificity and sensitivity for distinguishing insomnia patients and controls [25,27].

2.4. Statistical Analysis

The C-FFQ calculates a total caffeine value and caffeine values for beverage and food subcategories as mg/day. All data were checked for normality and caffeine variables were found to be positively skewed. Log transformation of total caffeine intake allowed correction to a normal distribution; however, due to the skew of caffeine from individual beverage and food categories they could not be transformed. Data extracted from the PSQI included subscales of sleep information and from these a global score was calculated. Good sleepers were determined by a global score of less than or equal to 5 and poor sleepers were determined by a global score of above 5 as described by Buysse, Reynolds, Monk, Berman and Kupfer [25]. Sleep variables were non-normal and could not be transformed to normal.

Mean, standard deviation, median, interquartile range, and range was calculated for caffeine values to describe the population. Participants were broken into age groups similar to the Australian Bureau of Statistics categorization [5] to allow for comparison. All outliers for the sleep and caffeine variables (>3 SD above the mean) were clarified with the participant completing the questionnaire, and all variables were subsequently considered to be accurate and viable. To determine differences between groups both parametric and non-parametric tests were used. For parametric data independent samples *t*-tests were used, for the data which could not be transformed and were non normal Mann Whitney *U* tests were used, and for categorical comparisons chi square tests were used.

For further analysis, non-parametric (Spearman) correlations were utilised to assess relationships with caffeine and sleep variables. Finally, to determine if there were differences between PSQI categorical sleep variables and total caffeine consumption a one-way ANOVA were undertaken. The ANOVA dependent variables included subjective sleep quality, sleep disturbances, use of sleep medication, and daytime dysfunction. In all tests, significance was determined if $p < 0.05$.

3. Results

3.1. Study Participants

Of the 104 people who were provided with study information, 90 participants consented to the study and 84 participants returned the questionnaires. The final data set for analyses included 80 participants with four questionnaires having missing data (Figure 1). The final sample consisted of 54 females and 26 males, aged 19–94 years (mean $\pm$ SD 38.9 $\pm$ 19.3 years), with a mean caffeine intake of 164.9 mg/day. Most of the participants (85%) reported their sleep quality to be either very or fairly good and 86% of the participants had not taken medications to help them sleep over the past month (prescribed or over the counter). Of the sample, 80% stated that they had disturbed sleep less than once a week. Finally, 83% of the sample had minimal problems during the day due to their sleepiness (further measures of caffeine and sleep are reported in Table 1). There was no difference in age between the good sleepers (PSQI global score < 5) and poor sleepers (PSQI global score > 5) and age had no relationship with sleep efficiency ($p = 0.0574$), sleep onset latency ($p = 0.756$), however as age increased so did time in bed ($p = 0.030$).

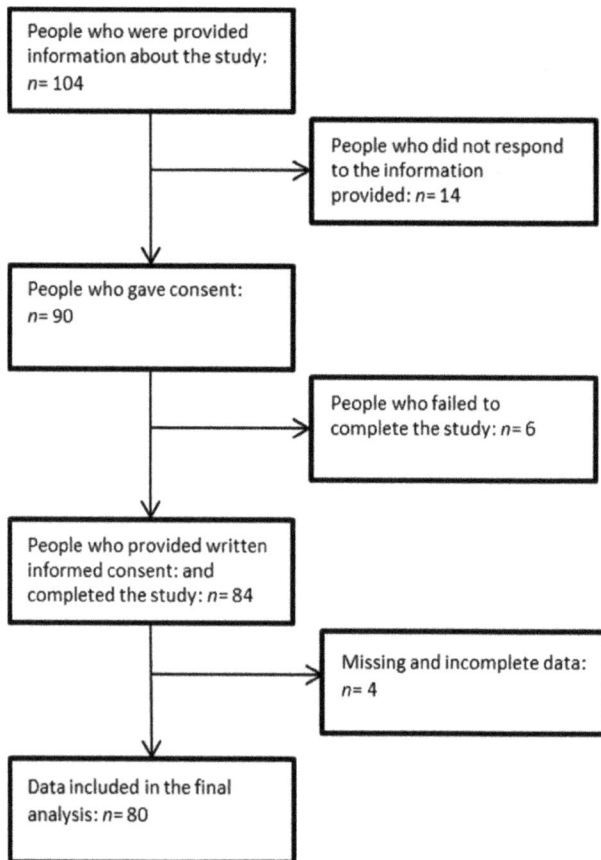

Figure 1. Description of participant flow throughout the study.

Table 1. Caffeine consumption and sleep measures for participants.

	Mean (SD)	Median (IQR)	Range
Total caffeine (mg)	165.1 (105.3)	133.4 (120.1)	41.6–726.6
Coffee (mg)	109.9 (99.4)	87.2 (82.3)	0.0–646.6
Tea (mg)	38.0 (56.2)	13.6 (50.9)	0.0–271.4
Chocolate (mg)	3.5 (4.6)	1.7 (4.3)	0.0–20.6
Soft Drink (mg)	9.0 (24.0)	0.0 (8.6)	0.0–182.4
Energy drink (mg)	4.9 (20.4)	0.0 (0.0)	0.0–135.0
PSQI global score	5.3 (2.5)	5.0 (4.0)	0.0–21.0
SOL (min)	18.8 (11.8)	20.0 (20.0)	1.0–60.0
SE (%)	88.3 (9.3)	89.1 (13.7)	55.6–100.0
TIB (h)	8.0 (1.0)	8.0 (1.0)	6.0–13.3

Abbreviations: SD, standard deviation; PSQI, Pittsburgh Sleep Quality Index; IQR, interquartile range; mg, milligrams; SOL, sleep onset latency; SE, sleep efficiency; TIB, time in bed; global score, PSQI total score; %, percentage. Notes: Chocolate includes both food and drink.

3.2. Types of Foods/Beverages That Contribute to Caffeine Intake by Gender

There were no differences in total caffeine consumption between men and women $t(78) = 0.60$, $p = 0.548$. Further, Mann Whitney U tests were undertaken to determine any differences in caffeine consumption from different caffeine sources between genders and showed no differences in caffeine consumption from coffee, tea, soft drink and chocolate between genders. However, males consumed more caffeine from energy drinks compared with females ($U = 589.50$, $z = -2.36$, $p = 0.018$; Male median (IQR): 0.0 (0.0) mg, range: 0.0–135.0 mg; Female median (IQR): 0.0 (0.0) mg, range: 0.0–22.4 mg). Due to the small intake of energy drinks consumed overall in this sample the differences between gender in overall caffeine consumption was not considered to impact the results and males and females were analysed together.

3.3. Types of Foods/Beverages That Contribute to Caffeine Intake by Age

There was no significant correlation between total caffeine consumption and age ($r = 0.167$, $p = 0.145$), with similar mean intakes across age groups and a wide variation within age groups (18–30 years: 174.6 ($\pm$139.4) mg; 31–50 years: 149.1 ($\pm$74.6) mg; 51–92 years: 184.4 ($\pm$72.4) mg). Energy drink consumption significantly decreased with age ($r = -0.297$, $p = 0.008$). Tea consumption increased with age ($r = 0.217$, $p = 0.056$) and soft drink consumption decreased with age ($r = -0.221$, $p = 0.052$), however these effects were only trends. Coffee intake and chocolate intake was not correlated with age (Figure 2).

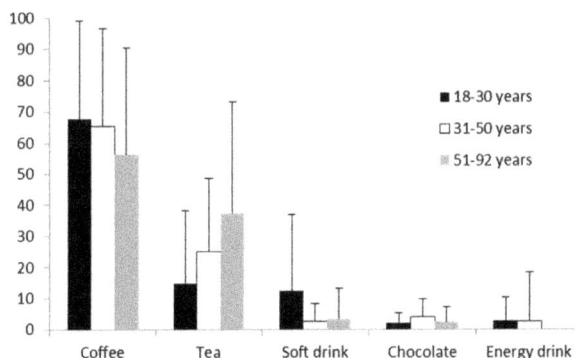

Figure 2. Percent of caffeine intake from different sources by age groups. Total $n = 80$; 18–30 years: $n = 32$, 31–50 years: $n = 31$, 51–92 years: $n = 16$. Notes: Chocolate includes beverages and food.

3.4. Impact of Caffeine on Sleep Quality

Sleep onset latency (Figure 3A) and sleep efficiency (Figure 3B) were not significantly correlated with caffeine (Figure 3). Time in bed was significantly related to total caffeine intake ($r = -0.229$, $p = 0.041$) with time in bed increasing with decreasing caffeine consumption (Figure 3C). Furthermore, caffeine consumption was not significantly associated with other sleep factors (subjective sleep quality, medications needed to sleep, sleep disturbance, and daily dysfunction due to sleepiness).

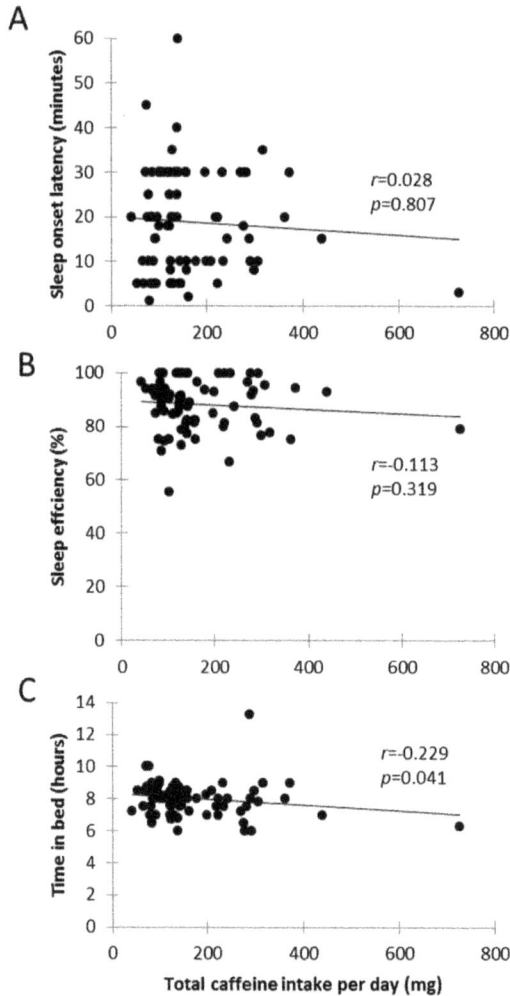

Figure 3. Scatterplots showing the relationship between total caffeine consumed and sleep variables: sleep efficiency, time in bed and sleep onset latency. (**A**) represents total caffeine intake versus sleep onset latency, $r = 0.028$; (**B**) shows total caffeine intake versus sleep efficiency, $r = -0.113$; (**C**) shows total caffeine intake versus time in bed, $r = -0.229$.

3.5. Caffeine Intake between Self-Reported Good and Poor Sleepers

To determine if caffeine consumption differed between good and poor sleepers, caffeine variables were compared between participants who reported a PSQI global score $\geqslant 5$ (poor sleep quality) and

PSQI < 5 (good sleep quality). On average, poor sleepers reported greater total caffeine consumption (mean ± SD: 192.1 ± 122.5 mg) compared to good sleepers (mean ± SD: 130.0 ± 62.6 mg; mean difference = 62.2 mg, $t(78) = -2.73$, $p = 0.008$, $d = 0.64$).

Furthermore, caffeine from coffee intake was significantly less in good sleepers (median = 66.5, IQR = 83.1) than poor sleepers (median = 99.2, IQR = 83.3), $U = 1028.50$, $z = 2.34$, $p = 0.019$, $r = 0.26$. While caffeine from tea ($p = 0.874$), chocolate ($p = 0.658$), soft drink ($p = 0.368$) and energy drinks ($p = 0.395$) showed no differences found between groups (Table 2).

Table 2. A descriptive table showing the means, standard deviations, medians, and interquartile ranges for all variables for good and poor sleepers as indicated from the PSQI. The table also shows p values comparing good and poor sleepers using either independent samples t-test. Mann Whitney U test and chi square tests. Participants with good sleep quality had PSQI global scores of less than 5 and participants with poor sleep quality had PSQI global scores of greater than 5.

	Good Sleep Quality $n = 35$		Poor Sleep Quality $n = 45$		p Values
	Mean (SD)	Median (IQR)	Mean (SD)	Median (IQR)	
Total caffeine (mg)	130.0 (62.6)	123.2 (58.2)	192.1 (122.5)	140.4 (160.6)	0.008 [I]
Coffee (mg)	81.7 (68.5)	66.5 (83.1)	132.2 (115.0)	99.2 (83.3)	0.019 [M]
Tea (mg)	35.4 (48.4)	13.6 (54.3)	39.5 (61.5)	13.6 (55.0)	0.874 [M]
Chocolate (mg)	3.6 (4.0)	1.7 (4.5)	3.5 (4.9)	1.7 (4.5)	0.658 [M]
Soft Drink (mg)	6.5 (13.2)	0.0 (5.2)	10.9 (29.2)	0.0 (10.4)	0.368 [M]
Energy drink (mg)	2.9 (15.4)	0.0 (0.0)	6.0 (23.0)	0.0 (0.0)	0.395 [M]
SOL (min)	11.4 (7.6)	10.0 (13.0)	24.3 (11.0)	30.0 (15.0)	0.000 [C]
SE (%)	95.0 (4.6)	94.1 (8.6)	82.9 (8.8)	82.4 (11.1)	0.239 [M]
TIB (h)	7.9 (0.7)	8.0 (1.3)	8.2 (1.2)	8.0 (1.1)	0.000 [C]

Abbreviations: SD, standard deviation; PSQI, Pittsburgh Sleep Quality Index; IQR, interquartile range; mg, milligrams; SOL, sleep onset latency; SE, sleep efficiency; TIB, time in bed; global score, PSQI total score; %, percentage; [I], Independent samples t-test was used; [M], Mann-Whitney U test was used; [C], Chi-square test was used. Notes: Chocolate includes both food and drink.

4. Discussion

The current study found that caffeine consumption did not change dramatically across the lifespan, with only energy drinks changing significantly across age groups. Furthermore, decreased time in bed was associated with increased caffeine consumption, and people with poor self-reported sleep quality consumed significantly more caffeine than people with good self-reported sleep quality scores.

The first aim of the study was to identify the sources of caffeine that contribute to an adult's total caffeine intake using the newly validated C-FFQ. It was found that the average consumption of caffeine in this population was 165.1 mg per day. National data, obtained using an intensive 24 h recall process on two occasions, suggests Australian adults consume approximately 103–183 mg of caffeine per day [5]. This is similar to that found in the current study additionally, the sources of caffeine across age groups were also similar in amounts to the national data [5]. In the current study the percentage of caffeine from tea was highest in the 51–92 years age group; in the previous national data it steadily rose across the lifespan and was highest in the 71 years and over age group. Furthermore, the current sample showed that as people age they are significantly less likely to consume caffeine from energy drinks and consume less soft drinks. Finally, the percentage of caffeine from chocolate remained steady across the lifespan in both our sample and the previous national data. There was, however, a difference in percentage of caffeine from coffee between the current data and the previous national data. The current study consumed less caffeine from coffee intake in the 31–50 years age bracket when compared to the national data, with the percentage of caffeine from coffee remaining equal from 18 to 50 years and declining in the oldest age group.

The second aim of the study was to determine the relationship between caffeine and sleep quality (variables from the subscales of the PSQI). The current study showed that total caffeine consumption had a small negative correlation with time in bed. This result is similar to a previous cross sectional survey study [17] however, in contrast with Sanchez-Ortuno and colleagues [17] total caffeine consumption was not correlated with sleep efficiency. The contrast in findings could be explained by the differences in measuring caffeine. The current study used a validated food frequency questionnaire to estimate total caffeine intake and not a generic "cups per day" or "number of drinks in the last week" question as in other studies [17–19,23], nor did it rely on participants knowing what beverages they consume contain caffeine. Furthermore, the mean caffeine intake value is greater in the study by Sanchez-Ortuno and colleagues [17] (mean caffeine intake across the day: 225 mg) and perhaps is large enough to impact sleep compared to the current study which recorded an average of 165.1 mg per day.

The current study showed that total caffeine consumption was not correlated with subjective sleep quality, medicinal sleep aids, sleep disturbance, or daily dysfunction due to sleepiness, similar to other studies [18,23]. However, this is different to experimental laboratory studies that have found caffeine consumption negatively impacts sleep quality [11,14]. This could be explained by the dose of caffeine consumed, as laboratory studies tend to give higher amounts of caffeine to participants than the habitual amount recorded in the current study. For example Carrier et al. [13] gave 100 mg three hours before bed followed by an additional 100 mg one hour before bed time. Additionally, given that the time of caffeine consumption was not recorded in this study it is possible that it was consumed earlier in the day and therefore had less of an effect on sleep. Finally, the results of the current study indicate a global relationship between sleep and caffeine consumption and it is highly possibly that poor or short sleep drives caffeine consumption rather than the other way around. It would be beneficial for future studies to measure the timing of caffeine consumption to further investigate if habitual caffeine consumption interferes with sleep.

The third aim of the study was to determine the difference in caffeine consumption between good and poor sleepers as measured by the PSQI global score (a score which included all the variables to determine an overall score of sleep quality). There was a significant difference in caffeine consumption between participants who were classified as good sleepers and those classified as poor sleepers. Good sleepers on average consumed 67 mg less caffeine per day; approximately one cup of instant coffee. However other field studies [18,19,23] have found that the PSQI global score was not related to the amount of caffeine consumed. The contrast in findings could be explained by the differences in the ways caffeine consumption was measured as discussed above. The strength of the current study is that it measured all sources of caffeine and examined a broad population with a wide age range throughout the year, i.e., not specifically medical students [23] or students during exam period [19].

The current study provides an overview of the average daily caffeine habits of adults across the lifespan and compares it to the sleep habits. However, some limitations need to be taken into consideration. Firstly, we did not record the participants' weight or height measurements to calculate the body mass index. The relationship between sleep and weight is well documented [8], with shorter sleep and poorer sleep quality associated with obesity. Secondly, the general population sample means that the results may not be generalizable to groups who consume more caffeine such as shift workers. Therefore, it is not possible to generalise this information to shift workers as they have different sleep and wake patterns which would potentially increase caffeine use and worsen sleep quality. Furthermore, there are limitations to self-report sleep compared to objective measures such as Actiwatches and Polysomnography. While objective measures are preferred, observational studies have widely used subjective measures previously due to cost and logistics. In adults it has been shown that subjective measures of sleep is equal to objective measures of sleep [28,29].

5. Conclusions

This study demonstrates the importance of accurately measuring caffeine sources as patterns of consumption can differ across the lifespan. Additionally, while this study found higher amounts of caffeine consumed related to decreased time in bed there was no association between subjective sleep

Nutrients **2016**, *8*, 479

quality and the amount of caffeine consumed. This could be due to the fact daily caffeine consumption was, on average, low to moderate or it could be because caffeine was not consumed close to bed time. This should be the focus of future research. With caffeine being consumed by a wide range of the population and found in many beverages and foods, it is necessary to understand the full health implications and how it may interfere with our daily behaviours such as sleep.

Acknowledgments: We would like to thank all the participants and Louise Massie who helped make this research possible. E.W. was funded through a University of South Australia Post Graduate Award; otherwise this research received no specific grant from any funding agency, commercial or not-for-profit sectors.

Author Contributions: E.W. developed the project, carried out the study, collected data, undertook analysis and prepared the first draft of the manuscript. A.C., M.K. and S.B. assisted in developing the project, analysis and revising the manuscript as well as supervising the study.

Conflicts of Interest: The authors declare no conflict of interest.

Abbreviations

The following abbreviations are used in this manuscript:

TST	Total Sleep Time
TIB	Time in Bed
FFQ	Food Frequency Questionnaire
PSQI	Pittsburgh Sleep Quality Index
SOL	Sleep Onset Latency
C-FFQ	Caffeine food frequency questionnaire
SE	Sleep Efficiency

References

1. Dorrian, J.; Paterson, J.; Dawson, D.; Pincombe, J.; Grech, C.; Rogers, A.E. Sleep, stress and compensatory behaviors in Australian nurses and midwives. *Rev. Saude Publica* **2011**, *45*, 922–930. [CrossRef] [PubMed]
2. Porkka-Heiskanen, T.; Strecker, R.E.; Thakkar, M.; Bjørkum, A.A.; Greene, R.W.; McCarley, R.W. Adenosine: A mediator of the sleep-inducing effects of prolonged wakefulness. *Science* **1997**, *276*, 1265–1268. [CrossRef] [PubMed]
3. Strecker, R.E.; Morairty, S.; Thakkar, M.M.; Porkka-Heiskanen, T.; Basheer, R.; Dauphin, L.J.; Rainnie, D.G.; Portas, C.M.; Greene, R.W.; McCarley, R.W. Adenosinergic modulation of basal forebrain and preoptic/anterior hypothalamic neuronal activity in the control of behavioral state. *Behav. Brain Res.* **2000**, *115*, 183–204. [CrossRef]
4. Brice, C.; Smith, A. The effects of caffeine on simulated driving, subjective alertness and sustained attention. *Hum. Psychopharmacol. Clin. Exp.* **2001**, *16*, 523–531. [CrossRef] [PubMed]
5. Australian Bureau of Statistics Australian Health Survey: Nutrition First Results—Foods and Nutrients, 2011–12. Available online: http://www.abs.gov.au/ausstats/abs@.nsf/Lookup/by%20Subject/4364.0.55.007~2011-12~Main%20Features~Non-alcoholic%20beverages~701 (accessed on 15 December 2015).
6. Hirshkowitz, M.; Whiton, K.; Albert, S.M.; Alessi, C.; Bruni, O.; DonCarlos, L.; Hazen, N.; Herman, J.; Hillard, P.J.A.; Katz, E.S. National sleep foundation's updated sleep duration recommendations: Final report. *Sleep Health* **2015**, *1*, 233–243. [CrossRef]
7. Cappuccio, F.P.; D'Elia, L.; Strazzullo, P.; Miller, M.A. Quantity and quality of sleep and incidence of type 2 diabetes a systematic review and meta-analysis. *Diabetes Care* **2010**, *33*, 414–420. [CrossRef] [PubMed]
8. Cappuccio, F.P.; Taggart, F.M.; Kandala, N.; Currie, A.; Peile, E.; Stranges, S.; Miller, M.A. Meta-analysis of short sleep duration and obesity in children and adults. *Sleep* **2008**, *31*, 619–626. [PubMed]
9. Jennings, J.; Muldoon, M.; Hall, M. Self-reported sleep quality is associated with the metabolic syndrome. *Sleep* **2007**, *30*, 219–223. [PubMed]
10. Xie, L.; Kang, H.; Xu, Q.; Chen, M.J.; Liao, Y.; Thiyagarajan, M.; O'Donnell, J.; Christensen, D.J.; Nicholson, C.; Iliff, J.J. Sleep drives metabolite clearance from the adult brain. *Science* **2013**, *342*, 373–377. [CrossRef] [PubMed]

11. Shilo, L.; Sabbah, H.; Hadari, R.; Kovatz, S.; Weinberg, U.; Dolev, S.; Dagan, Y.; Shenkman, L. The effects of coffee consumption on sleep and melatonin secretion. *Sleep Med.* **2002**, *3*, 271–273. [CrossRef]
12. Drapeau, C.; Hamel-Hebert, I.; Robillard, R.; Selmaoui, B.; Filipini, D.; Carrier, J. Challenging sleep in aging: The effects of 200 mg of caffeine during the evening in young and middle-aged moderate caffeine consumers. *J. Sleep Res.* **2006**, *15*, 133–141. [CrossRef] [PubMed]
13. Carrier, J.; Fernandez-Bolanos, M.; Robillard, R.; Dumont, M.; Paquet, J.; Selmaoui, B.; Filipini, D. Effects of caffeine are more marked on daytime recovery sleep than on nocturnal sleep. *Neuropsychopharmacology* **2007**, *32*, 964–972. [CrossRef] [PubMed]
14. Hindmarch, I.; Rigney, U.; Stanley, N.; Quinlan, P.; Rycroft, J.; Lane, J. A naturalistic investigation of the effects of day-long consumption of tea, coffee and water on alertness, sleep onset and sleep quality. *Psychopharmacology* **2000**, *149*, 203–216. [CrossRef] [PubMed]
15. Grant, D.M.; Tang, B.K.; Kalow, W. Variability in caffeine metabolism. *Clin. Pharmacol. Ther.* **1983**, *33*, 591–602. [CrossRef] [PubMed]
16. Regestein, Q.; Natarajan, V.; Pavlova, M.; Kawasaki, S.; Gleason, R.; Koff, E. Sleep debt and depression in female college students. *Psychiatry Res.* **2010**, *176*, 34–39. [CrossRef] [PubMed]
17. Sanchez-Ortuno, M.; Moore, N.; Taillard, J.; Valtat, C.; Leger, D.; Bioulac, B.; Philip, P. Sleep duration and caffeine consumption in a French middle-aged working population. *Sleep Med.* **2005**, *6*, 247–251. [CrossRef] [PubMed]
18. Lund, H.G.; Reider, B.D.; Whiting, A.B.; Prichard, J. Sleep patterns and predictors of disturbed sleep in a large population of college students. *J. Adolesc. Health* **2010**, *46*, 124–132. [CrossRef] [PubMed]
19. Zunhammer, M.; Eichhammer, P.; Busch, V. Sleep quality during exam stress: The role of alcohol, caffeine and nicotine. *PLoS ONE* **2014**, *9*, e109490. [CrossRef] [PubMed]
20. Whittier, A.; Sanchez, S.; Castaneda, B.; Sanchez, E.; Gelaye, B.; Yanez, D.; Williams, M.A. Eveningness chronotype, daytime sleepiness, caffeine consumption, and use of other stimulants among Peruvian university students. *J. Caffeine Res.* **2014**, *4*, 21–27. [CrossRef] [PubMed]
21. Kant, A.K.; Graubard, B.I. Association of self-reported sleep duration with eating behaviors of American adults: NHANES 2005–2010. *Am. J. Clin. Nutr.* **2014**, *100*, 938–947. [CrossRef] [PubMed]
22. Reid, A.; Baker, F.C. Perceived sleep quality and sleepiness in South African university students. *S. Afr. J. Psychol.* **2008**, *38*, 287–303. [CrossRef]
23. Brick, C.A.; Seely, D.L.; Palermo, T.M. Association between sleep hygiene and sleep quality in medical students. *Behav. Sleep Med.* **2010**, *8*, 113–121. [CrossRef] [PubMed]
24. Watson, E.; Kohler, M.; Banks, S.; Coates, A. Development of an Australian caffeine food frequency questionnaire. *Nutrients* **2016**, under review.
25. Buysse, D.J.; Reynolds, C.F.; Monk, T.H.; Berman, S.R.; Kupfer, D.J. The Pittsburgh sleep quality index: A new instrument for psychiatric practice and research. *Psychiatry Res.* **1989**, *28*, 193–213. [CrossRef]
26. Cole, J.C.; Motivala, S.J.; Buysse, D.J.; Oxman, M.N.; Levin, M.J.; Irwin, M.R. Validation of a 3-factor scoring model for the Pittsburgh sleep quality index in older adults. *Sleep* **2006**, *29*, 112–116. [PubMed]
27. Backhaus, J.; Junghanns, K.; Broocks, A.; Riemann, D.; Hohagen, F. Test–retest reliability and validity of the Pittsburgh sleep quality index in primary insomnia. *J. Psychosom. Res.* **2002**, *53*, 737–740. [CrossRef]
28. Armitage, R.; Trivedi, M.; Hoffmann, R.; Rush, A.J. Relationship between objective and subjective sleep measures in depressed patients and healthy controls. *Depression Anxiety* **1997**, *5*, 97–102. [CrossRef]
29. Zinkhan, M.; Berger, K.; Hense, S.; Nagel, M.; Obst, A.; Koch, B.; Penzel, T.; Fietze, I.; Ahrens, W.; Young, P. Agreement of different methods for assessing sleep characteristics: A comparison of two actigraphs, wrist and hip placement, and self-report with polysomnography. *Sleep Med.* **2014**, *15*, 1107–1114. [CrossRef] [PubMed]

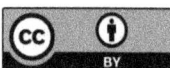

nutrients

MDPI

Article

Exploring the Effect of Lactium™ and *Zizyphus* Complex on Sleep Quality: A Double-Blind, Randomized Placebo-Controlled Trial

Andrew Scholey [1,*], Sarah Benson [1], Amy Gibbs [1], Naomi Perry [1], Jerome Sarris [1,2] and Greg Murray [3]

1   Centre for Human Psychopharmacology, Swinburne University of Technology, Hawthorn VIC 3122, Australia; sarahbenson@swin.edu.au (S.B.); Amygibbs57@gmail.com (A.G.); naomiperry21@gmail.com (N.P.); jsarris@unimelb.edu.au (J.S.)
2   ARCADIA Mental Health Research Group, The Professorial Unit, The Melbourne Clinic, Department of Psychiatry, Melbourne University, Richmond VIC 3121, Australia
3   Psychological Sciences and Statistics, Swinburne University of Technology, Hawthorn VIC 3122, Australia; gwm@swin.edu.au
*   Correspondence: andrew@scholeylab.com; Tel.: +61-392-148-932

Received: 26 July 2016; Accepted: 13 February 2017; Published: 17 February 2017

Abstract: Acute, non-clinical insomnia is not uncommon. Sufferers commonly turn to short-term use of herbal supplements to alleviate the symptoms. This placebo-controlled, double-blind study investigated the efficacy of LZComplex3 (lactium™, *Zizyphus*, *Humulus lupulus*, magnesium and vitamin B6), in otherwise healthy adults with mild insomnia. After a 7-day single-blind placebo run-in, eligible volunteers ($n = 171$) were randomized (1:1) to receive daily treatment for 2 weeks with LZComplex3 or placebo. Results revealed that sleep quality measured by change in Pittsburgh Sleep Quality Index (PSQI) score improved in both the LZComplex3 and placebo groups. There were no significant between group differences between baseline and endpoint on the primary outcome. The majority of secondary outcomes, which included daytime functioning and physical fatigue, mood and anxiety, cognitive performance, and stress reactivity, showed similar improvements in the LZComplex3 and placebo groups. A similar proportion of participants reported adverse events (AEs) in both groups, with two of four treatment-related AEs in the LZComplex3 group resulting in permanent discontinuation. It currently cannot be concluded that administration of LZComplex3 for 2 weeks improves sleep quality, however, a marked placebo response (despite placebo run-in) and/or short duration of treatment may have masked a potential beneficial effect on sleep quality.

Keywords: lactium; *Zizyphus*; *Humulus lupulus*; nutritional supplements; complementary medicines; sleep disturbance; insomnia; LZComplex3; clinical trial

1. Introduction

Insomnia is defined by disturbances in sleep quality together with impairment of daytime functioning, for example fatigue and low mood [1]. Disturbances in sleep quality include difficulty getting to sleep, staying asleep or experiencing non-restorative sleep despite adequate opportunity for sleep [1]. An estimated 13%–33% of Australians experience some form of insomnia, similar to the estimated rates of insomnia in Western countries including Canada and the United States and in low-income countries across Africa and Asia [2–4]. Insomnia can occur as an acute episode, usually triggered by factors such as ill health, change of medication or circumstances, or stress [5]. Such sleep disturbances generally resolve without treatment once the trigger is eliminated. However, people can also turn to short-term use of medications (typically hypnotics such as a benzodiazepine) or herbal supplements during these episodes of insomnia [5–7]. In contrast, long-term or chronic insomnia can involve the development of maladaptive behaviors and a different treatment approach is required [5].

Commonly used herbal supplements for insomnia often include single or combined formulations of lemon balm (*Melissa officinalis*), chamomile (*Matricaria recutita*), valerian (*Valeriana* spp.), hops (*Humulus lupulus*), passionflower (*Passiflora incanata*), lactium™ (α_{S1}-casein hydrolysate) and sour date (*Zizyphus jujube var. spinosa*) [8]. A new combined formulation, LZComplex3, contains lactium, sour date and hops, plus magnesium and vitamin B6 (pyridoxine) to provide nutritional support for metabolic pathways involved in sleep regulation. The rationale for the use of lactium as a sleeping aid originates from the observation that milk calms and soothes newborns [9]. The milk compound thought to be responsible for the calming or anxiolytic effects is a hydrolysate of α_{S1}-casein, the bioactive peptide α-casozepine [10]. Lactium is the manufactured form of α_{S1}-casein hydrolysate containing the α-casozepine peptide. Clinical studies have demonstrated that lactium reduces some symptoms related to stress [11,12]. Lactium has also been shown to have anxiolytic effects and to improve stress-induced sleep disturbance in animal studies [10,13,14].

Sour date (*Zizyphus jujube var. spinosa*; alternative spelling *Ziziphus*) is a fruit used in traditional Chinese medicine for its mild sedative and calming properties, to relieve irritability and aid sleep [15,16]. In combination with other herbs, it has been reported to improve mood and performance in individuals with anxiety and to improve sleep quality and a sense of well-being in individuals with sleep disorders [17,18]. Hops (*Humulus lupulus*) have been used in traditional western medicine for the treatment of mood disturbances such as restlessness and anxiety and in sleep disturbances due to reported calming and sleep-promoting properties [19–24]. Magnesium is involved in more than 300 metabolic reaction pathways including the production of melatonin, which regulates the sleep cycle [25]. Human and animal studies have implicated magnesium in the modulation of sleep [26–31]. Vitamin B6 may indirectly promote sleep quality through its role in the synthesis of a number of neurotransmitters involved in sleep regulation, including dopamine, serotonin, glutamate, γ-aminobutyric acid (GABA), and histamine [32,33].

Although the individual components in LZComplex3 have been studied with respect to their effects on sleep and/or stress (a common cause of sleeping difficulties), the efficacy of the combined formulation as a treatment for sleep disturbance has not been investigated. We report here the results of a clinical trial the primary objective of which was to investigate the short-term effect of LZComplex3 on sleep quality, mood and cognitive function in individuals with sleeping difficulties not caused by a primary sleeping disorder or other diagnosed condition.

2. Materials and Methods

2.1. Trial Design

This study was a placebo-controlled, double-blind, randomized, parallel group phase III trial with a single blind placebo run-in period (Figure 1). The trial was conducted at the Centre for Human Psychopharmacology, Swinburne University of Technology, Hawthorn, Victoria, Australia between 6 January 2014 and 23 December 2014. Ethical approval was granted by Bellberry Ltd., Eastwood, SA, Australia. The trial is registered with the Australian New Zealand Clinical Trials Registry (number ACTRN: 12613001363774) and was performed in accordance with the requirements for the conduct of clinical studies set by the Clinical Trial Notification (CTN) scheme of the Australian Therapeutic Goods Administration (TGA) and the Declaration of Helsinki.

Assessments of sleep quality, daytime functioning and physical fatigue, mood and anxiety, stress-reactivity, and cognitive function were completed by participants during the baseline and end of treatment visits, as well as during a final follow-up visit one week after the end of treatment. All assessment visits followed a procedure identical to that used at the baseline visit. In addition, participants completed all subjective sleep, daytime functioning, physical fatigue, mood and anxiety assessments at home 1, 3 and 7 days after baseline. All participant data were collected either at the study site (at screening, baseline, end of treatment, and final follow-up visits) or at the participants' homes (interim assessments between baseline and end of treatment).

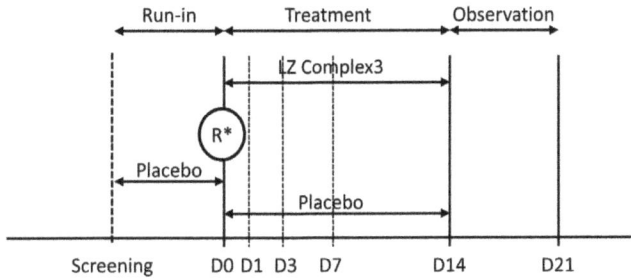

Figure 1. Study design. **R*** = randomization; D = study day.

2.2. Study Participants and Randomization

Potentially eligible participants were identified in an initial telephone screen. Participant eligibility was confirmed at the initial screening visit; each eligible participant was allocated a unique participant number as soon as written informed consent was obtained and prior to any screening assessments. Mood questionnaires including the Hospital Anxiety and Depression Scale (HADS) [34] and State-Trait Anxiety Inventory Trait subscale (STAI-T) [35] were completed and participants were required to familiarize themselves with all the study assessments and procedures in order to reduce errors at baseline and practice effects.

Eligible participants were healthy adults aged 18–65 years with no significant diagnosed diseases (as judged by the Investigator) who had self-reported sleeping difficulties over one month prior to the screening call. Following accepted practice [36], sleeping difficulties were defined as a Pittsburgh Sleep Quality Index (PSQI) Score >5 (PSQI scores range from 0 to 21 and higher scores indicate worse sleep quality). Participants with a primary sleep disorder (sleep apnoea-hypopnoea, periodic limb movement disorder, restless legs syndrome, narcolepsy, idiopathic hypersomnia, Kleine-Levin syndrome, as determined by subjective report and compilation of participants' medical history during the initial telephone screening assessment prior to randomization) were excluded. The full lists of inclusion and exclusion criteria are provided in Appendix A: Table A1.

Eligible participants entered a one-week single-blind placebo run-in period, during which a daily sleep questionnaire (Consensus Sleep Diary; CSD [37]) was used to establish baseline sleeping criteria and detect placebo responders. Placebo response was based on CSD scores, and defined as sleep efficiency above 85%, sleep onset latency below 31 min, and wake after sleep onset below 31 min.

At the baseline visit following the placebo run-in, placebo responders were excluded and all other participants were randomly assigned to treatment for two weeks (placebo or LZComplex3 in a 1:1 ratio) based on a randomization list generated centrally by an external independent third party. Participants and investigators were blinded to study treatment in the treatment phase and did not have access to the randomization codes except under exceptional medical circumstances.

Participants were invited at the baseline visit to wear an actiwatch to collect objective sleep data for exploratory cross-validation of the subjective sleep outcome measures. Participants who agreed were given an actiwatch to wear for the duration of the two-week treatment period.

2.3. Study Treatment

LZComplex3 tablets (Table 1) and placebo tablets were provided in blister packs and were matched for size, appearance, colour, smell and taste. The tablets were supplied to participants at the start of the placebo run-in and treatment phases in kit boxes. Each kit box contained sufficient blister packs of tablets to last for the duration of each phase of the trial plus an additional week to cover for any delays in attending the next scheduled visit. For the duration of each phase, participants were required to take two tablets daily, 30 min before retiring for sleep.

Table 1. LZComplex3 components.

Nutrient	Amount per Tablet
Lactium™ (hydrolysed milk protein; alpha casozepine enriched)	75 mg
Sour date (*Zizyphus jujube var. spinosa*) ext. equiv. to dry seed	4.5 g (4500 mg)
Hops (*Humulus lupulus*) ext. equiv. to dry flower	500 mg
Magnesium oxide (equivalent magnesium)	81.7 mg (52.5 mg)
Vitamin B6; pyridoxine hydrochloride (equivalent pyridoxine)	10 mg (8.23 mg)

2.4. Primary and Secondary Outcome Measurments

The primary outcome was the change in overall sleep quality after two weeks of daily supplementation with LZComplex3. The primary outcome was measured by the change in PSQI scores from baseline to end of treatment at day 14. Secondary outcomes were the safety of LZComplex3 and the change in sleep quality, daytime functioning and physical fatigue, mood and anxiety, cognitive performance, and stress reactivity at 1, 3, 7 and 14 days after treatment with LZComplex3 and after one week post-treatment. The secondary outcomes were measured using validated assessments as outlined in Table 2. Objective measurement of sleep efficiency and time asleep using actigraph data from a subset of up to 90 participants was a pre-specified exploratory outcome designed to assess the use of actigraphy as a means of cross-validation of the primary and secondary endpoints. The Mini-Mitter Actiwatch-L (Respironics, Inc., Bend, Oregon) was used to collect actigraph data. Adverse Events (AEs), including Serious Adverse Events (SAEs) and Adverse Events of Special Interest (AESI), were collected at every visit. The AE observation period commenced the day of consent and finished at the final follow-up visit.

Table 2. Outcome measures.

Outcome	Measurements
Primary outcome	
Sleep quality	Pittsburgh Sleep Quality Index (PSQI) [38]
Secondary outcome	
Sleep quality	Leeds Sleep Evaluation Questionnaire (LSEQ) [39] Epworth Sleepiness Scale (ESS) [40] Insomnia Severity Index (ISI) [41] Consensus Sleep Diary (CSD) [37]
Daytime functioning and physical fatigue	Burckhardt Quality of Life Scale (QoLS) [42] Chalder Fatigue Scale (CFS) [43]
Mood, anxiety and stress reactivity	Bond–Lader Visual Analogue Scales (Bond-Lader VAS) [44] State-Trait Anxiety Inventory (STAI) State subscale (STAI-S) [35] Stress and Fatigue Visual Analogue Mood Scales (VAMS)
Cognitive performance	Purple multi-tasking framework (MTF)

2.4.1. Screening Assessments

Screening assessments included the HADS, STAI-T, Leeds Sleep Evaluation Questionnaire (LSEQ), Bond-Lader Visual Analogue Scale (VAS), and the Stress and Fatigue Visual Analogue Mood Scales (VAMS). The HADS is a 14-item questionnaire designed to measure levels of anxiety and depression and was administered at screening to exclude participants with depression and/or anxiety [34]. The STAI-T comprises 20 different statements (e.g., "Some unimportant thought runs through my mind and bothers me") [35]. Participants indicate how they generally feel on a scale ranging from "almost never" to "almost always". Scores on the STAI-T range from 20 to 80, with higher scores indicating more anxiety. The Trait subscale of the STAI was to be used at screening to detect those participants who may have excessive levels of trait anxiety prior to commencing the study.

2.4.2. Treatment Assessments

Details of each assessment method are provided in Appendix A: Table A2.

2.5. Statistical Analyses

With an anticipated drop-out/non-compliance rate of 33%, it was estimated that a total of 170 participants would be required for 80% power to detect a medium effect size of approximately 0.5 at the 5% level of significance, with respect to the primary outcome. All analyses were conducted on a modified intention-to-treat (mITT) population, representing a per protocol/completer analysis and defined as all participants who were randomized and who had valid PSQI measures at both baseline and end of treatment. The primary outcome was also measured in the per protocol (PP) population, which included all participants in the mITT population who were at least 80% and less than 120% compliant with randomized treatment medication and had no major protocol deviations. Safety analyses were conducted on the safety population, which included all participants who were randomized and received at least one dose of study drug.

All measures were analyzed using SAS software (V9.4, SAS Statistical Institute, Cart, NC, USA). A general repeated measures mixed model was fitted to explore the difference between placebo and LZComplex3 in unadjusted change of total PSQI across all PSQI assessments for the mITT population. Day numbers and treatment group were included as fixed effects, participant as a random effect, the change in PSQI from baseline as the dependent variable and the baseline value of PSQI as a covariate. Secondary endpoints except ISI scores were analyzed in the same form as the primary endpoint. For the STAI-S, Bond-Lader VAS and VAMS scores, the mixed model also included time point (before and after administration of the MTF) as a fixed effect. A multinomial distribution and cumulative logit link function using PROC GLIMMIX was used to explore the difference between placebo and LZComplex3 in unadjusted change in ISI. The intended analysis of actigraphy data was not performed due to insufficient participant numbers ($n = 16$).

3. Results

3.1. Participant Characteristics

From a total of 241 participants, 171 were eligible for randomization following screening and the placebo run-in period. Eighty-five participants were allocated to the LZComplex3 group and 86 participants to the placebo group. After exclusions and losses, a total of 160 participants (LZComplex3, $n = 78$; placebo, $n = 82$) were eligible for analysis in the mITT population (Figure 2).

Participant demographics and other baseline characteristics are shown in Table 3. All characteristics were similar in the placebo and LZComplex3 groups. Most subjects were compliant during both the placebo run-in and treatment periods of the study. The mean compliance score, calculated as the percentage of study drug taken relative to the amount prescribed in the protocol, was 83.0 (standard deviation; SD 17.6) during the run-in period. The mean compliance scores in the LZComplex3 and placebo groups during the treatment period were 98.3 (SD 8.6) and 100.5 (SD 7.3) respectively.

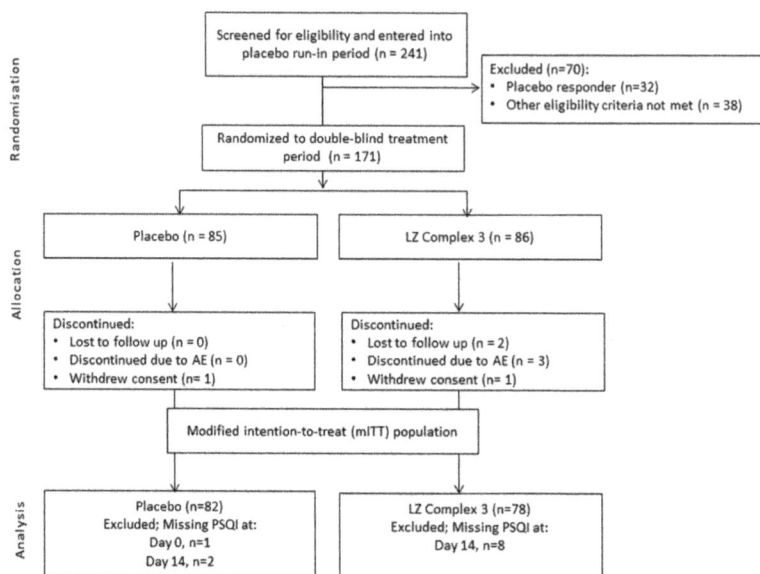

Figure 2. Participant flow. AE = adverse event, PSQI = Pittsburgh Sleep Quality Index

Table 3. Demographic and other baseline characteristics (safety population; n = 170).

Characteristic	Placebo (n = 85)	LZComplex3 (n = 85)
Gender		
Male, n (%)	38 (44.7)	36 (42.4)
Female, n (%)	47 (55.3)	49 (57.6)
Ethnicity		
Caucasian/White, n (%)	61 (71.8)	58 (68.2)
Black, n (%)	0 (0.0)	1 (1.2)
Asian/Oriental, n (%)	13 (15.3)	13 (15.3)
Other, n (%)	11 (12.9)	13 (15.3)
Age in years, mean (SD)	31.0 (10.5)	29.6 (9.05)
Height in cm, mean (SD)	172.6 (9.9)	171.2 (10.4)
Weight in kg, mean (SD)	71.3 (12.6)	70.0 (13.9)
Years of education, mean (SD)	16.6 (2.5)	17.0 (2.6)

SD = Standard deviation.

3.2. Primary Outcome

The mean change in total PSQI across time in the mITT population is presented in Figure 3a. Over the 2-week treatment period, the mITT population showed a gradual reduction in mean total PSQI from baseline to end of treatment (day 14) in both the LZComplex3 and placebo groups. Negative change scores indicate improved sleep quality in both groups, thus the change in both groups is in the direction of improved sleep. A mixed models analysis of covariance found a significant effect of day on PSQI ($F_{4,517}$ = 30.40, $p < 0.001$) but no effect of treatment ($F_{1,157}$ = 0.14, $p = 0.713$) and no interaction between treatment and day ($F_{4,517}$ = 1.13, $p = 0.340$) in the mITT population. The results were similar in the PP population, with a significant effect of day ($F_{4,499}$ = 29.63, $p < 0.001$), no effect of treatment ($F_{1,150}$ = 0.17, $p = 0.685$) and no interaction between treatment and visit ($F_{4,499}$ = 1.06, $p = 0.374$). The unadjusted PSQI scores between baseline and end of treatment are presented in Table 4.

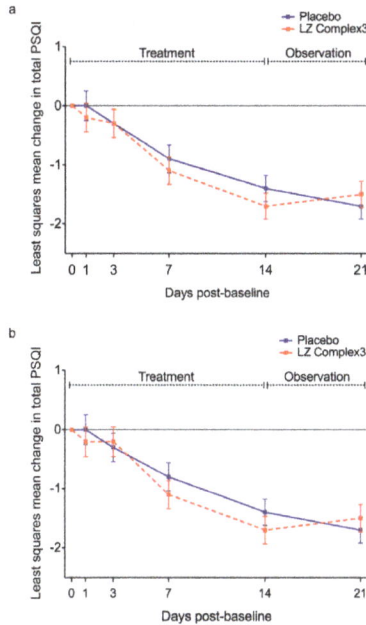

Figure 3. Least squares mean change in total Pittsburgh Sleep Quality Index (PSQI) between baseline (day 0) and end of the observation period (day 21) by treatment group in: (**a**) the modified intention-to-treat (mITT) population and (**b**) the per protocol (PP) population.

Table 4. Total PSQI, mean (SD).

	mITT Population			PP Population		
	n	Mean PSQI	Change from Baseline	*n*	Mean PSQI	Change from Baseline
Baseline						
Placebo	82	9.0 (2.5)		81	9.0 (2.1)	
LZComplex3	78	9.4 (2.6)		72	9.5 (2.6)	
Day 1						
Placebo	56	9.0 (2.3)	0.0 (2.1)	55	8.9 (2.3)	0.0 (2.1)
LZComplex3	61	9.2 (2.6)	−0.2 (1.3)	59	9.1 (2.6)	−0.3 (1.2)
Day 3						
Placebo	60	8.7 (2.3)	−0.4 (1.8)	59	8.7 (2.3)	−0.4 (1.8)
LZComplex3	60	9.2 (2.6)	−0.3 (1.4)	58	9.1 (2.6)	−0.3 (1.3)
Day 7						
Placebo	62	8.0 (2.4)	−0.9 (1.9)	61	8.0 (2.4)	−0.8 (1.9)
LZComplex3	67	8.2 (2.8)	−1.2 (2.1)	62	8.2 (2.7)	−1.2 (2.1)
Day 14						
Placebo	82	7.7 (2.7)	−1.3 (2.4)	81	7.7 (2.7)	−1.3 (2.5)
LZComplex3	78	7.6 (2.8)	−1.8 (2.1)	72	7.7 (2.8)	−1.8 (2.0)
Day 21						
Placebo	82	7.3 (2.5)	−1.7 (2.8)	81	7.3 (2.5)	−1.7 (2.8)
LZComplex3	77	7.9 (3.0)	−1.5 (2.3)	72	7.9 (3.0)	−1.6 (2.3)

mITT = modified intention-to-treat, PP = per protocol, PSQI = Pittsburgh Sleep Quality Index, SD = standard deviation.

3.3. Secondary Outcomes

Similar to the primary outcome measure, the majority of secondary outcome measures showed similar changes in the placebo and LZComplex3 groups across the study period (Figures S1–S9, Table S1). A significant effect of day was found across all secondary outcomes measures except CSD domains, "Alertness" and "Calmness" components of the Bond-Lader VAS, and "Stress" and "Fatigue" components of the VAMS. A cumulative logit link function in PROC GLIMMIX found a significant effect of treatment on ISI between baseline and end of the study. A between-group difference was detected in the proportions of participants with improved, worsened, or no change in ISI at day 3 compared with baseline (Figure S3). A mixed models analysis of covariance found a significant effect of treatment on STAI-S total scores that was due to a significant difference between the placebo and LZComplex3 groups in change in STAI-S total scores from pre- to post-administration of the MTF at day 0 and day 14 (Figure S7). There were no significant treatment effects detected across any other secondary outcome measures. Time point (before or after administration of the MTF) was found to have a significant independent effect on STAI-S total score, Bond-Lader VAS "Calmness" and "Contentedness" components, and VAMS "Stress" and "Fatigue" components (Figures S7–S9).

3.4. Safety

There were 25 AEs (19 mild, 5 moderate and 1 severe) reported during the run-in period, none of which were serious (defined as any experience which was fatal or life-threatening, was permanently disabling, required hospitalisation or prolongation of hospitalisation, was a congenital anomaly, or was an important medical event that could jeopardize the subject or require intervention to prevent one of those outcomes). Overall, 25 AEs were reported during the treatment period (Table 5). The proportion of participants reporting an AE was similar in each treatment group (placebo, $n = 9$ (10.6%; LZComplex3, $n = 11$ (12.9%); $p = 0.8125$; Table 5). The most common AEs were infections (placebo, $n = 6$; LZComplex3, $n = 7$) and gastrointestinal disorders (placebo, $n = 0$; LZComplex3, $n = 4$). There were no deaths or other serious adverse events. Two of the 4 AEs related to treatment in the LZComplex3 group led to permanent discontinuation. There were two hospitalizations reported, both in the LZComplex3 group, neither of which fulfilled the criteria of a serious AE.

Table 5. Summary of adverse events (AEs) reported during the treatment period (safety population).

Type	Placebo ($n = 85$)	LZComplex3 ($n = 85$)
AEs, n	11	14
Mild	5	5
Moderate	5	4
Severe	1	5
Patients reporting AEs, n (%)	9 (10.6)	11 (12.9)
Mild	5 (5.9)	5 (5.9)
Moderate	4 (4.7)	4 (4.7)
Severe	1 (1.2)	4 (4.7)
AEs leading to discontinuation, n	0	2
Abdominal pain	0 (0.0)	1 (1.2)
Dyspepsia	0 (0.0)	1 (1.2)
Serious AEs, n	0	0
AEs of special interest, n	0	0
AEs related to study treatment, n	0	4
Abdominal pain	0 (0.0)	1 (1.2)
Dyspepsia	0 (0.0)	1 (1.2)
Gastritis	0 (0.0)	1 (1.2)
Gastroenteritis	0 (0.0)	1 (1.2)

4. Discussion

This study evaluated the efficacy of LZComplex3 in improving sleep quality in otherwise-well individuals with sleeping difficulties. There were no group differences in the primary outcome. Improvements in sleep quality were seen over a two-week treatment period with LZComplex3, however a persistent placebo response was observed and there was no significant treatment effect compared with placebo. Although the study included a one-week placebo run-in period designed to identify and exclude placebo-responders, it appears that that the run-in period may not have been of sufficient length. It is also possible that the persistent placebo response occurring after randomization may have been due to participants' increased focus on overall sleep hygiene as a result of study visits and assessments, filling in a daily sleep diary and observing the protocol-mandated study parameters regarding stimulant use and sleep times. This degree of attention was not required in the placebo run-in phase. It has previously been suggested that having a patient keep a sleep diary for 2 weeks will aid with identification of behaviors that may worsen insomnia, thus providing a useful behavioral intervention [45]. Participants were required to fill in the CSD daily for the duration of the run-in and treatment periods, which may have contributed to the improvements in sleep quality observed in both treatment groups.

An improvement in sleep quality with LZComplex3 was expected, as previous studies have supported the use of individual components of the formulation as an aid for sleeping difficulties or insomnia (see Introduction). However, rigorous clinical studies are lacking. Effects of lactium on sleep quality have been investigated in a double-blind, controlled, parallel study of 32 Japanese patients experiencing poor sleep as determined by a global PSQI score greater than 4 [46]. As in the current study, improvements in sleep quality were observed over 4 weeks within the lactium group, however there were no significant differences between the placebo and lactium groups for any of the sleep components evaluated. It is possible that an effect of lactium was not detected due to a placebo response and the small sample size. Clinical evidence for the anxiolytic effects of lactium is more supportive. In a double-blind, randomized, controlled study of 42 healthy men treated with 3 doses each 12 h apart, experimental stress-induced elevations in blood pressure were significantly lower in the lactium group compared with the placebo group, supporting an anti-stress activity of lactium. As stress is a common cause of sleeping difficulties, it is thought that lactium may promote good quality sleep through its anti-stress activity.

The efficacy of sour date (*Zizyphus jujube var. spinosa*) in treating insomnia has been investigated in one clinical trial in the form of suanzaorentang [17,47], a popular Chinese herbal formula consisting of sour date (*Zizyphus jujube var. spinosa*), Fu Ling (mushroom) (*Poria cocos*), szechuan lovage (*Ligusticum wallichii*), Zhi Mu (*Anemarrhenae rhizoma*), and liquorice root (*Glycyrrhizae radix*) in a ratio of 7:5:2:1:1 [48]. The study compared self-rated measures of sleep quality in 60 participants with insomnia who received placebo for one week, followed by suanzaorentang for two weeks, followed by another week of placebo. All ratings of sleep quality significantly improved during the suanzaorentang treatment phase compared with the placebo periods. A number of trials evaluating the efficacy of suanzaorentang using benzodiazepines as the comparator showed favorable results for suanzaorentang in improving sleep, although the studies lacked methodological rigor [47].

Hops (*Humulus lupulus*) is considered to be a sedative agent, a view that originated from the observation of sleepiness in European hops-pickers [49]. It is commonly used in combination preparations with other herbs such as valerian (*Valeriana* spp.) and passionflower (*Passiflora incanata*) [50,51]. Although hops (*Humulus lupulus*) is listed as an approved herb for mood disturbances including sleep disturbances in The Complete German Commission E Monographs [52], there are no randomized controlled trials investigating the efficacy of hops (*Humulus lupulus*) alone in the treatment of insomnia. Thus it remains unclear whether hops (*Humulus lupulus*) has independent sedative effects, works as a synergist, or lacks sedative activity.

The rationale for inclusion of magnesium and vitamin B6 in LZComplex3 is based on in vitro and animal studies suggesting they may promote sleep quality by supporting metabolic pathways involved in sleep regulation, rather than due to any direct sedative activity [26–33]. Given the current clinical evidence base for the individual components in LZComplex3, it is difficult to determine whether the primary endpoint of this study was not met because of an absence of sedative activity, unknown complex pharmacokinetic interaction between the individual active ingredients, or because of methodological factors.

It is possible that the two-week treatment duration in our study was not long enough to observe a treatment effect, and/or the one-week placebo run-in period was not long enough to eliminate all placebo responders. Another possibility is that the study population may have included individuals with chronic insomnia, which unlike brief or acute insomnia generally requires a cognitive behavioral approach to treatment [5]. The study population was selected based on a global PSQI score greater than 5, which indicates poor sleep [38]. However, individual's responses on the PSQI questionnaire could not be used to differentiate between acute and chronic insomnia. Conversely, our ability to detect a treatment effect may be due to eligibility here being set at a minor level of sleeping difficulties, while individuals with more severe insomnia would be expected to benefit most from treatment.

Overall, the secondary outcome measures did not support a benefit of LZComplex3 over placebo during the two week treatment period. Participants completed a battery of questionnaires assessing various aspects of sleep quality, daytime functioning and physical fatigue, mood and anxiety, cognitive performance, and stress. Poor sleep can contribute to impairment of daytime functioning and physical fatigue thus these outcomes were anticipated to improve with better quality sleep. However, given that no significant difference between LZComplex3 and placebo was detected with respect to improvement in sleep quality as measured by the PSQI, it is not surprising that daytime functioning and physical fatigue were also not significantly different between the treatment groups. An improvement in ISI at day 3 favoring LZComplex3 and a between-group difference in stress reactivity as measured by change in STAI-S total score from pre- to post-administration of the MTF which appeared to be due to a slight increase in stress reactivity in the placebo group at baseline and at day 14 were the only significant treatment effects detected. Potential improvements in mood, anxiety and stress with LZComplex3 were anticipated as there is evidence that they may be positively impacted by some of the individual components of the formulation [10–14,17–24]. In our study, a clinically significant treatment effect may not have been detected for the same reasons as described for the primary outcome measure.

The safety data collected in this study indicate that LZComplex3 is well-tolerated at the dose of two tablets prior to sleep. Overall the safety profile of LZComplex3 was similar to placebo, with similar proportions of patients reporting AEs in both groups, the majority of which were mild or moderate and none of which were serious. There were more severe AEs reported in the LZComplex3 group and only two were considered possibly, probably or definitely related to treatment (both gastrointestinal disorders).

5. Conclusions

Despite finding a negative primary efficacy outcome, this study demonstrated an improvement in the PSQI and other measures of sleep quality for patients taking LZComplex3 with no deficits in cognitive or psychomotor function and a benign safety profile. These findings, taken into context with the marked placebo effect, short treatment duration and methodological limitations, suggest that further investigation of LZComplex3 is warranted.

Supplementary Materials: The following are available online at http://www.mdpi.com/2072-6643/9/2/154/s1, Figure S1: Adjusted mean change in Leeds Sleep Evaluation Questionnaire (LSEQ) scores, Figure S2: Adjusted mean change in Epworth Sleepiness Scale (ESS) scores, Figure S3: Adjusted mean change in Insomnia Severity Index (ISI), Figure S4: Adjusted mean change in Consensus Sleep Diary (CSD) scores, Figure S5: Adjusted mean change in the Chalder Fatigue Scale (CFS) total score, Figure S6: Adjusted mean change in the Burckhardt Quality of Life Scale (QoLS) total score, Figure S7: Adjusted mean change in the State-Trait Anxiety Inventory State subscale (STAI-S) score, Figure S8: Adjusted mean change in Bond-Lader Visual Analogue Scale (VAS) scores, Figure S9: Adjusted mean change in Visual Analogue Mood Scale (VAMS) scores, Table S1: Adjusted change in multi-tasking framework (MTF) total and component scores.

Acknowledgments: The authors would like to thank the study participants. This study was sponsored by Sanofi Consumer Healthcare Pty Ltd. (Macquarie Park, NSW, Australia). Jim Sockler of Datapharm Australia Pty Ltd. (Drummoyne, NSW, Australia) developed the statistical analysis plan and analysed the data. Editorial assistance in the preparation of this manuscript was provided by Adrianna Kalous and Hazel Palmer, ISMPP CMPP™ of Scripitx Pty Ltd. (Freshwater, NSW, Australia) and sponsored by Sanofi Consumer Healthcare Pty Ltd. The authors were responsible for all content, interpretation of the data and the decision to publish the results; they received no honoraria related to the development of this manuscript.

Author Contributions: A.S. and G.M. conceived and designed the experiments; A.S., S.B., A.G., N.P. and G.M. performed the experiments; A.S., G.M. and J.S. analyzed the data; all authors contributed reagents/materials/analysis tools; A.S. and J.S. wrote the paper.

Conflicts of Interest: A.S. has received presentation honoraria, travel support and/or clinical trial grants from Abbott Nutrition, Arla Foods, Australian Wine Research Institute, Barilla, Bayer Healthcare, Blackmores, Cognis, Cyvex, Dairy Health Innovation Consortium, Danone, Ginsana, GlaxoSmithKline Healthcare, Masterfoods, Martek, Naturex, Nestlé, Novartis, Red Bull, Sanofi, Unilever, Verdure Sciences, Wrigley. J.S. is supported by a CR Roper Fellowship at The University of Melbourne. J.S. reports no specific direct conflict of interest; general disclosures involve presentation honoraria, travel support, clinical trial grants, or book royalties from Integria Healthcare & MediHerb, Pfizer, Taki Mai, Bioceuticals & Blackmores, Soho-Flordis, Healthworld, HealthEd, Elsevier, Chaminade University, International Society for Affective Disorders, Complementary Medicines Australia, ANS, Society for Medicinal Plant and Natural Product Research, Omega-3 Centre, and the National Health and Medical Research Council. The sponsor was involved in the design of the study. G.M., S.B., A.G. and N.P. report having no specific direct conflicts of interest".

Abbreviations

The following abbreviations are used in this manuscript:

AE	adverse event
CFS	Chalder Fatigue Scale
CSD	Consensus Sleep Diary
EOT	end of treatment
ESS	Epworth sleepiness scale
HADS	Hospital Anxiety And Depression Scale
ISI	Insomnia Severity Scale
LSEQ	Leeds Sleep Evaluation Questionnaire
mITT	Modified intention-to-treat
MTF	Multi-tasking framework
PP	per protocol
PSQI	Pittsburgh Sleep Quality Index
QoLS	Quality of Life Scale
STAI-S	State-Trait Anxiety Inventory State subscale
STAI-T	State-Trait Anxiety Inventory Trait subscale
VAMS	Visual Analogue Mood Scale

Appendix A

Table A1. Participant inclusion and exclusion criteria.

Inclusion Criteria
• Individuals (male and female) with no significant diagnosed diseases by the judgment of the Investigator, who self-report sleeping difficulties over one month prior to the screening call.
• Age 18–65 years.
• Body mass index 18–30 kg/m².
• Normal vital signs (blood pressure less than 140/90 mmHg (i.e., systolic blood pressure less than 140 mmHg and a diastolic blood pressure less than 90 mmHg, and a heart rate between 60–100 bpm).
• Pittsburgh Sleep Quality Index Score >5.
• Typical bedtime between 9 p.m. and 12 a.m.
• Symptoms consistent with Primary Insomnia established at Screening.
• Signed written informed consent.

Table A1. *Cont.*

Exclusion Criteria
• Hospital Anxiety And Depression Scale depression score >8 and/or anxiety score >12 (assessed at Screening)
• Regular use of illicit drugs, excessive or inappropriate use of over the counter or prescription drugs or excessive use of alcohol (assessed by the Investigator or delegate and/or reported by the volunteers).
• Smoking more than 10 cigarettes a day.
• Consumption of more than 10 cups of tea or coffee (or equivalent of other caffeine containing drinks) and/or consumption of these drinks after 5 p.m.
• Allergy to milk proteins, latex or LZComplex3 ingredients.
• Primary sleep disorder (sleep apnoea-hypopnoea, periodic limb movement disorder, restless legs syndrome, narcolepsy, idiopathic hypersomnia, Kleine-Levin syndrome).
• Use of medicinal products for sleep disorders (e.g., hypnotic agents, anxiolytics, herbal remedies, homeopathy for hypnotic purposes) in the month prior to inclusion, or exhibiting withdrawal symptoms from the use of medicinal products for sleep disorders at Screening.
• On-going non-pharmacological treatment of sleep disorders (e.g., cognitive behavioral therapy, relaxation therapy)
• Expected sleep disturbance from external sources during the study period (such as young children or other household disturbance).
• Previous failure on prescription sleep medication.
• Pregnancy or lactation.
• Current sleep disturbance due to pain or a general medical condition including but not limited to pain, cystitis, urinary frequency, heart burn or others by the judgment of the Investigator that would preclude participation in the study.
• Sleep Efficiency >85% AND Sleep Onset Latency below 31 min AND Wake after Sleep Onset below 31 min (assessed during week 1 using the Consensus Sleep Diary).
• Participants who withdraw consent during screening (participants who are not willing to continue or fail to return).

Table A2. Treatment assessments.

Sleep quality	The PSQI is a 19-item questionnaire that produces a global sleep quality score and the following seven component scores: sleep quality, sleep latency, sleep duration, habitual sleep efficiency, sleep disturbance, use of sleeping medications, and daytime dysfunction [38]. Scores range from 0 to 21 and are designed to differentiate between good and poor sleep quality. Higher score indicates worse sleep quality.
	The LSEQ is a standardised self-reporting instrument comprising ten 100 mm visual analogue scales that pertain to the ease of getting to sleep, quality of sleep, ease of awakening from sleep and alertness and behavior following wakefulness [39].
	The ESS is an 8-item questionnaire asking subjects to rate their probability of falling asleep on a scale of increasing probability from 0–3 for eight different situations that most people engage in during their daily lives, though not necessarily every day (e.g., sitting and reading, as a passenger in a car for an hour without a break) [40]. A score between 0 and 9 is considered to be normal while a score between 10 and 24 could indicate sleep problems.
	The ISI is a 7-item questionnaire that addresses the degree of distress or concern caused by different sleep problems including sleep-onset and sleep maintenance problems, satisfaction with current sleep pattern, interference with daily functioning, noticeability of impairment attributed to the sleep problem [41]. Total score ranges from 0 to 28, with a higher score suggesting more severe sleep problems.
	The CSD is a standardised sleep diary that measures sleep efficiency, wake after sleep onset, and sleep onset latency [37].

Table A2. *Cont.*

Daytime functioning and physical fatigue	The Burckhardt QoLS is a 16-item scale that measures six conceptual domains of quality of life: material and physical well-being; relationships with other people; social, community and civic activities; personal development and fulfilment; recreation, and independence, the ability to do for yourself [42]. Each domain is scored on a 7-point "delighted-terrible" scale, with a higher total quality of life score indicating better quality of life. The CFS is an 11-item self-rating measure of fatigue severity for both physical and mental symptoms. The total score is derived from the number of items in which the participant responded "Worse than usual" or "Much worse than usual", with higher scores indicating greater fatigue, and negative change values indicating less fatigue [43].
Mood and anxiety	The Bond-Lader VAS comprises a total of 16 lines (approximately 100 mm) anchored at either end by antonyms (e.g., alert–drowsy, calm–excited), on which participants indicate their current subjective position [44]. Individual item scores are calculated as the percentage distance along the line. The Bond-Lader VAS was collapsed into three category scales of "alertness", "contentedness", and "calmness". The STAI-S measures fluctuating levels of anxiety on a 20-item subscale [35]. Scores range from 20 to 80, with higher scores indicating more anxiety. Stress and Fatigue VAMS are single visual analogue scales aimed to gauge subjective mood experience at the present moment relating to stress and fatigue. The Bond-Lader VAS, STAI-S and Stress and Fatigue VAMS were each administered before and after the MTF in order to measure acute levels of anxiety in response to an experimental stressor.
Cognitive performance and stress reactivity	The purple MTF consists of two tasks assessing executive function (mathematical processing and stroop colour-word), a psychomotor task that has a set time limit for completion (target tracker), and a working memory task that presents stimuli at 10 s intervals (memory search), all conducted simultaneously. The MTF can be used to elicit acute psychological stress in laboratory settings to assess stress reactivity.

CFS = Chalder Fatigue Scale; CSD = Consensus Sleep Diary; ESS = Epworth Sleepiness Scale; ISS = Insomnia Severity Index; LSEQ = Leeds Sleep Evaluation Questionnaire; MTF = multi-tasking framework; PSQI = Pittsburgh Sleep Quality Index Score; QoLS = Quality of Life Scale; STAI-S = State-Trait Anxiety Inventory State subscale; VAMS = Visual Analogue Mood Scales; VAS = Visual Analogue Scales.

References

1. Association, A.P. *Diagnostic and Statistical Manual of Mental Disorders*, 5th ed.; American Psychiatric Publishing: Arlington, MA, USA, 2013.

2. Bartlett, D.J.; Marshall, N.S.; Williams, A.; Grunstein, R.R. Sleep Health New South Wales: Chronic Sleep Restriction and Daytime Sleepiness. *Intern. Med. J.* **2008**, *38*, 24–31. [CrossRef] [PubMed]

3. Lack, L.; Miller, W.; Turner, D. A Survey of Sleeping Difficulties in an Australian Population. *Community Health Stud.* **1988**, *12*, 200–207. [CrossRef] [PubMed]

4. Stranges, S.; Tigbe, W.; Gomez-Olive, F.X.; Thorogood, M.; Kandala, N.B. Sleep Problems: An Emerging Global Epidemic? Findings from the Indepth Who-Sage Study among more than 40,000 Older Adults from 8 Countries across Africa and Asia. *Sleep* **2012**, *35*, 1173–1181. [CrossRef] [PubMed]

5. Cunnington, D.; Junge, M.F.; Fernando, A.T. Insomnia: Prevalence, Consequences and Effective Treatment. *Med. J. Aust.* **2013**, *199*, S36–S40. [CrossRef] [PubMed]

6. Pearson, N.J.; Johnson, L.L.; Nahin, R.L. Insomnia, Trouble Sleeping, and Complementary and Alternative Medicine: Analysis of the 2002 National Health Interview Survey Data. *Arch. Intern. Med.* **2006**, *166*, 1775–1782. [CrossRef] [PubMed]

7. Sanchez-Ortuno, M.M.; Belanger, L.; Ivers, H.; Leblanc, M.; Morin, C.M. The Use of Natural Products for Sleep: A Common Practice? *Sleep Med.* **2009**, *10*, 982–987. [CrossRef] [PubMed]

8. Sarris, J.; Panossian, A.; Schweitzer, I.; Stough, C.; Scholey, A. Herbal Medicine for Depression, Anxiety And Insomnia: A Review of Psychopharmacology and Clinical Evidence. *Eur. Neuropsychopharmacol.* **2011**, *21*, 841–860. [CrossRef] [PubMed]

9. The Origins of Lactium®. Available online: http://www.lactium.com/what-is-lactium%C2%AE/the-origins-of-lactium%C2%AE.html (accessed on 1 March 2016).

10. Miclo, L.; Perrin, E.; Driou, A.; Papadopoulos, V.; Boujrad, N.; Vanderesse, R.; Boudier, J.F.; Desor, D.; Linden, G.; Gaillard, J.L. Characterization of Alpha-Casozepine, a Tryptic Peptide From Bovine Alpha(S1)-Casein with Benzodiazepine-Like Activity. *FASEB J.* **2001**, *15*, 1780–1782. [PubMed]

11. Messaoudi, M.; Lefranc-Millot, C.; Desor, D.; Demagny, B.; Bourdon, L. Effects of a Tryptic Hydrolysate From Bovine Milk Alphas1-Casein on Hemodynamic Responses in Healthy Human Volunteers Facing Successive Mental and Physical Stress Situations. *Eur. J. Nutr.* **2005**, *44*, 128–132. [CrossRef] [PubMed]
12. Kim, J.H.; Desor, D.; Kim, Y.T.; Yoon, W.J.; Kim, K.S.; Jun, J.S.; Pyun, K.H.; Shim, I. Efficacy of Alphas1-Casein Hydrolysate on Stress-Related Symptoms in Women. *Eur. J. Clin. Nutr.* **2007**, *61*, 536–541. [PubMed]
13. Violle, N.; Messaoudi, M.; Lefranc-Millot, C.; Desor, D.; Nejdi, A.; Demagny, B.; Schroeder, H. Ethological Comparison of the Effects of a Bovine Alpha S1-Casein Tryptic Hydrolysate and Diazepam on the Behaviour of Rats in Two Models of Anxiety. *Pharmacol. Biochem. Behav.* **2006**, *84*, 517–523. [CrossRef] [PubMed]
14. Guesdon, B.; Messaoudi, M.; Lefranc-Millot, C.; Fromentin, G.; Tome, D.; Even, P.C. A Tryptic Hydrolysate from Bovine Milk Alphas1-Casein Improves Sleep in Rats Subjected to Chronic Mild Stress. *Peptides* **2006**, *27*, 1476–1482. [CrossRef] [PubMed]
15. Adzu, B.; Amos, S.; Amizan, M.B.; Gamaniel, K. Evaluation of the Antidiarrhoeal Effects of *Zizyphus Spina-Christi* Stem Bark in Rats. *Acta Trop.* **2003**, *87*, 245–250. [CrossRef]
16. Jiang, J.G.; Huang, X.J.; Chen, J.; Lin, Q.S. Comparison of the Sedative and Hypnotic Effects of Flavonoids, Saponins, and Polysaccharides Extracted From Semen Ziziphus Jujube. *Nat. Prod. Res.* **2007**, *21*, 310–320. [CrossRef] [PubMed]
17. Chen, H.C.; Hsieh, M.T. Clinical Trial of Suanzaorentang in the Treatment of Insomnia. *Clin. Ther.* **1985**, *7*, 334–337. [PubMed]
18. Chen, H.C.; Hsieh, M.T.; Shibuya, T.K. Suanzaorentang versus Diazepam: A Controlled Double-Blind Study in Anxiety. *Int. J. Clin. Pharmacol. Ther. Toxicol.* **1986**, *24*, 646–650. [PubMed]
19. Braun, L.; Cohen, M. *Hops. Herbs & Natural Supplements: An Evidence Based Guide*, 2nd ed.; Elsevier: Chatswood, Australia, 2007.
20. Scientific Committee of the British Herbal Medicine Association. *British Herbal Pharmacopoeia*, 2nd ed.; British Herbal Medicine Association: Bournemouth, UK, 1983; pp. 111–112.
21. Bradley, P.R. (Ed.) *British Herbal Compendium Volume 1: A Handbook of Scientific Information on Widely Used Plant Drugs*; British Herbal Medicine Association: Dorset, UK, 1992.
22. European Scientific Cooperative on Phytotherapy. *Escop Monographs: The Scientific Foundation for Herbal Medicinal Products*; Escop: Exeter, UK, 2003; pp. 306–311.
23. Newal, A.C.; Anderson, L.A.; Phillipson, J.D. *Hops. Herbal Medicines. A Guide for Healthcare Professionals*, 1st ed.; Pharmaceutical Press: London, UK; Chicago, IL, USA, 1996; pp. 162–163.
24. Ulbricht, C.; Basch, E. (Eds.) Hops (*Humulus Lupulus* L.). Natural Standard Database. Available online: https://naturalmedicines.therapeuticresearch.com (accessed on 26 February 2009).
25. Altura, B.M. Basic Biochemistry and Physiology of Magnesium: A Brief Review. *Magnes. Trace Elem.* **1991**, *10*, 167–171. [PubMed]
26. Chollet, D.; Franken, P.; Raffin, Y.; Henrotte, J.G.; Widmer, J.; Malafosse, A.; Tafti, M. Magnesium Involvement in Sleep: Genetic and Nutritional Models. *Behav. Genet.* **2001**, *31*, 413–425. [CrossRef] [PubMed]
27. Dralle, D.; Bodeker, R.H. Serum Magnesium Level and Sleep Behavior of Newborn Infants. *Eur. J. Pediatr.* **1980**, *134*, 239–243. [CrossRef] [PubMed]
28. Depoortere, H.; Francon, D.; Llopis, J. Effects of a Magnesium-Deficient Diet on Sleep Organization in Rats. *Neuropsychobiology* **1993**, *27*, 237–245. [CrossRef] [PubMed]
29. Poenaru, S.; Rouhani, S.; Durlach, J.; Aymard, N.; Belkahla, F.; Rayssiguier, Y.; Iovino, M. Vigilance States and Cerebral Monoamine Metabolism in Experimental Magnesium Deficiency. *Magnesium* **1984**, *3*, 145–151. [PubMed]
30. Hornyak, M.; Haas, P.; Veit, J.; Gann, H.; Riemann, D. Magnesium Treatment of Primary Alcohol-Dependent Patients during Subacute Withdrawal: An Open Pilot Study with Polysomnography. *Alcohol. Clin. Exp. Res.* **2004**, *28*, 1702–1709. [CrossRef] [PubMed]
31. Held, K.; Antonijevic, I.A.; Kunzel, H.; Uhr, M.; Wetter, T.C.; Golly, I.C.; Steiger, A.; Murck, H. Oral Mg(2$^+$) Supplementation Reverses Age-Related Neuroendocrine and Sleep Eeg Changes in Humans. *Pharmacopsychiatry* **2002**, *35*, 135–143. [CrossRef] [PubMed]
32. Holst, S.C.; Valomon, A.; Landolt, H.P. Sleep Pharmacogenetics: Personalized Sleep-Wake Therapy. *Annu. Rev. Pharmacol. Toxicol.* **2016**, *56*, 577–603. [CrossRef] [PubMed]
33. Clayton, P.T. B6-Responsive Disorders: A Model of Vitamin Dependency. *J. Inherit. Metab. Dis.* **2006**, *29*, 317–326. [CrossRef] [PubMed]

34. Zigmond, A.S.; Snaith, R.P. The Hospital Anxiety and Depression Scale. *Acta Psychiatr. Scand.* **1983**, *67*, 361–370. [CrossRef] [PubMed]

35. Spielberger, C.D.; Gorsuch, R.L.; Lushene, R.; Vagg, P.R.; Jacobs, G.A. *Manual for the State-Trait Anxiety Inventory*; Consulting Psychologists Press, Inc.: Palo Alto, CA, USA, 1983.

36. Grandner, M.A.; Kripke, D.F.; Yoon, I.Y.; Youngstedt, S.D. Criterion Validity of the Pittsburgh Sleep Quality Index: Investigation in a Non-Clinical Sample. *Sleep Biol. Rhythm.* **2006**, *4*, 129–139. [CrossRef] [PubMed]

37. Carney, C.E.; Buysse, D.J.; Ancoli-Israel, S.; Edinger, J.D.; Krystal, A.D.; Lichstein, K.L.; Morin, C.M. The Consensus Sleep Diary: Standardizing Prospective Sleep Self-Monitoring. *Sleep* **2012**, *35*, 287–302. [CrossRef] [PubMed]

38. Buysse, D.J.; Reynolds, C.F., 3rd; Monk, T.H.; Berman, S.R.; Kupfer, D.J. The Pittsburgh Sleep Quality Index: A New Instrument for Psychiatric Practice and Research. *Psychiatry Res.* **1989**, *28*, 193–213. [CrossRef]

39. Parrott, A.C.; Hindmarch, I. The Leeds Sleep Evaluation Questionnaire in Psychopharmacological Investigations—A Review. *Psychopharmacology* **1980**, *71*, 173–179. [CrossRef] [PubMed]

40. Johns, M.W. A New Method for Measuring Daytime Sleepiness: The Epworth Sleepiness Scale. *Sleep* **1991**, *14*, 540–545. [CrossRef] [PubMed]

41. Bastien, C.H.; Vallieres, A.; Morin, C.M. Validation of the Insomnia Severity Index as an Outcome Measure for Insomnia Research. *Sleep Med.* **2001**, *2*, 297–307. [CrossRef]

42. Burckhardt, C.S.; Woods, S.L.; Schultz, A.A.; Ziebarth, D.M. Quality of Life of Adults with Chronic Illness: A Psychometric Study. *Res. Nurs. Health* **1989**, *12*, 347–354. [CrossRef] [PubMed]

43. Chalder, T.; Berelowitz, G.; Pawlikowska, T.; Watts, L.; Wessely, S.; Wright, D.; Wallace, E.P. Development of a Fatigue Scale. *J. Psychosom. Res.* **1993**, *37*, 147–153. [CrossRef]

44. Bond, A.J.; James, D.C.; Lader, M.H. Physiological and Psychological Measures in Anxious Patients. *Psychol. Med.* **1974**, *4*, 364–373. [CrossRef] [PubMed]

45. Thorndike, F.P.; Ritterband, L.M.; Saylor, D.K.; Magee, J.C.; Gonder-Frederick, L.A.; Morin, C.M. Validation of the Insomnia Severity Index as a Web-Based Measure. *Behav. Sleep Med.* **2011**, *9*, 216–223. [CrossRef] [PubMed]

46. De Saint-Hilaire, Z.; Messaoudi, M.; Desor, D.; Kobayashi, T. Effects of a Bovine Alpha S1-Casein Tryptic Hydrolysate (Cth) on Sleep Disorder in Japanese General Population. *Open Sleep J.* **2009**, *2*, 26–32. [CrossRef]

47. Xie, C.L.; Gu, Y.; Wang, W.W.; Lu, L.; Fu, D.L.; Liu, A.J.; Li, H.Q.; Li, J.H.; Lin, Y.; Tang, W.J.; et al. Efficacy and Safety of Suanzaoren Decoction for Primary Insomnia: A Systematic Review of Randomized Controlled Trials. *BMC Complement. Altern. Med.* **2013**, *13*, 18. [CrossRef] [PubMed]

48. Chung, K.F.; Lee, C.K. Over-the-counter Sleeping Pills: A Survey of Use in Hong Kong and a Review of Their Constituents. *Gen. Hosp. Psychiatry* **2002**, *24*, 430–435. [CrossRef]

49. Humulus Lupus. Monograph. Available online: http://www.altmedrev.com/publications/8/2/190.pdf (accessed on 16 February 2017).

50. Koetter, U.; Schrader, E.; Kaufeler, R.; Brattstrom, A. A Randomized, Double Blind, Placebo-Controlled, Prospective Clinical Study to Demonstrate Clinical Efficacy of a Fixed Valerian Hops Extract Combination (Ze 91019) in Patients Suffering from Non-Organic Sleep Disorder. *Phytother. Res.* **2007**, *21*, 847–851. [CrossRef] [PubMed]

51. Maroo, N.; Hazra, A.; Das, T. Efficacy and Safety of a Polyherbal Sedative-Hypnotic Formulation Nsf-3 in Primary Insomnia in Comparison to Zolpidem: A Randomized Controlled Trial. *Indian J. Pharmacol.* **2013**, *45*, 34–39. [CrossRef] [PubMed]

52. Blumenthal, M. *The Complete German Commission E Monograph: Therapeutic Guide to Herbal Medicines*; American Botanical Council: Austin, TX, USA, 1998; Volume 147.

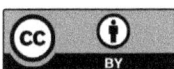

nutrients

MDPI

Article

Effect of Six-Month Diet Intervention on Sleep among Overweight and Obese Men with Chronic Insomnia Symptoms: A Randomized Controlled Trial

Xiao Tan [1,2], Markku Alén [2,3], Kun Wang [1], Jarkko Tenhunen [2], Petri Wiklund [1,2], Markku Partinen [4] and Sulin Cheng [1,2,*]

[1] Exercise Health and Technology Center, Shanghai Jiao Tong University, Shanghai 200240, China; xiao.tan@jyu.fi (X.T.); wangkunz@sjtu.edu.cn (K.W.); petri.wiklund@jyu.fi (P.W.)

[2] Department of Health Sciences, University of Jyväskylä, Jyväskylä 40014, Finland; markku.alen@jyu.fi (M.A.); tenhujar@gmail.com (J.T.)

[3] Department of Medical Rehabilitation, Oulu University Hospital and Center for Life Course Health Research, University of Oulu, Oulu 90220, Finland

[4] VitalMed Research Center, Helsinki Sleep Clinic and Department of Neurosciences, University of Helsinki, Helsinki 00380, Finland; markku.partinen@helsinki.fi

* Correspondence: sulin.cheng@jyu.fi; Tel.: +358-40-558-0209; Fax: +358-14-260-2011

Received: 14 September 2016; Accepted: 16 November 2016; Published: 23 November 2016

Abstract: Growing evidence suggests that diet alteration affects sleep, but this has not yet been studied in adults with insomnia symptoms. We aimed to determine the effect of a six-month diet intervention on sleep among overweight and obese (Body mass index, BMI $\geq$ 25 kg/m^2) men with chronic insomnia symptoms. Forty-nine men aged 30–65 years with chronic insomnia symptoms were randomized into diet ($n = 28$) or control ($n = 21$) groups. The diet group underwent a six-month individualized diet intervention with three face-to-face counseling sessions and online supervision 1–3 times per week; 300–500 kcal/day less energy intake and optimized nutrient composition were recommended. Controls were instructed to maintain their habitual lifestyle. Sleep parameters were determined by piezoelectric bed sensors, a sleep diary, and a Basic Nordic sleep questionnaire. Compared to the controls, the diet group had shorter objective sleep onset latency after intervention. Within the diet group, prolonged objective total sleep time, improved objective sleep efficiency, lower depression score, less subjective nocturnal awakenings, and nocturia were found after intervention. In conclusion, modest energy restriction and optimized nutrient composition shorten sleep onset latency in overweight and obese men with insomnia symptoms.

Keywords: insomnia symptoms; sleep; sleep onset; diet intervention; nutrient; overweight; obesity

1. Introduction

Insomnia is a highly prevalent sleep disorder and has become a significant health issue in many countries. The prevalence of chronic insomnia symptoms classified by the Diagnostic and Statistical Manual of Mental Disorders, 4th Edition (DSM-IV) criteria ranges between 15.2% and 22.1% of the general population in different regions of the world [1–3]. In Finland, nearly a quarter of the employed people are reported to suffer from insomnia [4]. Insomnia symptoms are risk factors of various adverse health consequences [5]. For instance, difficulty initiating sleep, the symptom represented by prolonged sleep onset latency (SOL), is independently associated with all-cause mortality among Finnish men [6].

A growing body of evidence suggests that overweight and obesity are significant risk factors for impaired sleep and insomnia [7–9]. Population-based study showed that obese adults had higher incidence of subjective sleep disturbances than non-obese ones [9]. Longitudinal studies suggested that both obesity and weight gain could predict future development of insomnia symptoms [7,8]. Diet is an important mediator between sleep and overweight/obesity. Growing evidence suggest that diet alterations can directly influence sleep parameters [10,11]. Furthermore, the associations between nutrients and insomnia symptoms have been reported by recent studies [12–14]. However, no previous study has investigated whether diet intervention leads to improved sleep parameters related to insomnia symptoms, such as sleep onset latency. There is also a lack of data regarding the effects of diet-induced weight loss on sleep among overweight and obese populations, especially in men, among which the combined prevalence of overweight and obesity is higher than women in Finland [15].

Thus, the present study aimed to investigate whether sleep parameters among overweight and obese men with chronic insomnia symptoms can be improved through a six-month diet intervention. We hypothesized that reduced energy intake and optimized nutrient composition can improve one or multiple objectively and subjectively measured sleep parameters.

2. Methods

The present randomized controlled trial forms part of a larger study with different lifestyle interventions on middle-aged men with sleep disorders (Monitoring and treatment of obesity-related sleep disorders, ISRCTN77172005). Results regarding the comparisons between exercise and control groups have been reported in an earlier publication [16]. In the present paper, we focus solely on the comparison between diet and control groups. However, to give an overall picture of the study, baseline characteristics and sleep outcomes at baseline and six months across the three groups are summarized in Tables S1 and S2. The study was approved by the Ethics Committee of the Central Finland Health Care District (7/2011). Informed consent was obtained from all participants prior to the baseline measurements and a copy of the signed consent form was archived.

2.1. Participants

Participants were 49 Finnish men aged 30–65 years with chronic (three months or longer) complaints of insomnia symptoms. Ninety-four percent (n = 46) of them had BMI $\geq$ 25 kg/m^2. Participants were voluntarily recruited through the outpatient clinics and public health care centers in the Central Finland Health Care District, or through advertising on the local radio news media and the Internet. The summary of participant flow is presented in Figure 1.

The modified Basic Nordic sleep questionnaire (BNSQ) [17], the health and behavior questionnaire, and participant's medical history were collected and reviewed by a physician for screening. Insomnia symptoms were classified according to the DSM-IV-TR criteria (without the criterion of daytime consequences) from answers to the modified BNSQ. Individuals were considered to have chronic insomnia symptoms if one or more of the following symptoms had occurred at least three nights per week, during the past three months: (1) Difficulty initiating sleep (subjective SOL $\geq$ 30 min); (2) Difficulty maintaining sleep (awakening during sleep $\geq$3 times/night, or difficulty in falling asleep after nocturnal awakening with total wake after sleep onset $\geq$30 min); (3) Early morning awakenings (wake up $\geq$30 min earlier than desired in the morning and unable to fall asleep again); (4) Non-restorative sleep [18,19].

Exclusion criteria were: (1) other sleep disorders include moderate or severe apnea (Apnea-hypopnea index, AHI $\geq$ 15), restless leg syndrome and periodic leg movement disorder (periodic leg movement arousal index > 15), narcolepsy, REM behavior disorder, and circadian rhythm disorder; (2) Medical history during the past three years related to diseases such as cardiovascular disease, heart failure, liver disease, and cancer; (3) Current diagnosis of major depression; (4) History of other major mental illness or substance abuse; (5) History of cognitive impairment and major neurological disorders; (6) History of eating disorders; (7) Taking special diet at the moment; (8) Chronic pain conditions; (9) Regular use of sedatives, hypnotics, and painkillers; (10) Shift work [12].

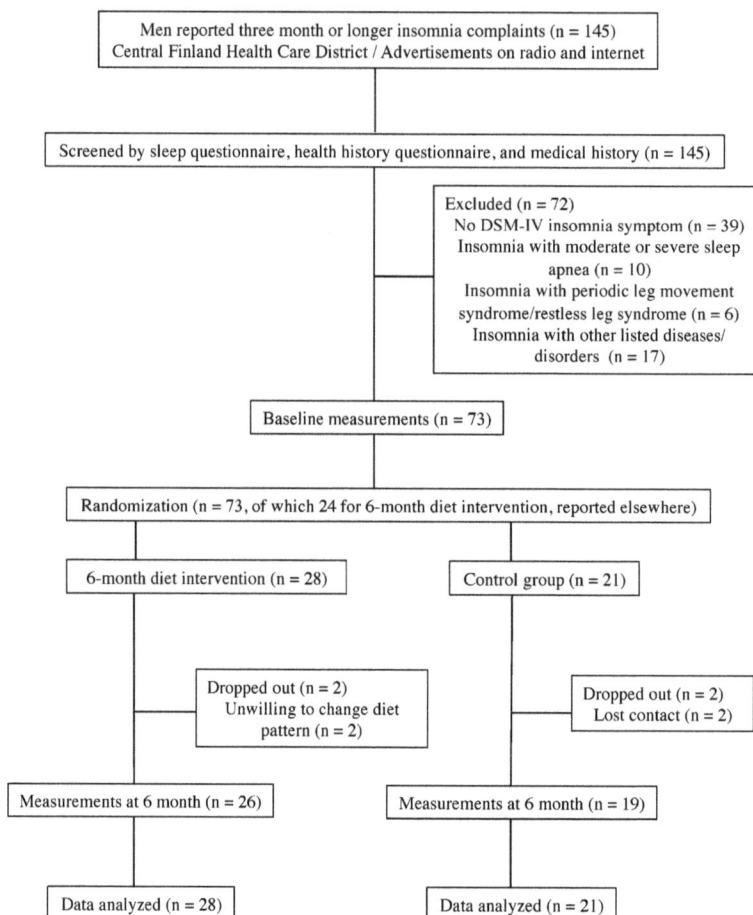

Figure 1. Participant flow of the study.

2.2. Measurements

All measurements were carried out before randomization, and after the six-month intervention period. In addition, nutrient intake and anthropometry were measured at three months.

2.2.1. Descriptive Characteristics

Age, education, employment, and smoking habits were elicited at baseline with the health and behavior questionnaire. Age of onset of insomnia and occurrences of insomnia symptoms were elicited with the baseline modified BNSQ.

2.2.2. Energy Consumption and Nutrients Intake

A three-day diet diary (two weekdays and one weekend) collected the type, item, and estimated portion of all food and drink intake during each day. Archiving of diet information, calculation of nutrients intake, total calories, and proportions of energy-yielding nutrients in total calories (E%) were carried out by the Micro-Nutrica software (The Social Insurance Institution of Finland, Turku, Finland).

2.2.3. Anthropometry and Fat Mass

All anthropometric measurements were performed after overnight fasting (12 h). Height was measured to the nearest 0.5 cm using a fixed wall scale. Weight was determined to the nearest 0.1 kg using a calibrated physician weight scale. BMI was calculated as weight (kg) per height^2 (m^2). Neck, chest, waist, and hip circumferences were determined to the nearest 0.1 cm by a measuring tape using standardized procedures, and the average value of three measurements was taken for analysis. Blood pressure were measured using an oscillometric monitor in sitting position after five-minute resting, average value of three measurements was retained. Fat mass was determined using dual energy X-ray densitometry (DXA; Prodigy, GE Lunar, Madison, WI, USA).

2.2.4. Energy Expenditures

A seven-day physical activity diary was collected on the same days as sleep measurements. The diary recorded primary living activity at 30-min intervals over 24 h. Energy expenditures were calculated as metabolic equivalent multiplied by minutes per day (MET min/day), according to the 2011 Compendium of Physical Activities [20]. Expenditures were categorized into exercise and recreational activity (e.g., walking a dog, berry picking), livelihood physical activity (e.g., personal care, housework, commuting, occupational activities), as well as sedentary behaviors (METs $\leq$ 1.5 while in a sitting or reclining posture) and sleep [21].

2.2.5. Objective Sleep Measurement

Home-based objective sleep data were collected by an unobtrusive online sleep monitoring system (Beddit pro; Beddit Ltd., Espoo, Finland). The system included a piezoelectric bed sensor. Ballistocardiographic signals were sampled by the piezoelectric sensor at 140 Hz and simultaneously uploaded to a web server through the Internet, where sleep/wake status was classified in 30-s epochs based on heart rate variability, respiration rate variability, and binary actigram [22]. An ambient brightness sensor, included in the system, was placed in the bedroom for determining lights-out time. For participants who had a bed partner, sensor attachment was considered to avoid overlapping measurements. Participants were instructed to mention conditions that might have affected the measurements, such as children and pets in the bedroom, in the sleep diary. Measurement was set automatically to start each evening at 18:00, and end at noon the next day. Total sleep time (TST), SOL (determined as the duration from being present in bed with lights out to the first five minutes of consecutive sleep) [23], wakefulness after sleep onset (WASO), and sleep efficiency (SE) were obtained for each night. Sleep was measured for seven nights, including two weekends. Measurements were taken within 14 days both before and after the six-month study period. For analyses, average values across the nights were used; at least five nights' valid data at both baseline and six months were needed. Validation of the sleep/wake in 30-s epochs was carried out against two-night polysomnography measurement (31 subjects with insomnia complaints, age ($\pm$SD) = 51.8 $\pm$ 8.4 years, BMI = 30.9 $\pm$ 4.8 kg/m^2). Correlations in sleep outcomes were obtained as follow: TST (Pearson's r = 0.85, p < 0.001), SOL (Pearson's r = 0.81, p < 0.001), WASO (Kendall's tau-b = 0.74, p < 0.001), SE (Kendall's tau-b = 0.68, p < 0.001) [16].

2.2.6. Sleep Diary and Modified BNSQ

The seven-night sleep diary was collected on same nights with objective sleep measurement. Items included time of going to bed, estimated time of falling asleep, number of nocturnal awakenings, final waking-up time, morning-rated subjective sleep quality, fatigue upon awakening, nap duration, and other issues related with sleep. The average values for the recorded nights were used for analyses. Epworth sleepiness scale (ESS) score [24], Rimon's brief depression scale score [25], insomnia symptom frequency, and other subjective sleep assessment results were elicited by the modified BNSQ.

2.3. Randomization

After the baseline measurements, participants were randomized and allocated into the diet intervention or control group, by an external statistician. Randomization was stratified by age and BMI ($\leq$ or >medians) with a block size of 5, using SAS v. 9.2, (SAS Institute, Cary, NC, USA).

2.4. Interactive Diet Intervention

A six-month individualized diet intervention program was made according to the three-day diet diary results and BMI at baseline. Individualized programs were introduced to each participant face-to-face by study nutritionists on the first day of intervention. Diet suggestions were made according to the Finnish Nutrition Recommendations [26]. Suggested proportions of energy-yielding nutrients were: 40%–45% of carbohydrate in total daily energy intake (E%) with <5 E% sucrose; 35–40 E% total fat with $\leq$10 E% saturated fatty acids (SFA), 15–20 E% monounsaturated fatty acids (MUFA), and 5–10 E% polyunsaturated fatty acids (PUFA); and 20 E% protein [26]. In addition, greater consumption of dietary fiber, vitamin A, vitamin D, vitamin E, B vitamins, vitamin C, magnesium, and potassium was recommended through selected food options (cereals, vegetables, fruits, berries, nuts, legumes, mushrooms, etc.). Participants with overweight and obesity ($n = 27$) were advised to gradually reduce their daily energy intake by 300–500 kcal during the first three months, with a target of reducing body weight by 3 kg. After this period, calorie intake was suggested to remain at the reduced level. Two intermediate face-to-face counseling sessions were held in the first and the fourth month of the intervention. Each intermediate session involved individualized diet counseling with a nutritionist, and a cooking course in which examples of meals that fulfilled the nutritional criteria of this study were introduced.

During the intervention, an online diet and nutrition counseling service (MealTracker, Wellness Foundry Holding Ltd., Helsinki, Finland) was utilized for supervising individuals' dietary intake and providing diet suggestions. Participants were instructed to photograph all daily dietary intakes (including drinks) using a smartphone or a digital camera, and upload all photos to the server 1–3 days per week during the intervention. The photos were uploaded via a mobile application, or through the service's website. According to the uploaded photos, a nutritionist assessed each individual's daily calorie intake and consumptions of nutrients. Individualized feedback including dietary intake facts and instructions for diet adjustment in the upcoming days was thus formulated and sent to participants via mobile text message and e-mail each day with uploaded information. Diet photos were saved in each participant's account in the server, which was only accessible to the participant and the nutritionist. A training session for taking and uploading diet photos was held prior to the intervention. All participants in the diet group were able to use the service correctly.

2.5. Control Group

Controls were instructed to keep their habitual, pre-recruitment lifestyle for six months. They were given an opportunity to participate in the diet plus exercise intervention program for three months after the study period.

2.6. Statistical Analysis

The estimated change of the objective SOL was based on published data [16,27]. Statistical power was over 80% to detect a 30% lowered SOL in the diet group from baseline, and no change of SOL in the control group, with the unbalanced allocation of 28 and 21 participants in each randomized group.

Analyses were carried out following the intention-to-treat principle. For participants with missing or incomplete values at follow-ups, the last observed values were carried forward. All analyses were performed using IBM SPSS statistics version 20 (SPSS, Inc., Chicago, IL, USA). All tests were two-tailed; a p value less than 0.05 was set as significant. The Shapiro–Wilk W test and Levene's test were used to examine the normality and homogeneity, respectively. Skewed data were transformed by natural logarithm. Baseline differences between groups were evaluated by one-way analysis of variance (ANOVA), or Pearson's χ^2 test. Time-by-group differences were evaluated by analysis of covariance (ANCOVA), controlling for the baseline values. Within-group differences were evaluated by repeated measures ANOVA, followed with Bonferroni corrections for multiple comparisons. In addition, Pearson's correlation coefficients were calculated between changes from baseline to six months for selected variables.

3. Results

Baseline descriptive characteristics by group are given in Table 1. Retention rates between diet and control groups were comparable (Diet = 26/28, Control = 19/21, p = 0.579, Fisher's exact test).

Table 1. Descriptive characteristics at baseline.

	Diet (n = 28)	Control (n = 21)	p #
	Mean (95% CI)	Mean (95% CI)	
Age (year)	51.0 (47.3 to 54.8)	52.6 (48.0 to 57.2)	0.592
Age when insomnia complaint started (year)	37.4 (33.1 to 41.6)	39.8 (33.7 to 46.0)	0.482
Height (cm)	178.9 (177.0 to 180.8)	178.3 (175.6 to 180.9)	0.696
Weight (kg)	93.8 (89.2 to 98.4)	93.1 (85.2 to 100.9)	0.860
BMI (kg/m^2)	29.4 (27.9 to 30.8)	29.2 (27.2 to 31.2)	0.879
Systolic blood pressure (mmHg)	142.8 (139.0 to 146.6)	140.7 (135.2 to 146.3)	0.513
Diastolic blood pressure (mmHg)	88.8 (84.9 to 92.6)	91.4 (86.7 to 96.1)	0.363
Occurrences	**Percentage**	**Percentage**	
Difficulty initiating sleep	42.9	42.9	1.000
Difficulty maintaining sleep	57.1	76.2	0.166
Early morning awakenings	32.1	23.8	0.523
Non-restorative sleep	39.3	42.9	0.801
Smoking presently	14.3	19.0	0.655
At least tertiary degree education	82.1	95.2	0.166
Employed	82.1	71.4	0.374

One-way ANOVA or Pearson's χ^2 test.

3.1. Compliance with Diet Interventions

On average, participants in the diet group who attended the six-month follow-up measurements uploaded 1.9 ± 1.1 (SD) days per week during intervention. All of these participants attended all three counseling sessions. Two participants dropped out during the first month of the study, both due to the unwillingness to change diet. There were no diet photos uploaded from the participants who dropped out.

3.2. Energy Consumption and Nutrient Intake

Within the diet group, total energy intake was reduced at six months compared to baseline (p = 0.006, Figure 2); however, changes in other nutrients were not detected. Total energy intake was reduced at three months in both groups (p = 0.001 and 0.012, respectively). Proportions of energy-yielding nutrients in total calories did not show significant change in either group. Compared to the controls, the diet group had greater intakes of potassium (2158 vs. 1806 mg/1000 kcal, p = 0.029, ANCOVA controlling for baseline) and magnesium (219 vs. 193 mg/1000 kcal, p = 0.036, ANCOVA controlling for baseline) at three months (not shown in figure).

Total calorie intake per day (kcal)

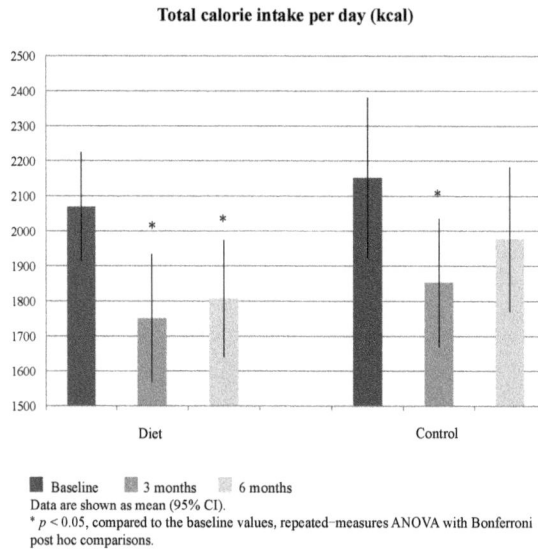

■ Baseline ▓ 3 months ░ 6 months
Data are shown as mean (95% CI).
* $p < 0.05$, compared to the baseline values, repeated–measures ANOVA with Bonferroni
post hoc comparisons.

Figure 2. Daily calorie intake by three-day diet diary at baseline vs. three and six months.

3.3. Anthropometry, Fat Mass, and Energy Expenditures

Body weight, total fat mass, and waist circumference decreased significantly in the diet group compared to the control group ($p = 0.043$ to 0.009, Table 2). No significant changes in physical activity, sedentary time, or total energy expenditure were found in either group during the intervention.

Table 2. Anthropometry, fat mass, and energy expenditures at baseline and follow-ups.

	Diet			Control		
	Baseline	3 Months	6 Months	Baseline	3 Months	6 Months
Anthropometry						
Weight (kg)	93.8 (89.2 to 98.4)	92.7 (88.3 to 97.0) [#]	92.7 (88.1 to 97.4) [#]	93.1 (85.2 to 100.9)	93.5 (85.5 to 101.5) [#]	94.4 (86.3 to 102.5) *,[#]
Neck circumference (cm)	42.0 (41.0 to 43.0)	41.9 (40.9 to 43.0)	42.2 (41.3 to 43.2)	41.9 (40.6 to 43.3)	42.0 (40.5 to 43.4)	42.6 (41.2 to 44.0) *
Chest circumference (cm)	109.4 (106.8 to 112.0)	109.2 (106.5 to 111.9)	109.7 (106.9 to 112.5)	107.7 (102.6 to 112.9)	108.0 (102.9 to 113.1)	109.5 (104.5 to 114.5) *
Waist circumference (cm)	106.6 (102.9 to 110.2)	106.1 (102.7 to 109.4)	105.9 (102.4 to 109.4) [#]	105.0 (99.9 to 110.1)	105.4 (99.9 to 110.8)	106.7 (101.3 to 112.2) *,[#]
Hip circumference (cm)	104.5 (101.9 to 107.1)	103.1 (100.1 to 106.1)	103.5 (100.4 to 106.7)	102.7 (98.6 to 106.7)	103.5 (99.6 to 107.3)	104.0 (100.0 to 108.1)
Fat mass						
Total fat mass (kg)	27.5 (24.2 to 30.7)	n/a	26.8 (23.5 to 30.2) [#]	28.0 (23.6 to 32.5)	n/a	28.9 (24.0 to 33.8) *,[#]
Trunk fat mass (kg)	17.6 (15.6 to 19.6)	n/a	17.2 (15.1 to 19.3)	17.7 (14.5 to 20.8)	n/a	18.2 (14.9 to 21.5) *
Energy expenditures						
Total expenditure (MET min/day)	2346.1 (2254.9 to 2437.3)	n/a	2398.8 (2299.7 to 2498.0)	2341.1 (2224.0 to 2458.1)	n/a	2322.6 (2210.0 to 2435.3)
Exercise and recreational physical activity (MET min/day)	226.7 (150.8 to 302.6)	n/a	292.5 (194.5 to 390.4)	249.5 (145.2 to 353.8)	n/a	254.3 (151.9 to 356.7)
Household physical activity (MET min/day)	840.9 (675.4 to 1006.5)	n/a	845.4 (689.9 to 1000.9)	803.0 (631.5 to 974.5)	n/a	751.6 (548.6 to 954.6)
Sedentary behaviors (MET min/day)	846.7 (739.0 to 954.4)	n/a	801.7 (706.1 to 897.3)	824.6 (737.1 to 912.1)	n/a	845.0 (758.3 to 931.7)

Data are shown as mean (95% CI); [#] $p < 0.05$, compared to the other group, analyses of covariance controlling for baseline values; * $p < 0.05$, compared to the baseline values, repeated measures ANOVA with Bonferroni post hoc comparisons.

3.4. Objective Sleep Parameters

At baseline, the valid objective sleep data for analyzing were on average 6.4 ± 1.1 and 6.8 ± 0.6 nights in diet and control groups, respectively. At six months, the corresponding numbers were 6.4 ± 0.9 and 6.6 ± 0.7. There was no between-group difference in the number of nights analyzed at baseline or six months ($p = 0.110$ and 0.613, respectively, one-way ANOVA). Nights marked by participants as being subject to significant disturbance in the measurement process (such as a pet sleeping in the bed) were excluded. Results of the objective sleep measurements are given in Figure 3. Compared to the control group, the diet group showed shorter SOL ($p < 0.001$) after intervention. Within the diet group, prolonged TST ($p = 0.004$), curtailed SOL ($p < 0.001$), and increased sleep efficiency were found ($p = 0.004$) through intervention. In the diet group, change of objective SOL through intervention did not correlate with changes in body weight or fat mass (both $p > 0.05$, Pearson's r).

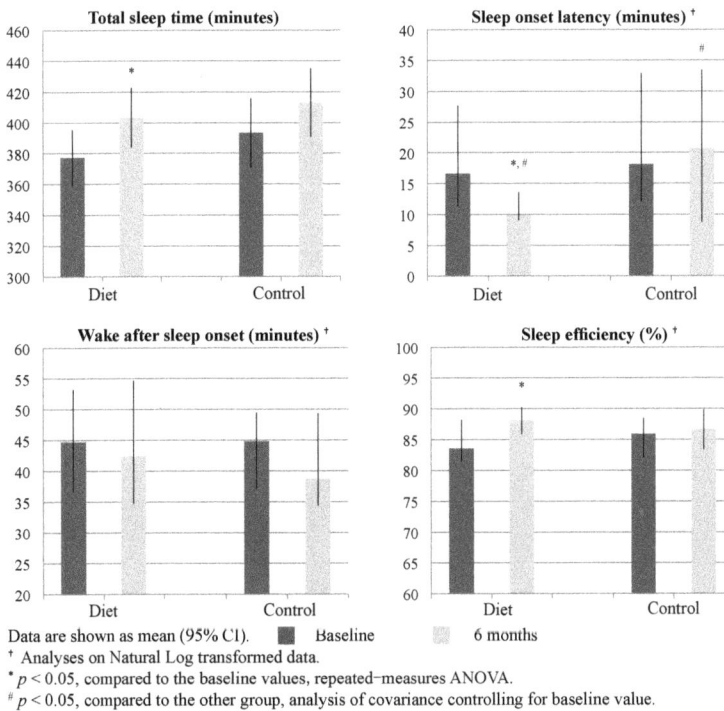

Data are shown as mean (95% CI). ■ Baseline   ▨ 6 months
[†] Analyses on Natural Log transformed data.
[*] $p < 0.05$, compared to the baseline values, repeated-measures ANOVA.
[#] $p < 0.05$, compared to the other group, analysis of covariance controlling for baseline value.

Figure 3. Sleep outcomes by piezoelectric system at baseline and six months.

3.5. Subjective Sleep Assessments

No time-by-group difference was detected among subjective sleep parameters (Table 3). Within the diet group, nocturnal awakenings ($p = 0.035$), number of nocturia ($p = 0.001$), and Rimon's depression score ($p = 0.029$) were reduced compared to the baseline values.

Table 3. Sleep outcomes by sleep diary and sleep questionnaire at baseline and six months.

	Diet			Control			Time by Group
	Baseline	6 Months	p	Baseline	6 Months	p	p [#]
Sleep diary							
Sleep onset latency (min) [†]	21.0 (13.5 to 31.0)	20.0 (13.3 to 23.8)	0.122	21.5 (17.3 to 41.8)	25.0 (15.0 to 42.5)	0.463	0.255
Nocturnal awakenings (numbers/night)	2.3 (1.8 to 2.9)	1.8 (1.3 to 2.4)	0.035	2.6 (1.8 to 3.4)	2.3 (1.8 to 2.8)	0.293	0.305
Nocturia (times/night)	0.8 (0.6 to 1.1)	0.5 (0.3 to 0.6)	0.001	0.7 (0.4 to 0.9)	0.5 (0.3 to 0.8)	0.080	0.075
Morning-rated sleep quality (1–4) [a]	2.4 (2.1 to 2.7)	2.7 (2.4 to 2.9)	0.094	2.4 (2.2 to 2.5)	2.4 (2.2 to 2.6)	0.785	0.153
Fatigue upon awakening (1–4) [b]	2.2 (2.0 to 2.4)	2.0 (1.7 to 2.2)	0.062	1.9 (1.6 to 2.1)	2.0 (1.8 to 2.2)	0.300	0.292
Nap (min/day) [*]	17.1 (11.2 to 23.1)	14.0 (8.1 to 19.9)	0.388	12.5 (4.4 to 20.6)	11.9 (2.2 to 21.6)	0.885	0.957
Sleep questionnaire							
Difficulty initiating sleep (1–5) [c]	2.5 (2.0 to 3.0)	2.3 (1.9 to 2.7)	0.227	2.8 (2.2 to 3.3)	2.7 (2.1 to 3.2)	0.540	0.376
Early morning awakenings (1–5) [c]	3.0 (2.5 to 3.5)	2.8 (2.2 to 3.3)	0.246	3.0 (2.5 to 3.5)	3.1 (2.5 to 3.7)	0.452	0.182
Sleep less than 5 h in last month (1–6) [d]	2.9 (2.4 to 3.3)	2.6 (2.1 to 3.1)	0.355	3.0 (2.3 to 3.6)	2.8 (2.2 to 3.3)	0.384	0.718
Habitual sleep duration (h)	6.6 (6.1 to 7.1)	6.7 (6.2 to 7.2)	0.706	6.7 (6.2 to 7.2)	6.6 (6.1 to 7.1)	0.545	0.658
Desired sleep duration (h)	7.9 (7.5 to 8.4)	7.8 (7.3 to 8.3)	0.398	8.1 (7.6 to 8.5)	7.9 (7.5 to 8.3)	0.117	0.776
Epworth sleepiness scale score	6.6 (5.2 to 8.0)	6.3 (4.9 to 7.7)	0.612	8.3 (6.2 to 10.5)	7.4 (5.2 to 9.7)	0.056	0.679
Rimon's depression score [†]	5.0 (4.0 to 7.0)	4.0 (1.3 to 6.0)	0.029	4.0 (3.0 to 7.5)	3.0 (2.5 to 5.5)	0.187	0.358

Data are shown as mean (95% CI) unless specified otherwise; [†] Comparisons under Natural Log transformed data, values are shown as the medians and 25th through 75th percentiles; [#] Analyses of covariance controlling for baseline values; [*] Diet (n = 19), Control (n = 12); [a] 1 = Very poor; 2 = Quite poor; 3 = Good; 4 = Very good; [b] 1 = Not fatigued at all; 2 = A little fatigued; 3 = Quite fatigued; 4 = Very fatigued; [c] 1 = Never/less than once per month; 2 = Less than once per week; 3 = 1–2 days per week; 4 = 3–5 days per week; 5 = daily or almost daily; [d] 1 = 0 night; 2 = 1–5 nights; 3 = 6–10 nights; 4 = 11–15 nights; 5 = 16–20 nights; 6 = more than 20 nights.

4. Discussion

In this study we found that a six-month diet intervention was associated with reduced body weight, fat mass, and curtailed objective sleep onset latency among overweight and obese men with chronic insomnia symptoms.

Previous studies have investigated whether adjusting total energy intake may alter sleep parameters. A recent study reported that one-week ad libitum feeding with increased calorie density (high fat diet) resulted in increased sleep/wake fragmentation in mice [11], which indicates a link between excessive energy consumption and disturbed sleep. A human study of acute diet alteration in normal sleepers has shown that, compared to limited total energy intake, sleep after ad libitum feeding was characterized by longer SOL and shorter slow wave sleep [10]. By suggesting controlled total calorie intake for a period of six months, our study further infers the association between energy restriction and improved nocturnal sleep parameters such as SOL in individuals with insomnia symptoms.

Nonetheless, it is not known whether total energy intake or the relative proportion of energy-yielding nutrients plays the more important role in mediating the effect of diet on sleep. In this study, subjects who received diet intervention reported significantly reduced total energy intake. However the proportions of the major categories of energy-yielding nutrients (carbohydrates, fat, protein) were not significantly changed through intervention. Hence energy reduction per se with negative energy balance may contribute to faster sleep onset among overweight individuals. More studies are needed in order to identify whether altering energy proportions without changing the total calories in the diet has the same effect on sleep among humans. So far, only a few studies have tested the effects of isocaloric diets with different nutrient composition on sleep and sleepiness. These studies suggested an association between macronutrient proportion and sleep-related parameters, but the results are inconclusive due to the small sample size and the non-randomized study nature. A study dating back to 1975 found less slow wave sleep following a two-day high-carb-low-fat diet than after a two-day low-carb-high-fat diet [28]. Another study compared the acute effect of high-carb/low-fat and low-carb/high-fat diets on sleepiness, and found a stronger feeling of sleepiness at 2–3 h following the former dietary pattern [29].

The mechanisms underlying the association between reduced energy intake and improved nocturnal sleep parameters remain to be revealed. It is known that diet among overweight and obese individuals is characterized by a larger proportion of fat in total energy consumption [12]. One study has shown that chronic high fat feeding reduces prepro-orexin level in hypothalamus in obese mice [30]. Since orexin is an important neuropepitide for maintaining wakefulness and regulating energy balance, we hypothesize that by reducing total energy intake, orexin signaling in the hypothalamus is strengthened, which induces more stable wakefulness and less sleep duration during the daytime. Less daytime sleep may further contribute to better nocturnal sleep, with higher sleep efficiency [31,32]. In addition, orexin neurons showed impaired thermo-sensitivity after high calorie density feeding [33], which prolonged sleep onset according to the mechanism that thermo downregulation triggers sleep. Therefore, we assume that lowering calorie intake may also recover the blunted thermo response of orexin neurons.

In the present study, we found that subjects in the diet intervention group had a greater intake of potassium and magnesium than the controls. This was partially in line with earlier reports that intakes of non-energy-yielding nutrients such as fiber, Vitamin D, potassium, and magnesium are associated with sleep [10,13,34–36]. Although the mechanisms regarding the role of potassium and magnesium on sleep regulation are not yet understood, these results suggest we should pay attention to micronutrients that may affect sleep.

Another noteworthy point in this study is that diet intervention led to lower body weight, fat mass, and waist circumference, and such contrasts were not just the result of weight and fat mass reductions in the diet group, but also, more significantly, of increased weight and fat mass among the controls. These results, together with other evidence, indicate that chronic insomnia symptoms contribute to weight gain [37–43]. This process is possibly caused by diet-induced positive energy balance. We also tested whether diet-induced weight change was associated with changes in objective sleep parameters; however, no significant correlation was found among dieters in our study. This might either be due to the small sample size (n = 28 in the diet group) or to the fact that the amount of body weight alteration is not necessarily related to absolute changes in objective sleep parameters.

The present study was subject to several limitations. First, apart from the objective sleep onset latency, no time-by-treatment difference was observed in the sleep parameters. Thus, in comparison with other non-pharmaceutical methods for mitigating insomnia symptoms, such as cognitive behavioral treatment and aerobic exercise [16,23,27,44], diet intervention may have a weaker treatment efficacy for insomnia. Nevertheless, as the average weight reduction did not achieve the goal (3 kg) under such a diet intervention protocol, stricter calorie intake control should be introduced in order to test the effects of diet on sleep in this population. Moreover, diet information was only recorded at baseline, three months, and six months, which limited information on actual nutrient intake during intervention. Finally, we did not exclude participants with mild sleep apnea ($5 \leq$ AHI < 15) due to the high prevalence of this symptom among overweight and obese men (up to 61.4%) [45]. Hence, it is possible that the improvement in sleep was partially due to improvements in sleep breathing.

To our knowledge, this is the first randomized controlled study investigating the effects of diet intervention on sleep among individuals with insomnia symptoms. The results suggest that a six-month diet intervention with reduced energy intake and recommended nutrient composition reduces objective SOL among overweight and obese men with chronic insomnia symptoms. The findings of the present study provide new evidence for the potential role of dietary interventions in overweight and obese men with insomnia.

5. Conclusions

Modest energy restriction and optimized nutrient composition shorten sleep onset latency in overweight and obese men with insomnia symptoms.

Supplementary Materials: The following are available online at http://www.mdpi.com/2072-6643/8/11/751/s1, Table S1: Descriptive characteristics of three groups at baseline; Table S2: Sleep outcomes of three groups at baseline and six months.

Acknowledgments: The authors are grateful to Shu Mei Cheng, Tuija M. Mikkola, Arja Lyytikäinen, Samu Martinmäki, and Aki Rahikainen for their contribution to data collection or diet intervention. This study was financially supported by the Finnish Funding Agency for Technology and Innovation (TEKES 2206/31/2010), the Chair Professor Program of Shanghai Jiao Tong University Zhiyuan Foundation (CP2014013), and the State General Administration of Sport of China (2015B062). The first author received financial support from the Juho Vainio Foundation and the Finnish Cultural Foundation. The study sponsors played no role in the design, methods, data management, or data analyses of the study, nor in the decision to publish.

Author Contributions: S.C., X.T., M.A. and M.P. designed the research. X.T., K.W., P.W., J.T., M.A. and S.C. conducted the research. X.T., M.P. and S.C. performed statistical analysis. X.T., M.A., K.W., P.W., J.T., M.P. and S.C. wrote the paper.

Conflicts of Interest: The authors declare no conflict of interest.

References

1. Roth, T.; Coulouvrat, C.; Hajak, G.; Lakoma, M.D.; Sampson, N.A.; Shahly, V.; Shillington, A.C.; Stephenson, J.J.; Walsh, J.K.; Kessler, R.C. Prevalence and perceived health associated with insomnia based on DSM-IV-TR; International Statistical Classification of Diseases and Related Health Problems, Tenth Revision; and Research Diagnostic Criteria/International Classification of Sleep Disorders, Second Edition criteria: Results from the America Insomnia Survey. *Biol. Psychiatry* **2011**, *69*, 592–600. [PubMed]
2. Pallesen, S.; Sivertsen, B.; Nordhus, I.H.; Bjorvatn, B. A 10-year trend of insomnia prevalence in the adult Norwegian population. *Sleep Med.* **2014**, *15*, 173–179. [CrossRef] [PubMed]

3.   Chung, K.F.; Yeung, W.F.; Ho, F.Y.; Yung, K.P.; Yu, Y.M.; Kwok, C.W. Cross-cultural and comparative epidemiology of insomnia: The Diagnostic and statistical manual (DSM), International classification of diseases (ICD) and International classification of sleep disorders (ICSD). *Sleep Med.* **2015**, *16*, 477–482. [CrossRef] [PubMed]

4.   Lallukka, T.; Arber, S.; Rahkonen, O.; Lahelma, E. Complaints of insomnia among midlifeemployed people: The contribution of childhood and present socioeconomic circumstances. *Sleep Med.* **2010**, *11*, 828–836. [CrossRef] [PubMed]

5.   Sivertsen, B.; Lallukka, T.; Salo, P.; Pallesen, S.; Hysing, M.; Krokstad, S.; Øverland, S. Insomnia as a risk factor for ill health: Results from the large population-based prospective HUNT Study in Norway. *J. Sleep Res.* **2014**, *23*, 124–132. [CrossRef] [PubMed]

6.   Lallukka, T.; Podlipskytė, A.; Sivertsen, B.; Andruškienė, J.; Varoneckas, G.; Lahelma, E.; Ursin, R.; Tell, G.S.; Rahkonen, O. Insomnia symptoms and mortality: A register-linked study among women and men from Finland, Norway and Lithuania. *J. Sleep Res.* **2016**, *25*, 96–103. [CrossRef] [PubMed]

7.   Palm, A.; Janson, C.; Lindberg, E. The impact of obesity and weight gain on development of sleep problems in a population-based sample. *Sleep Med.* **2015**, *16*, 593–597. [CrossRef] [PubMed]

8.   Singareddy, R.; Vgontzas, A.N.; Fernandez-Mendoza, J.; Liao, D.; Calhoun, S.; Shaffer, M.L.; Bixler, E.O. Risk factors for incident chronic insomnia: A general population prospective study. *Sleep Med.* **2012**, *13*, 346–353. [CrossRef] [PubMed]

9.   Vgontzas, A.N.; Lin, H.M.; Papaliaga, M.; Calhoun, S.; Vela-Bueno, A.; Chrousos, G.P.; Bixler, E.O. Short sleep duration and obesity: The role of emotional stress and sleep disturbances. *Int. J. Obes.* **2008**, *32*, 801–809. [CrossRef] [PubMed]

10. St-Onge, M.P.; Roberts, A.; Shechter, A.; Choudhury, A.R. Fiber and saturated fat are associated with sleep arousals and slow wave sleep. *J. Clin. Sleep Med.* **2016**, *12*, 19–24. [CrossRef] [PubMed]

11. Perron, I.J.; Pack, A.I.; Veasey, S. Diet/energy balance affect sleep and wakefulness independent of body weight. *Sleep* **2015**, *38*, 1893–1905. [CrossRef] [PubMed]

12. Tan, X.; Alén, M.; Cheng, S.M.; Mikkola, T.M.; Tenhunen, J.; Lyytikäinen, A.; Wiklund, P.; Cong, F.; Saarinen, A.; Tarkka, I.; et al. Associations of disordered sleep with body fat distribution, physical activity and diet among overweight middle-aged men. *J. Sleep Res.* **2015**, *24*, 414–424. [CrossRef] [PubMed]

13. Grandner, M.A.; Jackson, N.; Gerstner, J.R.; Knutson, K.L. Sleep symptoms associated with intake of specific dietary nutrients. *J. Sleep Res.* **2014**, *23*, 22–34. [CrossRef] [PubMed]

14. Kurotani, K.; Kochi, T.; Nanri, A.; Eguchi, M.; Kuwahara, K.; Tsuruoka, H.; Akter, S.; Ito, R.; Pham, N.M.; Kabe, I.; et al. Dietary patterns and sleep symptoms in Japanese workers: The Furukawa Nutrition and Health Study. *Sleep Med.* **2015**, *16*, 298–304. [CrossRef] [PubMed]

15. Saaristo, T.E.; Barengo, N.C.; Korpi-Hyövälti, E.; Oksa, H.; Puolijoki, H.; Saltevo, J.T.; Vanhala, M.; Sundvall, J.; Saarikoski, L.; Peltonen, M.; et al. High prevalence of obesity, central obesity and abnormal glucose tolerance in the middle-aged Finnish population. *BMC Public Health* **2008**, *8*, 423. [CrossRef] [PubMed]

16. Tan, X.; Alén, M.; Wiklund, P.; Partinen, M.; Cheng, S. Effects of aerobic exercise on home-based sleep among overweight and obese men with chronic insomnia symptoms: A randomized controlled trial. *Sleep Med.* **2016**, *25*, 113–121. [CrossRef] [PubMed]

17. Partinen, M.; Gislason, T. Basic Nordic Sleep Questionnaire (BNSQ): A quantitated measure of subjective sleep complaints. *J. Sleep Res.* **1995**, *4*, 150–155. [CrossRef] [PubMed]

18. American Psychiatric Association. *Diagnostic and Statistical Manual of Mental Disorders*, 4th ed.; Text Revision; American Psychiatric Assiciation: Washington, DC, USA, 2000.

19. Ohayon, M.M.; Reynolds, C.F., III. Epidemiological and clinical relevance of insomnia diagnosis algorithms according to the DSM-IV and the International Classification of Sleep Disorders (ICSD). *Sleep Med.* **2009**, *10*, 952–960. [CrossRef] [PubMed]

20. Ainsworth, B.E.; Haskell, W.L.; Herrmann, S.D.; Meckes, N.; Bassett, D.R., Jr.; Tudor-Locke, C.; Greer, J.L.; Vezina, J.; Whitt-Glover, M.C.; Leon, A.S. 2011 Compendium of Physical Activities: A second update of codes and MET values. *Med. Sci. Sports Exerc.* **2011**, *43*, 1575–1581. [CrossRef] [PubMed]

21. Sedentary Behaviour Research Network. Letter to the editor: Standardized use of the terms "sedentary" and "sedentary behaviours". *Appl. Physiol. Nutr. Metab.* **2012**, *37*, 540–542.

22. Paalasmaa, J.; Waris, M.; Toivonen, H.; Leppäkorpi, L.; Partinen, M. Unobtrusive online monitoring of sleep at home. *Conf. Proc. IEEE Eng. Med. Biol. Soc.* **2012**, *2012*, 3784–3788. [PubMed]

23. Morin, C.M.; Vallières, A.; Guay, B.; Ivers, H.; Savard, J.; Mérette, C.; Bastien, C.; Baillargeon, L. Cognitive behavioral therapy, singly and combined with medication, for persistent insomnia: A randomized controlled trial. *JAMA* **2009**, *301*, 2005–2015. [CrossRef] [PubMed]

24. Johns, M.W. A new method for measuring daytime sleepiness: The Epworth sleepiness scale. *Sleep* **1991**, *14*, 540–545. [PubMed]

25. Keltikangas-Järvinen, L.; Rimon, R. Rimon's Brief Depression Scale, a rapid method forscreening depression. *Psychol. Rep.* **1987**, *60*, 111–119. [CrossRef] [PubMed]

26. The National Nutrition Council of Finland. *Suomalaiset Ravitsemussuositukset—Ravinto ja Liikunta Tasapainoon [The Finnish Nutrition Recommendations—Nutrition and Physical Balance]*; The National Nutrition Council of Finland: Helsinki, Finland, 2005.

27. Passos, G.S.; Poyares, D.; Santana, M.G.; D'Aurea, C.V.; Youngstedt, S.D.; Tufik, S.; de Mello, M.T. Effects of moderate aerobic exercise training on chronic primary insomnia. *Sleep Med.* **2011**, *12*, 1018–1027. [CrossRef] [PubMed]

28. Phillips, F.; Chen, C.N.; Crisp, A.H.; Koval, J.; McGuinness, B.; Kalucy, R.S.; Kalucy, E.C.; Lacey, J.H. Isocaloric diet changes and electroencephalographic sleep. *Lancet* **1975**, *2*, 723–725. [CrossRef]

29. Wells, A.S.; Read, N.W.; Uvnas-Moberg, K.; Alster, P. Influences of fat and carbohydrate on postprandial sleepiness, mood, and hormones. *Physiol. Behav.* **1997**, *61*, 679–686. [CrossRef]

30. Tanno, S.; Terao, A.; Okamatsu-Ogura, Y.; Kimura, K. Hypothalamic prepro-orexin mRNA level is inversely correlated to the non-rapid eye movement sleep level in high-fat diet-induced obese mice. *Obes. Res. Clin. Pract.* **2013**, *7*, e251–e257. [CrossRef] [PubMed]

31. Jakubowski, K.P.; Hall, M.H.; Lee, L.; Matthews, K.A. Temporal relationships between napping and nocturnal sleep in healthy adolescents. *Behav. Sleep Med.* **2016**, *14*, 1–13. [CrossRef] [PubMed]

32. Owens, J.F.; Buysse, D.J.; Hall, M.; Kamarck, T.W.; Lee, L.; Strollo, P.J.; Reis, S.E.; Matthews, K.A. Napping, nighttime sleep, and cardiovascular risk factors in mid-life adults. *J. Clin. Sleep Med.* **2010**, *6*, 330–335. [PubMed]

33. Belanger-Willoughby, N.; Linehan, V.; Hirasawa, M. Thermosensing mechanisms and their impairment by high-fat diet in orexin neurons. *Neuroscience* **2016**, *324*, 82–91. [CrossRef] [PubMed]

34. Tuomilehto, H.; Peltonen, M.; Partinen, M.; Lavigne, G.; Eriksson, J.G.; Herder, C.; Aunola, S.; Keinänen-Kiukaanniemi, S.; Ilanne-Parikka, P.; Uusitupa, M.; et al. Sleep duration, lifestyle intervention, and incidence of type 2 diabetes in impaired glucose tolerance: The Finnish Diabetes Prevention Study. *Diabetes Care* **2009**, *32*, 1965–1971. [CrossRef] [PubMed]

35. Massa, J.; Stone, K.L.; Wei, E.K.; Harrison, S.L.; Barrett-Connor, E.; Lane, N.E.; Paudel, M.; Redline, S.; Ancoli-Israel, S.; Orwoll, E.; et al. Vitamin D and actigraphic sleep outcomes in older community-dwelling men: The MrOS sleep study. *Sleep* **2015**, *38*, 251–257. [CrossRef] [PubMed]

36. Durlach, J.; Pagès, N.; Bac, P.; Bara, M.; Guiet-Bara, A. Biorhythms and possible central regulation of magnesium status, phototherapy, darkness therapy and chronopathological forms of magnesium depletion. *Magnes. Res.* **2002**, *15*, 49–66. [PubMed]

37. St-Onge, M.P.; Roberts, A.L.; Chen, J.; Kelleman, M.; O'Keeffe, M.; RoyChoudhury, A.; Jones, P.J. Short sleep duration increases energy intakes but does not change energy expenditure in normal-weight individuals. *Am. J. Clin. Nutr.* **2011**, *94*, 410–416. [CrossRef] [PubMed]

38. Calvin, A.D.; Carter, R.E.; Adachi, T.; Macedo, P.G.; Albuquerque, F.N.; van der Walt, C.; Bukartyk, J.; Davison, D.E.; Levine, J.A.; Somers, V.K. Effects of experimental sleep restriction on caloric intake and activity energy expenditure. *Chest* **2013**, *144*, 79–86. [CrossRef] [PubMed]

39. Hursel, R.; Gonnissen, H.K.; Rutters, F.; Martens, E.A.; Westerterp-Plantenga, M.S. Disadvantageous shift in energy balance is primarily expressed in high-quality sleepers after a decline in quality sleep because of disturbance. *Am. J. Clin. Nutr.* **2013**, *98*, 367–373. [CrossRef] [PubMed]

40. Markwald, R.R.; Melanson, E.L.; Smith, M.R.; Higgins, J.; Perreault, L.; Eckel, R.H.; Wright, K.P., Jr. Impact of insufficient sleep on total daily energy expenditure, food intake, and weight gain. *Proc. Natl. Acad. Sci. USA* **2013**, *110*, 5695–5700. [CrossRef] [PubMed]

41. Shechter, A.; O'Keeffe, M.; Roberts, A.L.; Zammit, G.K.; RoyChoudhury, A.; St-Onge, M.P. Alterations in sleep architecture in response to experimental sleep curtailment are associated with signs of positive energy balance. *Am. J. Physiol. Regul. Integr. Comp. Physiol.* **2012**, *303*, R883–R889. [CrossRef] [PubMed]

42. Rahe, C.; Czira, M.E.; Teismann, H.; Berger, K. Associations between poor sleep quality and different measures of obesity. *Sleep Med.* **2015**, *16*, 1225–1228. [CrossRef] [PubMed]

43. Cheng, F.W.; Li, Y.; Winkelman, J.W.; Hu, F.B.; Rimm, E.B.; Gao, X. Probable insomnia is associated with future total energy intake and diet quality in men. *Am. J. Clin. Nutr.* **2016**, *104*, 462–469. [CrossRef] [PubMed]

44. Reid, K.J.; Baron, K.G.; Lu, B.; Naylor, E.; Wolfe, L.; Zee, P.C. Aerobic exercise improves self-reported sleep and quality of life in older adults with insomnia. *Sleep Med.* **2010**, *11*, 934–940. [CrossRef] [PubMed]

45. Peppard, P.E.; Young, T.; Barnet, J.H.; Palta, M.; Hagen, E.W.; Hla, K.M. Increased prevalence of sleep-disordered breathing in adults. *Am. J. Epidemiol.* **2013**, *177*, 1006–1014. [CrossRef] [PubMed]

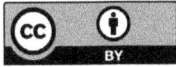

MDPI AG

St. Alban-Anlage 66

4052 Basel, Switzerland

Tel. +41 61 683 77 34

Fax +41 61 302 89 18

http://www.mdpi.com

Nutrients Editorial Office

E-mail: nutrients@mdpi.com

http://www.mdpi.com/journal/nutrients

www.ingramcontent.com/pod-product-compliance
Lightning Source LLC
Chambersburg PA
CBHW051314020426
42333CB00028B/3339